DR. ~~REINHART KLUGE~~
AM SPORTPLATZ 3
14558 FAHLHORST

D1692674

METHODS IN MOLECULAR BIOLOGY™

Series Editor
**John M. Walker
School of Life Sciences
University of Hertfordshire
Hatfield, Hertfordshire, AL10 9AB, UK**

For further volumes:
http://www.springer.com/series/7651

Animal Models in Diabetes Research

Edited by

Hans-Georg Joost

Department of Pharmacology, German Institute of Human Nutrition Potsdam-Rehbrücke, Nuthetal, Germany

Hadi Al-Hasani

German Diabetes Centre Clinical Biochemistry & Pathobiochemistry, Heinrich Heine University, Düsseldorf, Germany

Annette Schürmann

Department of Experimental Diabetology, German Institute of Human Nutrition Potsdam-Rehbrücke, Nuthetal, Germany

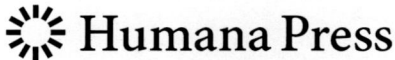

Editors
Hans-Georg Joost
Department of Pharmacology
German Institute of Human Nutrition
    Potsdam-Rehbrücke
Nuthetal, Germany

Hadi Al-Hasani
German Diabetes Centre Clinical
    Biochemistry and Pathobiochemistry
Heinrich Heine University
Düsseldorf, Germany

Annette Schürmann
Department of Experimental Diabetology
German Institute of Human Nutrition
    Potsdam-Rehbrücke
Nuthetal, Germany

ISSN 1064-3745   ISSN 1940-6029 (electronic)
ISBN 978-1-62703-067-0   ISBN 978-1-62703-068-7 (eBook)
DOI 10.1007/978-1-62703-068-7
Springer New York Heidelberg Dordrecht London

Library of Congress Control Number: 2012943831

© Springer Science+Business Media, LLC 2012
This work is subject to copyright. All rights are reserved by the Publisher, whether the whole or part of the material is concerned, specifically the rights of translation, reprinting, reuse of illustrations,recitation, broadcasting, reproduction on microfilms or in any other physical way, and transmission or information storage and retrieval, electronic adaptation, computer software, or by similar or dissimilar methodology now known or hereafter developed. Exempted from this legal reservation are brief excerpts in connection with reviews or scholarly analysis or material supplied specifically for the purpose of being entered and executed on a computer system, for exclusive use by the purchaser of the work. Duplication of this publication or parts thereof is permitted only under the provisions of the Copyright Law of the Publisher's location, in its current version, and permission for use must always be obtained from Springer. Permissions for use may be obtained through RightsLink at the Copyright Clearance Center. Violations are liable to prosecution under the respective Copyright Law.
The use of general descriptive names, registered names, trademarks, service marks, etc. in this publication does not imply, even in the absence of a specific statement, that such names are exempt from the relevant protective laws and regulations and therefore free for general use.
While the advice and information in this book are believed to be true and accurate at the date of publication, neither the authors nor the editors nor the publisher can accept any legal responsibility for any errors or omissions that may be made. The publisher makes no warranty, express or implied, with respect to the material contained herein.

Printed on acid-free paper

Humana Press is a brand of Springer
Springer is part of Springer Science+Business Media (www.springer.com)

Preface

Since the discovery of insulin by Banting and Best in 1922, diabetes mellitus is considered the paradigmatic disease where animal models have led to a therapeutic breakthrough. In addition, this breakthrough depended on earlier studies with animal experimentation by Claude Bernard (1849), Oskar Minkowski, and Joseph von Mehring (1889), indicating that diabetes mellitus is a failure of glucose homeostasis caused by a pancreatic malfunction. Furthermore, animal models have been indispensable for the elucidation of the cellular and molecular basis of both type 1 and type 2 diabetes in the second half of the last century. In spite of the enormous research progress made so far, diabetes is still a major life-shortening health threat. However, most of the experimentation needed for the invention and test of novel therapeutic approaches cannot be performed in humans. Thus, there is no alternative to appropriate animal models which are described in this volume.

In recent years, human studies have made enormous contributions towards an understanding of the genetic basis of diabetes mellitus. Genome wide association studies have identified numerous common gene polymorphisms that are associated with an increased risk to develop diabetes mellitus. Most of these polymorphisms are located in genes whose roles in the pathogenesis are almost completely unknown. Thus, animal models such as transgenic mice will be required for further progress in this area, and these mouse lines have to be characterized with accepted methods for the study of glucose homeostasis. In addition, the so far identified human genes explain only a small fraction of the total heredity of the disease. Thus, animal models with spontaneous diabetes mellitus may be useful to discover additional genes or pathways involved in the pathogenesis of the disease.

Research in humans has identified numerous factors that modify the risk of diabetes. Some of these factors such as environmental and nutritional variables have been identified by associations, and it is still necessary to establish their causality. Again, established and accepted animal models as well as validated procedures are required in order to test the efficacy of an intervention and to prove causality of associations. This volume therefore summarizes the current status of the most important models and procedures as a timely resource in experimental diabetology.

Animal Models in Diabetes Research is an unusual volume within the *Methods in Molecular Biology* series because its first two sections do not contain lab protocols but comprise a series of reviews on model strains. With these reviews, a comprehensive overview on our current knowledge of the pathogenesis and pathophysiology of diabetes is given. Models that are being used in the study of type 1 diabetes are the NOD mouse, the *Akita* mouse, and the BB rat (Part I). Major progress has been made in elucidating the polygenic pathogenesis of type 2 diabetes in the NZO and the TALLYHO mouse, and in the GK rat. With these strains, the strategy of positional cloning by mapping quantitative trait loci and subsequently identifying the responsible genes has proven to be very effective. It can be expected that future research employing this strategy will discover many more disease genes and malfunctioning pathways with relevance to the human disease.

Other well-characterized models that are described in Part II are the *db/db* mouse, the Zucker rat, and the sand rat *Psammomys obesus*. The pathogenesis and pathophysiology of these models is in part known, and allows targeted studies of preventive or therapeutic interventions. Thus, the chapters in the first two sections of the volume should help researchers to choose the appropriate model for their specific aims. As the closest model to human type 2 diabetes, spontaneously developing diabetes in non-human primates is described in Part III.

The fourth part of the volume contains established protocols that are employed in the characterization and study of animal models of diabetes. Key methods are the study of beta cell function (Chapters 12 and 13), of glucose homeostasis in vivo (Chapters 14 and 15) and in vitro (Chapter 16) as well as of beta cell autoimmunity (Chapter 17). In addition, models or protocols for the study of renal, cardiac, or retinal secondary complications are described in the Chapters 2, 3, and 19. Finally, two chapters are devoted to pancreatic stem cells.

All authors of this volume are distinguished experts in the field of diabetes research and have previously contributed original data with the models and/or methodology they have described here. I am deeply grateful for their contributions of excellent, informative, and comprehensive chapters. The credit for the success of the volume should be given to them. Also, I am grateful to my co-editors who have carefully reviewed and edited the chapters together with me; their input has enormously improved the volume. Finally, it is my hope that *Animal Models in Diabetes Research* will be an important resource to advance diabetes research in the years to come.

Nuthetal, Germany   *Hans-Georg Joost*

Contents

Preface v
Contributors ix

PART I RODENT MODELS OF TYPE 1 DIABETES

1 The Non-Obese Diabetic (NOD) Mouse as a Model of Human Type 1 Diabetes 3
Kritika Kachapati, David Adams, Kyle Bednar, and William M. Ridgway

2 Assessment of Diabetic Nephropathy in the Akita Mouse 17
Jae-Hyung Chang and Susan B. Gurley

3 The BB Rat as a Model of Human Type 1 Diabetes 31
Rita Bortell and Chaoxing Yang

PART II RODENT MODELS OF TYPE 2 DIABETES

4 Diabetes in Mice with Monogenic Obesity: The *db/db* Mouse and Its Use in the Study of Cardiac Consequences 47
Darrell D. Belke and David L. Severson

5 Pathophysiology and Genetics of Obesity and Diabetes in the New Zealand Obese Mouse: A Model of the Human Metabolic Syndrome 59
Reinhart Kluge, Stephan Scherneck, Annette Schürmann, and Hans-Georg Joost

6 The TALLYHO Mouse as a Model of Human Type 2 Diabetes 75
Jung Han Kim and Arnold M. Saxton

7 Diet-Induced Diabetes in the Sand Rat (*Psammomys obesus*) 89
Nurit Kaiser, Erol Cerasi, and Gil Leibowitz

8 Diabetes in Zucker Diabetic Fatty Rat 103
Masakazu Shiota and Richard L. Printz

9 The GK Rat: A Prototype for the Study of Non-overweight Type 2 Diabetes 125
Bernard Portha, Marie-Hélène Giroix, Cecile Tourrel-Cuzin, Hervé Le-Stunff, and Jamileh Movassat

10 Experimentally Induced Rodent Models of Type 2 Diabetes 161
Md. Shahidul Islam and Rachel Dorothy Wilson

Part III Other Species

11 Investigation and Treatment of Type 2 Diabetes
    in Nonhuman Primates.. 177
    Barbara C. Hansen

Part IV General Methodology

12 Determination of Beta-Cell Function: Insulin Secretion
    of Isolated Islets.. 189
    Michael Willenborg, Kirstin Schumacher, and Ingo Rustenbeck
13 Determination of Beta-Cell Function: Ion Channel
    Function in Beta Cells... 203
    Martina Düfer
14 Measurement of Glucose Homeostasis In Vivo: Glucose
    and Insulin Tolerance Tests.. 219
    Francesco Beguinot and Cecilia Nigro
15 Measurement of Glucose Homeostasis In Vivo: Combination
    of Tracers and Clamp Techniques.. 229
    Masakazu Shiota
16 Measurement of Insulin Sensitivity in Skeletal Muscle In Vitro........... 255
    Henrike Sell, Jørgen Jensen, and Juergen Eckel
17 Beta-Cell Autoimmunity... 265
    Yannick F. Fuchs, Kerstin Adler, and Ezio Bonifacio
18 Positional Cloning of Diabetes Genes..................................... 275
    Gudrun A. Brockmann and Christina Neuschl
19 Retinal Digest Preparation: A Method to Study Diabetic Retinopathy....... 291
    Nadine Dietrich and Hans-Peter Hammes
20 Lineage Tracing of Pancreatic Stem Cells and Beta Cell Regeneration...... 303
    Isabelle Houbracken, Iris Mathijs, and Luc Bouwens
21 Genetic Lineage Tracing of Beta Cell Neogenesis.......................... 317
    Iris Mathijs, Isabelle Houbracken, and Luc Bouwens

Index.. *323*

Contributors

DAVID ADAMS • *Division of Immunology, Allergy, and Rheumatology, University of Cincinnati College of Medicine, Cincinnati, OH, USA*
KERSTIN ADLER • *Forschergruppe Diabetes, Klinikum rechts der Isar, Technische Universität München, Munich, Germany*
KYLE BEDNAR • *Division of Immunology, Allergy, and Rheumatology, University of Cincinnati College of Medicine, Cincinnati, OH, USA*
FRANCESCO BEGUINOT • *Dipartimento di Biologia e Patologia Cellulare e Molecolare and Istituto di Endocrinologia ed Oncologia Sperimentale del CNR, Federico II University of Naples, Naples, Italy*
DARRELL D. BELKE • *The University of Calgary, Calgary, AB, Canada*
EZIO BONIFACIO • *Preclinical Approaches to Stem Cell Therapy/Diabetes, Technische Universität Dresden, DFG-Center for Regenerative Therapies Dresden, Cluster of Excellence, Dresden, Germany*
RITA BORTELL • *Program in Molecular Medicine, University of Massachusetts Medical School, Worcester, MA, USA*
LUC BOUWENS • *Cell Differentiation Lab, Vrije Universiteit Brussel, Brussels, Belgium*
GUDRUN A. BROCKMANN • *Breeding Biology and Molecular Genetics, Department for Crop and Animal Sciences, Humboldt-Universität zu Berlin, Berlin, Germany*
EROL CERASI • *Endocrinology and Metabolism Service, Department of Medicine, Hadassah—Hebrew University Medical Center, Jerusalem, Israel*
JAE-HYUNG CHANG • *Division of Nephrology, Department of Medicine, Duke University and Durham VA Medical Centers, Durham, NC, USA*
NADINE DIETRICH • *5th Medical Department, Universitätsmedizin Mannheim, University of Heidelberg, Mannheim, Germany*
MARTINA DÜFER • *Institute of Pharmacy, Department of Pharmacology, Toxicology, and Clinical Pharmacy, University of Tübingen, Tübingen, Germany*
JUERGEN ECKEL • *Paul-Langerhans-Group Integrative Physiology, German Diabetes Center, Düsseldorf, Germany*
YANNICK F. FUCHS • *Preclinical Approaches to Stem Cell Therapy/Diabetes, Technische Universität Dresden, DFG-Center for Regenerative Therapies Dresden, Cluster of Excellence, Dresden, Germany*
MARIE-HÉLÈNE GIROIX • *Laboratoire B2PE (Biologie et Pathologie du Pancréas Endocrine), Unité BFA (Biologie Fonctionnelle et Adaptive), Université Paris-Diderot, CNRS EAC 4413, Paris, France*
SUSAN B. GURLEY • *Division of Nephrology, Department of Medicine, Duke University and Durham VA Medical Centers, Durham, NC, USA*

HANS-PETER HAMMES • 5th Medical Department, Universitätsmedizin Mannheim, University of Heidelberg, Mannheim, Germany

BARBARA C. HANSEN • Departments of Internal Medicine and Pediatrics, University of South Florida, Tampa, FL, USA

ISABELLE HOUBRACKEN • Cell Differentiation Lab, Vrije Universiteit Brussel, Brussels, Belgium

MD. SHAHIDUL ISLAM • Department of Biochemistry, School of Biochemistry, Genetics and Microbiology, University of KwaZulu-Natal, Durban, South Africa

JØRGEN JENSEN • Department of Physical Performance, Norwegian School of Sport Sciences, Oslo, Norway

HANS-GEORG JOOST • Department of Pharmacology, German Institute of Human Nutrition Potsdam-Rehbrücke, Nuthetal, Germany

KRITIKA KACHAPATI • Division of Immunology, Allergy, and Rheumatology, University of Cincinnati College of Medicine, Cincinnati, OH, USA

NURIT KAISER • Endocrinology and Metabolism Service, Department of Medicine, Hadassah—Hebrew University Medical Center, Jerusalem, Israel

JUNG HAN KIM • Department of Pharmacology, Physiology and Toxicology, Marshall University School of Medicine, Huntington, WV, USA

REINHART KLUGE • Max-Rubner-Laboratory, German Institute of Human Nutrition Potsdam-Rehbrücke, Nuthetal, Germany

GIL LEIBOWITZ • Endocrinology and Metabolism Service, Department of Medicine, Hadassah—Hebrew University Medical Center, Jerusalem, Israel

HERVÉ LE-STUNFF • Laboratoire B2PE (Biologie et Pathologie du Pancréas Endocrine), Unité BFA (Biologie Fonctionnelle et Adaptive), Université Paris-Diderot, CNRS EAC 4413, Paris, France

IRIS MATHIJS • Cell Differentiation Lab, Vrije Universiteit Brussel, Brussels, Belgium

JAMILEH MOVASSAT • Laboratoire B2PE (Biologie et Pathologie du Pancréas Endocrine), Unité BFA (Biologie Fonctionnelle et Adaptive), Université Paris-Diderot, CNRS EAC 4413, Paris, France

CHRISTINA NEUSCHL • Breeding Biology and Molecular Genetics, Department for Crop and Animal Sciences, Humboldt-Universität zu Berlin, Berlin, Germany

CECILIA NIGRO • Dipartimento di Biologia e Patologia Cellulare e Molecolare and Istituto di Endocrinologia ed Oncologia Sperimentale del CNR, Federico II University of Naples, Naples, Italy

BERNARD PORTHA • Laboratoire B2PE (Biologie et Pathologie du Pancréas Endocrine), Unité BFA (Biologie Fonctionnelle et Adaptive), Université Paris-Diderot, CNRS EAC 4413, Paris, France

RICHARD L. PRINTZ • Department of Molecular Physiology and Biophysics, Vanderbilt University School of Medicine, Nashville, TN, USA

WILLIAM M. RIDGWAY • Division of Immunology, Allergy, and Rheumatology, University of Cincinnati College of Medicine, Cincinnati, OH, USA

INGO RUSTENBECK • Institute of Pharmacology and Toxicology, University of Braunschweig, Braunschweig, Germany

ARNOLD M. SAXTON • Department of Animal Science, The University of Tennessee, Knoxville, TN, USA

STEPHAN SCHERNECK • *Department of Experimental Diabetology, German Institute of Human Nutrition Potsdam-Rehbrücke, Nuthetal, Germany*

KIRSTIN SCHUMACHER • *Institute of Pharmacology and Toxicology, University of Braunschweig, Braunschweig, Germany*

ANNETTE SCHÜRMANN • *Department of Experimental Diabetology, German Institute of Human Nutrition Potsdam-Rehbrücke, Nuthetal, Germany*

HENRIKE SELL • *Paul-Langerhans-Group Integrative Physiology, German Diabetes Center, Düsseldorf, Germany*

DAVID L. SEVERSON • *Department of Physiology and Pharmacology, The University of Calgary, Calgary, AB, Canada*

MASAKAZU SHIOTA • *Department of Molecular Physiology and Biophysics, Vanderbilt University School of Medicine, Nashville, TN, USA*

CECILE TOURREL-CUZIN • *Laboratoire B2PE (Biologie et Pathologie du Pancréas Endocrine), Unité BFA (Biologie Fonctionnelle et Adaptive), Université Paris-Diderot, CNRS EAC 4413, Paris, France*

MICHAEL WILLENBORG • *Institute of Pharmacology and Toxicology, University of Braunschweig, Braunschweig, Germany*

RACHEL DOROTHY WILSON • *Department of Biochemistry, School of Biochemistry, Genetics and Microbiology, University of KwaZulu-Natal, Durban, South Africa*

CHAOXING YANG • *Program in Molecular Medicine, University of Massachusetts Medical School, Worcester, MA, USA*

Part I

Rodent Models of Type 1 Diabetes

Chapter 1

The Non-Obese Diabetic (NOD) Mouse as a Model of Human Type 1 Diabetes

Kritika Kachapati, David Adams, Kyle Bednar, and William M. Ridgway

Abstract

The non-obese diabetic (NOD) mouse spontaneously develops type 1 diabetes (T1D) and has thus served as a model for understanding the genetic and immunological basis, and treatment, of T1D. Since its initial description in 1980, however, the field has matured and recognized that prevention of diabetes in NOD mice (i.e., preventing the disease from occurring by an intervention prior to frank diabetes) is relatively easy to achieve and does not correlate well with curing the disease (after the onset of frank hyperglycemia). Hundreds of papers have described the prevention of diabetes in NOD mice but only a handful have described its actual reversal. The paradoxical conclusion is that preventing the disease in NOD mice does not necessarily tell us what caused the disease nor how to reverse it. The NOD mouse model is therefore best used now, with respect to human disease, as a way to understand the genetic and immunologic causes of and as a model for trying to reverse disease once hyperglycemia occurs. We describe how genetic approaches to identifying causative gene variants can be adapted to identify novel therapeutic agents for reversing new-onset T1D.

Key words: NOD mouse, Type 1 diabetes, Prevention of diabetes, Autoimmune, Quantitative trait loci, Insulin-dependent diabetes loci (*idd*), MHC genes, CD137, CTLA4

1. Introduction: The Problems Associated with Using NOD as a Model for Human T1D

Many good reviews have been published recently on NOD mice as a model of human disease, (1, 2) on the genetics of T1D in mice and humans (3, 4), on the outcome of human trials of autoantigenic approaches to disease (5), and on the immunology of NOD disease and comparison to human T1D (6). This review will assess some of the problematic aspects of the NOD model and suggest a more specific approach to using these mice in T1D research. After briefly reviewing the literature on the immunology and genetics of NOD T1D and its relevance to human T1D, we will focus on a genetic approach to gene discovery as a way to utilize the NOD model to develop new therapies relevant to human T1D. We will give examples of how a candidate gene approach can identify novel treatment targets. We will then show in depth how our lab has used this approach.

A Pubmed search with the keywords "type 1 diabetes NOD prevention" produces 952 articles. However, fewer than 20 articles have been published showing reversal of T1D in NOD mice (7–20). No therapy has yet reversed T1D in humans. It is important to understand these discrepancies and what they imply for productive research using the NOD model.

Diabetes in NOD mice is a complex, multigenic, and immunologically "delicate" disease. Pathogenic events begin at least as early as 3 weeks after birth with the presentation of islet antigens in the pancreatic lymph nodes, a process that has been related to the onset of weaning (21). Insulitis, or the gradual infiltration of islets with first antigen presenting cells (APCs, i.e., macrophages and dendritic cells) then lymphocytes, begins at this early time point and steadily progresses over the next 15 weeks (22). The initial infiltrating APCs, especially myeloid dendritic cells, present self-antigen to the autoantigenic CD4+ T cells that drive the disease (23). The final effector attack on the insulin-producing beta cells in the islets is thought to be mediated primarily by CD8 cells (24). Frank diabetes, i.e., blood glucose over 250 mg/dL, begins between 18 and 20 weeks. Thus the whole immune system acts in an orchestrated manner to mediate disease; CD4 and CD8 T cells are necessary for the disease, and B cells play an important role. In general, every immune cell is involved at some point. The hundreds of interventions that "prevent" diabetes in mice may therefore act at various time points and on various immune cell subsets to disrupt the development of disease.

It is not clear whether diabetes is similarly preventable in humans—this is unknown. It is easy to imagine that a larger proportion of the human population is susceptible to diabetes than the proportion that actually develops disease. Diabetes in humans might be prevented, just as in NOD mice, either by viral/bacterial infection or other stimulation of the immune system. This has clinical relevance if genetically "at risk" individuals (with a family history, disease-associated MHC genes, and the presence of serum autoantibodies to islet antigens such as GAD or insulin) (25) could be treated prior to disease onset (i.e., prior to the onset of hyperglycemia) with an immune modulatory agent that prevented the disease by diverting the immune system away from diabetes. However, this is a speculative concept and could only be addressed in large scale human trials.

Interventions in NOD mice that act to "prevent" diabetes could act via many different pathways, for example, some such interventions could cause immune activation by release of various cytokines that "retune" the immune system (26) at critical junctures and thus discourage autoreactivity. Shoda et al. undertook a comprehensive review of interventions that prevented diabetes in NOD mice from 1980 to 2004 (27). They identified 463 interventions and placed them into 8 general categories: (1) costimulation and adhesion, (2) cell infusions, (3) antigens, (4) cell surface and cells, (5) immunomodulatory, (6) pathogens, (7) cytokines and hormones, and (8) environmental. The full list of agents is found in the supplemental figures of their *Immunity* paper. They identify at least ten autoantigens that have prevented diabetes; over 15 immune costimulatory molecules, infusion of virtually any immune cell, multitudes of cell surface receptor modulators (e.g., anti-CD3, CD4, CD8, TCR). Some of their categories, such as "immunomodulatory" or "environmental" are very broadly defined and thus emphasize the point that deducing the pathogenesis of the disease from the approaches used to prevent it is not a productive approach. For example, the hundreds of "immunomodulatory", "pathogen," and "hormone" agents have no obvious common features. What to make of the meta-observation that androgens, testeosterone, and pregnancy all prevent diabetes? IFN-γ, TNF-α, IL-1, IL-4, IL-10, and IL-12 all prevent diabetes, is it possible to model this in a way that makes immunological sense? We suggest not—the proper interpretation of this massive literature is that pre-diabetic interventions are nonspecific and do not help us understand the detailed mechanisms of the disease process (nor help us predict what agents will be effective in human disease). How could it be possible that these therapeutic effects are not specific to the factors that "cause" type one diabetes? Depending on the intervention, there are multiple possible mechanisms of nonspecificity. For example, knocking out a variety of immune-related genes prevents diabetes—but knocking out these genes completely changes the immune system throughout its entire development (unless timed, tissue-specific knockout is performed) and thus could alter general immune pathways that play an important part in the final disease effector mechanisms. Similarly, release of various cytokines at critical times in the development of the immune system could completely change the genetically determined balance between T-cell subsets and thus prevent disease without telling us, for example, what caused the pathogenic subset balance to arise in the untreated NOD mouse in the first place.

Given the amount of published work on the NOD model the following maxim should be heeded by investigators: "strategies that prevent T1D in NOD have little predictive power for disease reversal." This point has been made previously (27–29) and may in fact have contributed to the increasing numbers of studies demonstrating reversal of new-onset diabetes. A corollary should also be considered: "proposed strategies to reverse established T1D in mice or humans should be directed to genes or immune mechanisms already shown to play a role in pathogenesis of the disease".

This point may be too obvious, or in fact wrong, but it is motivated by the huge literature wherein genes are knocked out that demonstrably play no role in the genetic constitution of the disease, or where nonspecific immunostimulants have been used. The point to realize is how easy it is to prevent diabetes but how difficult it is to treat T1D. There have been no published cures of human T1D and only modest modulation of disease. There may be many reasons for this intractability of T1D compared to other autoimmune diseases, for example, to rheumatoid arthritis where highly effective therapies have been developed. T1D is an organ-specific disease confined to a unique anatomic location that may restrict, or render ineffective, systemic therapies. T1D is also driven by a highly aggressive autoimmune response, that may require combinations of drugs (again, as is the case in Rheumatoid arthritis, where multiple drugs achieve better responses than monotherapy). Finally, the complexity of the disease process itself, and the fact that it is very far along in the natural history at the time of diagnosis, may limit the number of effective approaches that are even possible. A therapy directed to a genetically linked immune molecule will be useless if that gene plays a role only in the early stages, e.g., of insulitis. This leads us to a final criticism of our second maxim: it may be so broad as to be useless. If there are as many as 100 genes playing ever smaller roles in T1D pathogenesis, and the whole immune system is involved at some point during the disease—how can the possible therapeutic approaches be usefully limited?

Our lab has taken a highly focused approach to this problem. We have tried to identify immune molecules genetically linked to T1D in NOD that have also been associated with human T1D. In addition, we try to work on aspects of T1D immunogenetics that operate throughout the course of disease, not only in the early stages, so that they may become valid targets for therapy. In the next section we will briefly review T1D genetics in NOD and humans to give examples of how genetic studies can suggest immune targets. Then, we will go into detail about how we have tried to create a novel therapy directed to disease reversal based on this approach.

2. Using Genetics to Identify Disease-Related Causative Targets for Therapy/Treatment

T1D in the NOD mouse may be the most extensively genetically studied mammalian autoimmune disease, with comprehensive genetic studies performed over the 30 years (30, 31). T1D in the NOD mouse was probably the first murine autoimmune disease analyzed using microsatellite polymorphisms to perform genome-wide linkage studies (32). These approaches led to the discovery of quantitative trait loci (QTL), the so-called "insulin-dependent diabetes loci" (*Idd*) which are genetic intervals with one or more genes conferring susceptibility to the disease. We have recently reviewed the *Idd* loci in detail and tabulated over 40 *Idd* loci in the literature to date (4). The best resource for up-to-date information on all mouse and human genetic regions linked to T1D, as well as detailed information on orthologous regions between the species, possible shared genes, and full references to the literature, is T1Dbase (http://t1dbase.org/page/Welcome/display) (33). The genetic data can be viewed graphically or in list format. Importantly, T1Dbase includes a search function that allows one to ascertain if a gene of interest has been genetically linked to T1D. T1Dbase currently lists over 40 mouse and over 55 human regions genetically linked to T1D.

Linkage studies can be used to construct congenic mice, wherein *Idd* resistance intervals defined by the linkage analysis (from nondiabetic strains, such as B6/B10) are bred onto the NOD strain and diabetes incidence assessed. A drop in diabetes incidence in the congenic mouse confirms the presence of an *Idd* locus. Once established, congenic mice are bred to produce further recombinations in the *Idd* intervals, thus producing mice with a minimum segment length (the typical minimum practical length attainable by random recombination was around 1 megabase (34)) containing variable numbers of B6/B10 genes. This "congenic narrowing" approach has often resulted in the discovery of multiple Idd regions within a much larger segment. For example, the original "Idd9" congenic mouse, after congenic narrowing, produced three strains, Idd9.1-3, each contributory to decreased diabetes (35, 36).

Once a "minimal" interval congenic mouse is established, however, determining the genetic cause of resistance mediated by the genomic interval can be quite challenging. A classic example is Idd3, which was discovered in the initial genome scan (1991); il2 was a candidate gene from the earliest description of Idd3. The difficulty is that many other attractive immune genes were in the interval; il2 is adjacent to il21 on the genome and the two genes were not practically separable by breeding approaches. Various hypotheses concerning the mechanism of IL-2 disease prevention were explored and rejected over the years (37, 38). Ultimately, a very painstaking and beautiful body of work convincingly demonstrated that the NOD allele of il2 produced twofold less IL2 protein, and that an engineered haplodeficiency model in a TCR transgenic system mimicked the autoimmune manifestations of the NOD allele (39). The reduced peripheral IL2 resulted in T regulatory cell deficiencies, since Tregs are dependent on exogenous IL2 for survival (39).

Although the actual determination of the "causative" gene in an Idd interval can be problematic and difficult, this difficulty has been balanced by the remarkable success of genetic work on NOD mice in showing that many genes and immunogenetic pathways in T1D are shared between humans and mice. These have been identified by GWAS and other genetic approaches in humans, and by congenic narrowing strategies in mice. In particular, MHC genes (mouse Idd1), immune regulatory IL2/CD25 genes (40) (mouse Idd3), and T-cell signaling genes CTLA4 (mouse Idd5.1) and the tyrosine phosphatase LYP/PEP (human PTPN22) (mouse Idd18.2) have all been associated with both human and mouse disease (3). All of the candidate genes are immune related, suggesting that a similar overall immune pathway might be operating in human and mouse diabetes. These results justify further dual investigation to uncover shared genes, with the hope of further clarifying the similarities and differences in the immune basis for T1D in mice and humans.

CTLA4 is a fascinating example. CTLA4 was genetically linked to disease in both humans and mice, but the mechanism of the causative gene variant was different in the two species (41). In humans, the linked variant encoded lower levels of alternately spliced, soluble CTLA4. By engineering a mouse in which soluble CTLA4 levels were knocked down, Gerold et al. showed that soluble CTLA4 acted to downregulate dendritic cells (42). Decreased levels of soluble CTLA4 thus correlated with an increased level of immune activation and disease. In mice, the disease-associated variant (Idd5.1 (43)) encoded lower levels of a ligand-independent, alternately spliced CTLA4 variant. The ligand-independent form, although lacking a B71/2 binding domain, strongly inhibits T cell responses by binding and dephosphorylating the TcRzeta chain. Decreased levels of the ligand-independent splice variant therefore resulted in hyperactivated T cells, as did decreased levels of the human soluble form (44). In this case, research into both mouse and human CTLA4 mechanisms produced insights into disease and possible therapeutic approaches directed to regulatory elements that might act throughout the course of the disease. The fact that the actual genetic mechanism altering CTLA4 biology was different in the human and mice, actually strengthens the notion that a common immune pathway is operative in both species, and that it can be affected by a similar set of genetic and environmental modifications.

Our lab has focused on a different genetic pathway. NOD B10 *Idd*9.3 congenic mice have a 1.3 Mb region from nondiabetic B10 mice that reduces diabetes incidence by 40% and contains a *TNFRsf9* variant, encoding the 4-1bb (CD137) molecule, differing at three exonal SNPs from NOD (35, 36). The B10 allele signals more effectively in T cells, resulting in greater proliferation and IL-2 production (36). However, it has not been clear why a hypofunctional allele would result in increased diabetes in NOD mice. To address this conundrum, we began investigating the immunobiology of CD137 in NOD and NOD B10 *Idd*9.3 congenic mice.

An agonist antibody directed to CD137 prevented diabetes, by boosting Tregs after specifically binding to a constitutively CD137-positive Treg subset in vivo (45). This effect made some biological sense: if the disease-associated allele was hypofunctional, and expressed constitutively on a Treg subset, then hypofunctional Tregs could result in decreased immune regulation and increased autoimmunity (as in the case of CTLA4 above). Enhanced signaling directed specifically to the Treg subset (since only Tregs, not T cells, constitutively express CD137) could boost Treg function. These findings were promising; but what about the role of CD137 in human disease? Initial studies of CD137 did not find a linkage with human T1D (46). Subsequently, however, TNFAIP3 (A20) was linked to human diabetes (47), as well as to other autoimmune diseases such as lupus. One function of TNFAIP3 is to downregulate TRAF2 by transporting it to the lysosomal compartment, thus decreasing Traf2-mediated signaling (48). Since CD137 signals via TRAF2, there are direct links between CD137 and TNFAIP3 in modulating immune regulation (49). This led us to further explore the CD137 pathway and its impact on T1D immunity.

3. Role of CD137, solCD137, and CD137L in T1D

CD137 or 4-1BB is an inducible type 1 transmembrane protein of the TNF-receptor superfamily that functions as a costimulatory molecule (49). The CD137 glycoprotein exists as a 30-kDa monomer or a 55-kDa homodimer that is upregulated in T cells 48 h after in vitro activation (50, 51). Membrane-bound CD137 signals through TNF-receptor (TNFR)-associated factor 2 (TRAF2), which in turn activates NFκB and apoptosis signal-regulating kinase-1 (ASK-1), resulting in the upregulation of genes for cytokine production, effector function, and cell survival (49). Stimulation of CD137 either by agonistic anti-CD137 monoclonal antibody, soluble CD137L or in cell lines expressing CD137L in the presence of anti-TCR antibody, results in T-cell expansion, cytokine production, and upregulation of antiapoptotic genes that prevent activated-induced cell death (52, 53). Anti-CD137 mAb has also been shown to reduce the incidence and severity of different murine autoimmune diseases including experimental autoimmune encephalomyelitis, collagen-induced arthritis, and experimental allergic conjunctivitis (54–56).

Aside from the studies in congenic mice mentioned above, previous literature provided further clues for the role of CD137 in Tregs and T1D. Marson et al., in particular, showed that *Tnfrsf9* is one of a small set of genes directly upregulated by Foxp3 (57). The Mathis group, moreover, showed that Tregs isolated specifically from NOD pancreatic islets upregulated *Tnfrsf9* (58).

Cellular studies of the critical cell subset (CD4^{pos}CD25^{pos} T regulatory cells expressing CD137) in NOD and NOD.B10 *Idd9*.3 congenic mice helped us to further understand the role of CD137 in diabetes. We showed that the percentage of CD137^{pos} cells within CD4^{pos}CD25^{pos} T cells significantly declines with age in NOD spleen but not in NOD.B10 Idd9.3 spleen. These findings suggested that increased expression of CD137 on Tregs might enhance long-term survival of those cells, consistent with the previously published role of CD137 on CD8 and CD4 T-cell survival in vivo and in vitro (59–61). We constructed mixed bone marrow chimeras using NOD (CD45.2) and NOD.B10 Idd9.3 (CD45.1) bone marrow transferred into NOD.CD45.2 x NOD.B10 Idd9.3 (CD45.1) F1 mice to test whether the B10 CD137 allotype intrinsically mediated increased survival of CD137^{pos} Tregs. In the mixed bone marrow chimera mice, the percentage of peripheral (splenic or pancreatic lymph node) CD4^{pos}CD25^{pos}CD137^{pos} T cells expressing the B10 CD137 allotype was significantly increased compared to the NOD allotype. These results, in both unmanipulated mice and in mixed bone marrow chimeras, suggest the B10 CD137 allotype intrinsically and selectively mediates enhanced survival of CD137^{pos} Tregs.

To further understand the biology and importance of CD137^{pos} Tregs in diabetes, we performed in vitro suppression assays, and showed that CD137^{pos} Tregs are significantly more suppressive compared to CD137^{neg} in both contact-dependent and contact-independent conditions. When trying to understand the contact-independent suppression, we realized that alternate splicing produces two isoforms of CD137: *full length* CD137 that is expressed on the cell surface and *soluble* CD137 in which transmembrane exon 8 is spliced out (62). The production of soluble (sol) CD137 has been associated with decreased T-cell proliferation and increased T-cell death in human PBMC and mouse splenocytes, and its production has been hypothesized to serve as a negative feedback mechanism to control autoimmunity (63–65). We found that freshly isolated CD137^{pos} Tregs contained higher levels of soluble CD137 mRNA than CD137^{neg} Tregs, and that cultured CD137^{pos} Tregs produced higher levels of soluble CD137 protein than CD137^{neg} Tregs. We showed that in absence of APC, i.e., in a contact-independent culture, CD137L blockade abrogates the CD137^{pos} Treg-mediated suppression, suggesting that soluble CD137 suppressed via CD137L. Finally, soluble CD137-Fc chimeric protein directly suppressed CD4 T-cell proliferation in an APC and Treg independent assay. The presence of CD137L blocking antibody abrogated the suppression mediated by soluble CD137-Fc, further confirming the role of solCD137-CD137L interactions in mediating suppression. This hypothesis of a potential suppressive function of CD137L on lymphocytes is supported by studies showing that CD137 ligand signaling is essential to suppress B cell lymphomas; microarray analysis of the B cell lymphomas showed that lack of CD137L causes overexpression of molecules associated with cell growth (Stat-1, Elf-1, CIITA, AID, Bcl-10, and Rad21) and plasma cell differentiation (Bach-2, Spi-B, and Bcl-6) (66).

4. Approaches Towards Using CD137 as a Therapeutic Agent for T1D

The above experiments and literature show a rich biology involving CD137, CD137L, and solCD137. What struck us, however, was the selective production of solCD137 by Tregs and its clear down modulatory effects on immunity. While we were not sure how the disease-associated SNPs might affect solCD137 activity, it seemed likely that modulating this particular pathway might down modulate autoimmunity in diabetes. Moreover, since CD137L was upregulated at sites on inflammation (49), and solCD137 acted by interacting with CD137L on both T cells and APCs, we hypothesized that this could be an effective target, throughout the time course of disease and even at clinical onset (frank hyperglycemia) to down modulate autoimmunity in the islet. Given the general lack of success in systemic therapy for T1D, we did not think nonspecific systemic administration of solCD137 would be effective. Ideally we would like to overcome the problem of the anatomic "isolation" of pancreatic islets by using tissue-specific cellular therapy to deliver solCD137 to the site of inflammation, where it could bind to and downregulate CD137L in ligand-expressing islet cells. Given the recent demonstration that T-cell accumulation in the islets is largely driven by antigen specificity, i.e., that T cells lacking islet-specific TCRs do not accumulate (67), we decided to use a lentiviral approach and to use transduced BDC 2.5 T cells (specific for an islet autoantigen) to deliver the therapeutic agent. An alternate approach is to use retrogenically modified Tregs to deliver solCD137 locally.

To over-express the soluble B10 CD137 minigene, we used a retrogenic approach (68). The CD137-modified lentivirus, LeGO-iG2-sCD137, gave excellent transduction of bone marrow cells (allowing us to make retrogenic mice) and good transduction of T cells. Since we are using a self-inactivating (SIN) vector the virus lacks replicative potential (69, 70); this enhances safety and helps to avoid a host:virus immune response (71). The solCD137 minigene is expressed from an internal spleen focus-forming virus (SFFV) promoter in the sCD137 construct, and co-expression of enhanced green fluorescent protein (EGFP) reporter is driven from an internal ribosomal entry site (IRES). We used this vector first to transduce a fibroblast cell line, and confirmed by ELISA and western blotting that it produced large amounts of secreted soluble CD137.

Retrogenic mice (potentially useful as sources of sol CD137 expressing cell subsets for use in cellular therapy) were made by lethally irradiating NOD recipient and reconstituting with LeGO-iG2-sCD137-tranduced bone marrow cells or empty vector. Effective reconstitution is assessed by confirming the percent of EGFP-expressing cells in various cell subsets. To transfect BDC 2.5 cells, spleens were harvested from NOD BDC 2.5 TCR transgenic mice and cultured under similar permissive conditions. After 48 h, cells were analyzed by FACS to assess EGFP expression. EGFP+ CD4+ cells were sorted to use in cell transfer studies to reverse T1D. Restricting transgene expression to the BDC2.5 T cells is expected to further minimize any potential antitransgene immune response (71).

The above studies are still ongoing. We do not know at this point if solCD137 will be effective in reversing T1D. It may appear somewhat excessive to have gone to such lengths to try a therapy that may not work. However, the system presented here is highly flexible and allows us to test the effectiveness of multiple suspected genetic variants in modulating T1D. The lentiviral system described above is also highly modular, and will allow us to rapidly splice in and out different candidate genes, as well as test different cell types for gene delivery and therapeutic effectiveness. Hence it represents an excellent dual approach when used in conjunction with genetic studies oriented towards identifying potential candidate genes and their function. By focusing on genes implicated in immunopathogenesis of T1D, and by delivering variants of these genes to the islets in new-onset T1D, we hope to overcome some of the pitfalls in T1D mouse work described in this article.

5. Conclusion

The NOD mouse strain has been extensively analyzed both genetically and immunologically over the last 30 years. A main obstacle to its usefulness is the relative ease by which T1D is prevented in the model, making experiments showing prevention of T1D in NOD somewhat irrelevant to understanding the causes of the disease and how to reverse new-onset diabetes. One way around these problems is to use genetic studies to identify candidate genes/pathways playing a role in the actual pathogenesis of disease. An impressive number of such candidate genes/pathways identified to date have also been identified in human T1D. We can focus our therapeutic efforts and hypotheses to genes operating in common causal pathways in both humans and mice. By further restricting the therapeutic focus to immune genes that are likely active throughout the disease course (i.e., via stimulating ongoing inflammation or by ongoing, insufficient attempts at regulating inflammation) we can identify candidate genes to target for treatment of new-onset diabetes. Finally, by using a modular lentiviral approach expressed in tissue-specific cellular delivery systems, we can rapidly test different candidate genes for effectiveness.

Acknowledgments

This work was funded by a grant from the American Diabetes Association, grant ADA 1-11-BS-131 and from the VA, Merit review I01BX007080 from the Biomedical Laboratory Research & Development Service of the VA Office of Research and Development.

References

1. Driver JP, Serreze DV, Chen YG (2011) Mouse models for the study of autoimmune type 1 diabetes: a NOD to similarities and differences to human disease. Semin Immunopathol 33:67–87
2. Thayer TC, Wilson SB, Mathews CE (2010) Use of nonobese diabetic mice to understand human type 1 diabetes. Endocrinol Metab Clin North Am 39:541–561
3. Wicker LS, Clark J, Fraser HI, Garner VE, Gonzalez-Munoz A, Healy B, Howlett S, Hunter K, Rainbow D, Rosa RL, Smink LJ, Todd JA, Peterson LB (2005) Type 1 diabetes genes and pathways shared by humans and NOD mice. J Autoimmun 25(Suppl):29–33
4. Ridgway WM, Peterson LB, Todd JA, Rainbow DB, Healy B, Burren OS, Wicker LS (2008) Gene-gene interactions in the NOD mouse model of type 1 diabetes. Adv Immunol 100:151–175
5. Culina S, Boitard C, Mallone R (2011) Antigen-based immune therapeutics for type 1 diabetes: magic bullets or ordinary blanks? Clin Dev Immunol 2011:286248
6. Bluestone JA, Herold K, Eisenbarth G (2010) Genetics, pathogenesis and clinical interventions in type 1 diabetes. Nature 464:1293–1300
7. Oikawa Y, Shimada A, Yamada Y, Okubo Y, Katsuki T, Shigihara T, Miyazaki J, Narumi S, Itoh H (2010) CXC chemokine ligand 10 DNA vaccination plus Complete Freund's Adjuvant reverses hyperglycemia in non-obese diabetic mice. Rev Diabet Stud 7:209–224
8. Tarbell KV, Petit L, Zuo X, Toy P, Luo X, Mqadmi A, Yang H, Suthanthiran M, Mojsov S, Steinman RM (2007) Dendritic cell-expanded, islet-specific CD4+ CD25+ CD62L+ regulatory T cells restore normoglycemia in diabetic NOD mice. J Exp Med 204:191–201
9. Fiorina P, Vergani A, Dada S, Jurewicz M, Wong M, Law K, Wu E, Tian Z, Abdi R, Guleria I, Rodig S, Dunussi-Joannopoulos K, Bluestone J, Sayegh MH (2008) Targeting CD22 reprograms B-cells and reverses autoimmune diabetes. Diabetes 57:3013–3024
10. Parker MJ, Xue S, Alexander JJ, Wasserfall CH, Campbell-Thompson ML, Battaglia M, Gregori S, Mathews CE, Song S, Troutt M, Eisenbeis S, Williams J, Schatz DA, Haller MJ, Atkinson MA (2009) Immune depletion with cellular mobilization imparts immunoregulation and reverses autoimmune diabetes in nonobese diabetic mice. Diabetes 58:2277–2284
11. Hu CY, Rodriguez-Pinto D, Du W, Ahuja A, Henegariu O, Wong FS, Shlomchik MJ, Wen L (2007) Treatment with CD20-specific antibody prevents and reverses autoimmune diabetes in mice. J Clin Invest 117:3857–3867
12. Nikolic B, Takeuchi Y, Leykin I, Fudaba Y, Smith RN, Sykes M (2004) Mixed hematopoietic chimerism allows cure of autoimmune diabetes through allogeneic tolerance and reversal of autoimmunity. Diabetes 53:376–383
13. Jurewicz M, Yang S, Augello A, Godwin JG, Moore RF, Azzi J, Fiorina P, Atkinson M, Sayegh MH, Abdi R (2010) Congenic mesenchymal stem cell therapy reverses hyperglycemia in experimental type 1 diabetes. Diabetes 59:3139–3147
14. Tian L, Gao J, Hao J, Zhang Y, Yi H, O'Brien TD, Sorenson R, Luo J, Guo Z (2010) Reversal of new-onset diabetes through modulating inflammation and stimulating beta-cell replication in nonobese diabetic mice by a dipeptidyl

14. peptidase IV inhibitor. Endocrinology 151: 3049–3060
15. Suarez-Pinzon WL, Power RF, Yan Y, Wasserfall C, Atkinson M, Rabinovitch A (2008) Combination therapy with glucagon-like peptide-1 and gastrin restores normoglycemia in diabetic NOD mice. Diabetes 57:3281–3288
16. Grinberg-Bleyer Y, Baeyens A, You S, Elhage R, Fourcade G, Gregoire S, Cagnard N, Carpentier W, Tang Q, Bluestone J, Chatenoud L, Klatzmann D, Salomon BL, Piaggio E (2010) IL-2 reverses established type 1 diabetes in NOD mice by a local effect on pancreatic regulatory T cells. J Exp Med 207:1871–1878
17. Koulmanda M, Bhasin M, Hoffman L, Fan Z, Qipo A, Shi H, Bonner-Weir S, Putheti P, Degauque N, Libermann TA, Auchincloss H Jr, Flier JS, Strom TB (2008) Curative and beta cell regenerative effects of alpha1-antitrypsin treatment in autoimmune diabetic NOD mice. Proc Natl Acad Sci U S A 105:16242–16247
18. Bresson D, Fradkin M, Manenkova Y, Rottembourg D, von Herrath M (2010) Genetic-induced variations in the GAD65 T-cell repertoire governs efficacy of anti-CD3/GAD65 combination therapy in new-onset type 1 diabetes. Mol Ther 18:307–316
19. Godebu E, Summers-Torres D, Lin MM, Baaten BJ, Bradley LM (2008) Polyclonal adaptive regulatory CD4 cells that can reverse type I diabetes become oligoclonal long-term protective memory cells. J Immunol 181:1798–1805
20. Louvet C, Szot GL, Lang J, Lee MR, Martinier N, Bollag G, Zhu S, Weiss A, Bluestone JA (2008) Tyrosine kinase inhibitors reverse type 1 diabetes in nonobese diabetic mice. Proc Natl Acad Sci U S A 105:18895–18900
21. Hoglund P, Mintern J, Waltzinger C, Heath W, Benoist C, Mathis D (1999) Initiation of autoimmune diabetes by developmentally regulated presentation of islet cell antigens in the pancreatic lymph nodes. J Exp Med 189:331–339
22. Rosmalen JG, Leenen PJ, Katz JD, Voerman JS, Drexhage HA (1997) Dendritic cells in the autoimmune insulitis in NOD mouse models of diabetes. Adv Exp Med Biol 417:291–294
23. Saxena V, Ondr JK, Magnusen AF, Munn DH, Katz JD (2007) The countervailing actions of myeloid and plasmacytoid dendritic cells control autoimmune diabetes in the nonobese diabetic mouse. J Immunol 179:5041–5053
24. Wong FS, Janeway CA Jr (1997) The role of CD4 and CD8 T cells in type I diabetes in the NOD mouse. Res Immunol 148:327–332
25. Ziegler AG, Nepom GT (2010) Prediction and pathogenesis in type 1 diabetes. Immunity 32:468–478
26. Mueller DL (2003) Tuning the immune system: competing positive and negative feedback loops. Nat Immunol 4:210–211
27. Shoda LK, Young DL, Ramanujan S, Whiting CC, Atkinson MA, Bluestone JA, Eisenbarth GS, Mathis D, Rossini AA, Campbell SE, Kahn R, Kreuwel HT (2005) A comprehensive review of interventions in the NOD mouse and implications for translation. Immunity 23:115–126
28. Roep BO, Atkinson M, von Herrath M (2004) Satisfaction (not) guaranteed: re-evaluating the use of animal models of type 1 diabetes. Nat Rev Immunol 4:989–997
29. Atkinson MA, Leiter EH (1999) The NOD mouse model of type 1 diabetes: as good as it gets? Nat Med 5:601–604
30. Wicker LS, Todd JA, Peterson LB (1995) Genetic control of autoimmune diabetes in the NOD mouse. Annu Rev Immunol 13:179–200
31. Wicker LS, Miller BJ, Coker LZ, McNally SE, Scott S, Mullen Y, Appel MC (1987) Genetic control of diabetes and insulitis in the nonobese diabetic (NOD) mouse. J Exp Med 165:1639–1654
32. Todd JA, Aitman TJ, Cornall RJ, Ghosh S, Hall JR, Hearne CM, Knight AM, Love JM, McAleer MA, Prins JB et al (1991) Genetic analysis of autoimmune type 1 diabetes mellitus in mice. Nature 351:542–547
33. Burren OS, Adlem EC, Achuthan P, Christensen M, Coulson RM, Todd JA (2011) T1DBase: update 2011, organization and presentation of large-scale data sets for type 1 diabetes research. Nucleic Acids Res 39:D997–D1001
34. Ridgway WM, Healy B, Smink LJ, Rainbow D, Wicker LS (2007) New tools for defining the 'genetic background' of inbred mouse strains. Nat Immunol 8:669–673
35. Lyons PA, Hancock WW, Denny P, Lord CJ, Hill NJ, Armitage N, Siegmund T, Todd JA, Phillips MS, Hess JF, Chen SL, Fischer PA, Peterson LB, Wicker LS (2000) The NOD Idd9 genetic interval influences the pathogenicity of insulitis and contains molecular variants of Cd30, Tnfr2, and Cd137. Immunity 13:107–115
36. Cannons JL, Chamberlain G, Howson J, Smink LJ, Todd JA, Peterson LB, Wicker LS, Watts TH (2005) Genetic and functional association of the immune signaling molecule 4-1BB (CD137/TNFRSF9) with type 1 diabetes. J Autoimmun 25(1):13–20
37. Podolin PL, Wilusz MB, Cubbon RM, Pajvani U, Lord CJ, Todd JA, Peterson LB, Wicker LS, Lyons PA (2000) Differential glycosylation of interleukin 2, the molecular basis for the NOD Idd3 type 1 diabetes gene? Cytokine 12:477–482

38. Kamanaka M, Rainbow D, Schuster-Gossler K, Eynon EE, Chervonsky AV, Wicker LS, Flavell RA (2009) Amino acid polymorphisms altering the glycosylation of IL-2 do not protect from type 1 diabetes in the NOD mouse. Proc Natl Acad Sci U S A 106:11236–11240

39. Yamanouchi J, Rainbow D, Serra P, Howlett S, Hunter K, Garner VE, Gonzalez-Munoz A, Clark J, Veijola R, Cubbon R, Chen SL, Rosa R, Cumiskey AM, Serreze DV, Gregory S, Rogers J, Lyons PA, Healy B, Smink LJ, Todd JA, Peterson LB, Wicker LS, Santamaria P (2007) Interleukin-2 gene variation impairs regulatory T cell function and causes autoimmunity. Nat Genet 39:329–337

40. Rainbow DB, Esposito L, Howlett SK, Hunter KM, Todd JA, Peterson LB, Wicker LS (2008) Commonality in the genetic control of Type 1 diabetes in humans and NOD mice: variants of genes in the IL-2 pathway are associated with autoimmune diabetes in both species. Biochem Soc Trans 36:312–315

41. Ueda H, Howson JM, Esposito L, Heward J, Snook H, Chamberlain G, Rainbow DB, Hunter KM, Smith AN, Di Genova G, Herr MH, Dahlman I, Payne F, Smyth D, Lowe C, Twells RC, Howlett S, Healy B, Nutland S, Rance HE, Everett V, Smink LJ, Lam AC, Cordell HJ, Walker NM, Bordin C, Hulme J, Motzo C, Cucca F, Hess JF, Metzker ML, Rogers J, Gregory S, Allahabadia A, Nithiyananthan R, Tuomilehto-Wolf E, Tuomilehto J, Bingley P, Gillespie KM, Undlien DE, Ronningen KS, Guja C, Ionescu-Tirgoviste C, Savage DA, Maxwell AP, Carson DJ, Patterson CC, Franklyn JA, Clayton DG, Peterson LB, Wicker LS, Todd JA, Gough SC (2003) Association of the T-cell regulatory gene CTLA4 with susceptibility to autoimmune disease. Nature 423:506–511

42. Gerold KD, Zheng P, Rainbow DB, Zernecke A, Wicker LS, Kissler S (2011) The soluble CTLA-4 splice variant protects from type 1 diabetes and potentiates regulatory T-cell function. Diabetes 60:1955–1963

43. Wicker LS, Chamberlain G, Hunter K, Rainbow D, Howlett S, Tiffen P, Clark J, Gonzalez-Munoz A, Cumiskey AM, Rosa RL, Howson JM, Smink LJ, Kingsnorth A, Lyons PA, Gregory S, Rogers J, Todd JA, Peterson LB (2004) Fine mapping, gene content, comparative sequencing, and expression analyses support Ctla4 and Nramp1 as candidates for Idd5.1 and Idd5.2 in the nonobese diabetic mouse. J Immunol 173:164–173

44. Vijayakrishnan L, Slavik JM, Illes Z, Greenwald RJ, Rainbow D, Greve B, Peterson LB, Hafler DA, Freeman GJ, Sharpe AH, Wicker LS, Kuchroo VK (2004) An autoimmune disease-associated CTLA-4 splice variant lacking the B7 binding domain signals negatively in T cells. Immunity 20:563–575

45. Irie J, Wu Y, Kachapati K, Mittler RS, Ridgway WM (2007) Modulating protective and pathogenic CD4+ subsets via CD137 in type 1 diabetes. Diabetes 56:186–196

46. Maier LM, Smyth DJ, Vella A, Payne F, Cooper JD, Pask R, Lowe C, Hulme J, Smink LJ, Fraser H, Moule C, Hunter KM, Chamberlain G, Walker N, Nutland S, Undlien DE, Ronningen KS, Guja C, Ionescu-Tirgoviste C, Savage DA, Strachan DP, Peterson LB, Todd JA, Wicker LS, Twells RC (2005) Construction and analysis of tag single nucleotide polymorphism maps for six human-mouse orthologous candidate genes in type 1 diabetes. BMC Genet 6:9

47. Fung EY, Smyth DJ, Howson JM, Cooper JD, Walker NM, Stevens H, Wicker LS, Todd JA (2009) Analysis of 17 autoimmune disease-associated variants in type 1 diabetes identifies 6q23/TNFAIP3 as a susceptibility locus. Genes Immun 10:188–191

48. Li L, Soetandyo N, Wang Q, Ye Y (2009) The zinc finger protein A20 targets TRAF2 to the lysosomes for degradation. Biochim Biophys Acta 1793:346–353

49. Watts TH (2005) TNF/TNFR family members in costimulation of T cell responses. Annu Rev Immunol 23:23–68

50. Pollok KE, Kim YJ, Zhou Z, Hurtado J, Kim KK, Pickard RT, Kwon BS (1993) Inducible T cell antigen 4-1BB. Analysis of expression and function. J Immunol 150:771–781

51. Vinay DS, Kwon BS (1998) Role of 4-1BB in immune responses. Semin Immunol 10:481–489

52. Croft M (2003) Costimulation of T cells by OX40, 4-1BB, and CD27. Cytokine Growth Factor Rev 14:265–273

53. Croft M (2003) Co-stimulatory members of the TNFR family: keys to effective T-cell immunity? Nat Rev Immunol 3:609–620

54. Foell J, McCausland M, Burch J, Corriazzi N, Yan XJ, Suwyn C, O'Neil SP, Hoffmann MK, Mittler RS (2003) CD137-mediated T cell co-stimulation terminates existing autoimmune disease in SLE-prone NZB/NZW F1 mice. Ann N Y Acad Sci 987:230–235

55. Fukushima A, Yamaguchi T, Ishida W, Fukata K, Mittler RS, Yagita H, Ueno H (2005) Engagement of 4-1BB inhibits the development of experimental allergic conjunctivitis in mice. J Immunol 175:4897–4903

56. Sun Y, Lin X, Chen HM, Wu Q, Subudhi SK, Chen L, Fu YX (2002) Administration of

agonistic anti-4-1BB monoclonal antibody leads to the amelioration of experimental autoimmune encephalomyelitis. J Immunol 168: 1457–1465
57. Marson A, Kretschmer K, Frampton GM, Jacobsen ES, Polansky JK, MacIsaac KD, Levine SS, Fraenkel E, von Boehmer H, Young RA (2007) Foxp3 occupancy and regulation of key target genes during T-cell stimulation. Nature 445:931–935
58. Chen Z, Herman AE, Matos M, Mathis D, Benoist C (2005) Where CD4+CD25+ T reg cells impinge on autoimmune diabetes. J Exp Med 202:1387–1397
59. Bertram EM, Lau P, Watts TH (2002) Temporal segregation of 4-1BB versus CD28-mediated costimulation: 4-1BB ligand influences T cell numbers late in the primary response and regulates the size of the T cell memory response following influenza infection. J Immunol 168:3777–3785
60. Lee HW, Park SJ, Choi BK, Kim HH, Nam KO, Kwon BS (2002) 4-1BB promotes the survival of CD8+ T lymphocytes by increasing expression of Bcl-xL and Bfl-1. J Immunol 169:4882–4888
61. Kim J, Choi SP, La S, Seo JS, Kim KK, Nam SH, Kwon B (2003) Constitutive expression of 4-1BB on T cells enhances CD4+ T cell responses. Exp Mol Med 35:509–517
62. Setareh M, Schwarz H, Lotz M (1995) A mRNA variant encoding a soluble form of 4-1BB, a member of the murine NGF/TNF receptor family. Gene 164:311–315
63. Schwarz H, Blanco FJ, von Kempis J, Valbracht J, Lotz M (1996) ILA, a member of the human nerve growth factor/tumor necrosis factor receptor family, regulates T-lymphocyte proliferation and survival. Blood 87:2839–2845
64. Shao Z, Sun F, Koh DR, Schwarz H (2008) Characterisation of soluble murine CD137 and its association with systemic lupus. Mol Immunol 45:3990–3999
65. Michel J, Schwarz H (2000) Expression of soluble CD137 correlates with activation-induced cell death of lymphocytes. Cytokine 12:742–746
66. Middendorp S, Xiao Y, Song JY, Peperzak V, Krijger PH, Jacobs H, Borst J (2009) Mice deficient for CD137 ligand are predisposed to develop germinal center-derived B-cell lymphoma. Blood 114:2280–2289
67. Lennon GP, Bettini M, Burton AR, Vincent E, Arnold PY, Santamaria P, Vignali DA (2009) T cell islet accumulation in type 1 diabetes is a tightly regulated, cell-autonomous event. Immunity 31:643–653
68. Szymczak AL, Workman CJ, Wang Y, Vignali KM, Dilioglou S, Vanin EF, Vignali DA (2004) Correction of multi-gene deficiency in vivo using a single 'self-cleaving' 2A peptide-based retroviral vector. Nat Biotechnol 22:589–594
69. Miyoshi H, Blomer U, Takahashi M, Gage FH, Verma IM (1998) Development of a self-inactivating lentivirus vector. J Virol 72:8150–8157
70. Weber K, Bartsch U, Stocking C, Fehse B (2008) A multicolor panel of novel lentiviral "gene ontology" (LeGO) vectors for functional gene analysis. Mol Ther 16:698–706
71. Follenzi A, Santambrogio L, Annoni A (2007) Immune responses to lentiviral vectors. Curr Gene Ther 7:306–315

Chapter 2

Assessment of Diabetic Nephropathy in the Akita Mouse

Jae-Hyung Chang and Susan B. Gurley

Abstract

Akita mice have type 1 diabetes mellitus caused by a spontaneous point mutation in the *Ins2* gene which leads to misfolding of insulin, resulting in pancreatic β-cell failure. Akita mice develop pronounced and sustained hyperglycemia, high levels of albuminuria, and consistent histopathological changes, suggesting that these mice may be suitable as an experimental platform for modeling diabetic nephropathy. One key feature of diabetic kidney disease in Akita mice is that the severity of renal injury is significantly influenced by genetic background. In this chapter, we describe the Akita model and present some of the experimental studies utilizing Akita mice as a model of type 1 diabetes. For example, deficiency in bradykinin receptors, endothelial nitric oxide synthase, or angiotensin-converting enzyme 2 leads to development of functionally and structurally more advanced diabetic nephropathy in these mice, while ketogenic diet has been shown to reverse kidney injury associated with diabetes. This chapter also describes the application of 24-h urine collections from mice for careful measurement of urinary albumin excretion.

Key words: Mouse model of type I diabetes, Diabetic nephropathy, Genetic susceptibility, Albuminuria, Glomerular filtration rate, Bradykinin receptor, Endothelial nitric oxide synthase, Angiotensin-converting enzyme 2, Ketogenic diet, Mouse metabolic cage, 24-h urine collection

1. Introduction: The Akita Mouse as an Experimental Model of Diabetic Nephropathy

Diabetes mellitus is a serious public health problem with incidence reaching epidemic proportions in developed countries (1, 2). Among its complications, diabetic nephropathy (DN) is a leading cause of chronic kidney failure and end-stage renal disease (ESRD) worldwide (1–3). DN is characterized by microalbuminuria as the earliest detectable sign of glomerular injury followed by the development of macroalbuminuria and a progressive decline in glomerular filtration rate (GFR) (4). Histopathological hallmarks of the disease are glomerular mesangial matrix expansion, nodular glomerulosclerosis, and tubulointerstitial fibrosis (5). Consequently, much effort has been devoted to understanding disease mechanisms in DN with the goal of developing new treatment strategies for this devastating disorder. In this regard, mouse models of diabetes mellitus are useful for studying both pathogenesis and treatment of kidney disease, in particular because of the potential for genetic manipulation of the mouse genome (6). However, while significant progress has been made in the past few years, current mouse models still do not display the full spectrum of functional and pathological characteristics of human DN (6, 7).

The Akita mouse, which is a recently described genetic model of type 1 diabetes mellitus, shows promise in this regard (6, 8, 9). Akita mice harbor an autosomal dominant, spontaneous point mutation which was originally identified in a colony of C57BL/6 mice in Akita, Japan (10). This mutation introduces a Cys to Tyr substitution at the seventh amino acid in the A chain of mature insulin ($Ins2^{C96Y}$) and leads to a disruption of an intramolecular disulfide bond (11). This causes improper folding of the insulin protein resulting in selective proteotoxicity to the pancreatic β-cell (6, 11). Subsequently, islets from Akita mice are depleted of β-cells, and those remaining β-cells release very little mature insulin (11). While homozygosity for the mutation leads to perinatal lethality, mice heterozygous for the Akita mutation are viable and fertile, and develop spontaneous hyperglycemia around 3–4 weeks of age.

One clear finding from studies of Akita mice is that the renal phenotype of these mice is significantly influenced by their genetic background (6, 8, 9). The heterogeneity of disease severity across different strains suggests that genetic determinants might modulate susceptibility to kidney injury from diabetes in Akita mice as it has been previously shown to affect susceptibility to DN in humans (12). Thus far, a number of Akita mice on different inbred genetic background have been created and characterized, and studies using these mice have been performed to better understand pathogenic mechanisms of DN as well as to evaluate novel treatment strategies (8, 9). Table 1 provides a comparison of the DN-related features exhibited by these mouse models. In this chapter we present the key features of several experimental studies in DN that have been conducted using Akita mice as a model of kidney injury associated with type 1 diabetes mellitus and describe in detail our current protocol for 24-h urine collection in mice for urine albumin measurements, an important component of the renal phenotyping process.

1.1. Ins2-Akita Mutation Versus Streptozotocin-Induced Diabetes in Mice

STZ has been used widely to induce type 1 diabetes in rodents (6, 9, 13). Streptozotocin (STZ) causes diabetes in animals secondary to pancreatic β-cell failure, however, it may be toxic to a variety of other tissues which complicates interpretation of results (6) and also requires administration of a drug to animals. To investigate potential differences in the character of kidney injury between chemical and genetic models of type 1 diabetes, we compared C57BL/6 mice treated with STZ with C57BL/6 Akita mice (9).

Table 1
Summary of selected Akita mouse models used in diabetic nephropathy research

Mouse strains	Blood pressure	Blood glucose	Albuminuria[a]	Glomerular filtration rate	Renal structure	Primary references
C57BL/6	↑	↑	1+	↑	Mesangial expansion (mild)	(8, 9)
129/SvEv	↑	↑	3+	↑	Mesangial expansion (mild)	(8)
DBA/2	=	↑	7+	Not reported	Unchanged	(8)
FVB/NJ	↑	↑	10+	↑	Mesangial expansion (mild-to-moderate)	(Chang J. H. et al. unpublished)
F1(D2:B6)	↑	↑	5+	↑	Mesangial expansion (mild)	(8)

[a]Albuminuria scale 1+ ≈ 50 μg/day

Throughout the study period, male Akita mice developed hyperglycemia that was more pronounced and durable than that observed in the STZ model (518 ± 25 vs. 388 ± 50 mg/dL at 6 months of age). Male C57BL/6 Akita mice also developed mild hypertension and decrease in heart rates compared to their nondiabetic controls while C57BL/6 mice treated with STZ tended to have reduced BPs. Moreover, male Akita mice on C57BL/6 background developed more severe albuminuria, mesangial expansion, and renal and glomerular hypertrophy than the male mice with STZ-induced diabetes. These studies comparing both models on the same genetic background suggest that the Akita model offers advantages over chemical models of diabetes and thus, it may provide a better experimental platform for DN model development.

1.2. Impact of Genetic Background on Diabetic Kidney Injury in Akita Mice

In humans with diabetes, it is well established that there is a clear-cut genetic susceptibility to the development of kidney injury (12). Genetic background may also influence the development of diabetic renal complications in mice (8, 9, 13). In this regard, studies in mice with STZ-induced diabetes provided evidence for differential susceptibility to kidney injury among genetically distinct mouse lines (9, 13). To further test this hypothesis using the Akita model, we recently characterized renal manifestations of diabetes in several inbred strains of Akita mice (C57BL/6-$Ins2^{C96Y/+}$, DBA/2-$Ins2^{C96Y/+}$, and 129SvEv-$Ins2^{C96Y/+}$) (8). Male Akita mice on all three backgrounds developed marked and equivalent hyperglycemia compared with their respective wild-type controls. The marked levels of hyperglycemia were sustained through the 6-month study period. However, despite similar levels of hyperglycemia, there were significant differences in the magnitude of albuminuria among the three Akita strains at 6 months of age. While the absolute level of urinary albumin excretion was highest in the DBA/2-$Ins2^{C96Y/+}$ group (345 ± 110 μg/day), it was lowest in the C57BL/6-$Ins2^{C96Y/+}$ mice (40 ± 3 μg/day), and intermediate in the 129SvEv-$Ins2^{C96Y/+}$ group (151 ± 77 μg/day). Compared with their respective nondiabetic controls, there was a fivefold increase in urinary albumin excretion in the 129SvEv-$Ins2^{C96Y/+}$ animals (151 ± 77 μg/day (Akita) vs. 33 ± 20 μg/day (control); $P=0.03$), threefold increase in the DBA/2-$Ins2^{C96Y/+}$ group (345 ± 110 μg/day (Akita) vs. 116 ± 27 μg/day (control); $P=0.048$), and 2.8-fold increase in the C57BL/6-$Ins2^{C96Y/+}$ mice (40 ± 3 μg/day (Akita) vs. 14 ± 2 μg/day (control); $P<0.0001$). Similarly, estimated GFR was significantly higher in the 129SvEv-$Ins2^{C96Y/+}$ mice compared to the C57BL/6-$Ins2^{C96Y/+}$ group at 6 months of age (24.5 ± 1.9 μL/min/g body weight vs. 16.0 ± 1.3 μL/min/g body weight; $P=0.0004$). At this point in the disease process, increased GFR represents hyperfiltration. Examination of the kidneys by light microscopy revealed modest mesangial matrix expansion of similar severity in diabetic 129SvEv and C57BL/6 mice compared to their respective nondiabetic controls (2- to 2.5-fold increase in mesangial score) with preservation of normal morphology in the tubular and interstitial regions.

To assess the heritability of strain-specific modifiers affecting susceptibility to kidney injury associated with diabetes in Akita mice, we extended these studies to include a cohort of F1 intercross mice between the two strains, C57BL/6 and DBA/2 (8), with C57BL/6 being a strain resistant to developing DN and DBA/2 as a susceptible strain. These F1(DBA/2 × C57BL/6) $Ins2^{C96Y/+}$ animals developed robust and sustained hyperglycemia similar to the other strains examined in our study. Interestingly, however, the extent of albuminuria in the F1-$Ins2^{C96Y/+}$ mice was equivalent to the parental DBA/2-$Ins2^{C96Y/+}$ line (240 ± 54 μg/day vs. 345 ± 110 μg/day; $P=$ NS) while that of mesangial pathology was very similar to that seen in the parental C57BL/6-$Ins2^{C96Y/+}$ line. These studies suggest that there is a dominant pattern of susceptibility alleles for albuminuria from the DBA/2 strain. In a separate set of experiments, we determined the functional and structural characteristics of kidney disease in FVB/NJ Akita mice. In this study, male FVB/NJ Akita mice developed sustained hyperglycemia and albuminuria by 4 and 8 weeks of age, respectively. By 20 weeks of age, diabetic animals developed a tenfold increase in albuminuria (480 ± 73 μg/day (Akita) vs. 40 ± 7 μg/day (control); $P<0.0001$) as well as renal and glomerular hypertrophy. Levels of albuminuria in FVB/NJ Akita mice suggest a moderate to severe susceptibility to renal injury resulting from type 1 diabetes, with 24-h urinary albumin excretion values being greater than the strains reported by Gurley and coworkers (8, 9). Mild-to-moderate glomerular mesangial expansion was also observed in FVB/NJ Akita mice at 30 weeks of age (Chang J.H. et al., unpublished observation). Therefore, FVB/NJ Akita mice develop significant renal injury that may make this strain suitable for disease modeling.

Together, these findings provide evidence for strong genetic modifiers influencing kidney phenotypes associated with diabetes, such as albuminuria and mesangial pathology. Identification of these naturally occurring genetic modifiers among different genetic backgrounds may allow mapping of specific gene variants which can accelerate kidney injury associated with diabetes. Moreover, they are important considerations when selecting a model of type 1 diabetes.

1.3. Akita Mice as Type 1 Diabetes Models

Below are some examples of studies where the $Ins2^{C96Y/+}$ mutation is used to induce type 1 diabetes in mice, illustrating the utility for disease modeling with Akita mice.

1.3.1. Bradykinin B1 and B2 Receptor Deficiency in Akita Mice

Accumulating evidence suggests that kallikrein-kinin system (KKS) plays a key role in the pathogenesis of diabetic kidney disease (14–16). In this regard, the deletion (D) allele of the common insertion/deletion (I/D) polymorphism of the angiotensin-converting enzyme (ACE) gen in humans is associated with higher serum levels of ACE (17) with resultant-enhanced inactivation of bradykinin (14) and increased risk for type 1 DN. Additionally, ACE inhibitors have well-documented beneficial effects on diabetic kidney injury that are beyond those attributable to changes in BP (18, 19). One possibility to explain these findings is that bradykinin may partly mediate the renoprotective effects of ACE inhibitors (14, 16). In mammals, two receptors for bradykinin have been identified: B1R and B2R (14). While B2R is constitutively expressed in most tissues, B1R is expressed minimally under normal circumstances, but is induced by lipopolysaccharide (LPS) in kidney (14), diabetes in heart (20), inflammation in endothelial cells, fibroblasts, urothelial cells and sensory neurons (21–23), and in the absence of B2R in kidney and heart (24). In their studies, Kakoki and coworkers investigated the role of both bradykinin receptors in the development of DN using Akita mice on C57BL/6 background (15, 16). By 6 months of age, diabetic Akita mice lacking the B2R developed more severe kidney pathology than their diabetic littermates expressing B2R. BR knockout-Akita mice exhibited a fourfold increase in albuminuria, severe renal hypertrophy and mesangial sclerosis that closely resembles glomerular changes seen in humans with diabetic glomerulosclerosis. At 12 months of age, all of the renal diabetic phenotypes observed in Akita mice, including albuminuria, glomerulosclerosis, interstitial fibrosis, glomerular basement membrane (GBM) thickening, mitochondrial DNA deletions, and renal expression of fibrogenic genes (transforming growth factor (TGF)-β1, connective tissue growth factor, endothelin-1) were enhanced by lack of both B1R and B2R. Interestingly, diabetic Akita mice lacking both bradykinin receptors had more severe kidney injury than Akita mice lacking only B2R suggesting that expression of B1R may have beneficial effects in DN in the absence of constitutively expressed B2R. These results demonstrate the critical role of the bradykinin system in protecting kidney from damage caused by diabetes mellitus, and provide a clear example in how the Akita model can be used effectively to study the pathomechanisms of diabetic kidney injury in mice.

1.3.2. Endothelial Nitric Oxide Synthase Deficiency in Akita Mice

Endothelial dysfunction and damage are prevalent in patients with diabetes mellitus and contribute to the development of DN (25). Nitric oxide (NO) is a vasodilator that can modulate permeability in the vasculature (26), and besides its potency to control vascular tone and therefore BP, NO also inhibits platelet aggregation and smooth muscle cell proliferation. There are three different isoforms of nitric oxide synthase (NOS): endothelial, neuronal, and inducible (27). In endothelial cells, endothelial nitric oxide synthase (eNOS) is expressed constitutively and produces endothelial cell-derived NO (27). In humans, vascular eNOS activity can be altered in diabetes, and three functionally significant polymorphisms in the eNOS gene, *NOS3,* have been shown to lead to a decreased production of NO and are associated with the development of advanced DN in both patients with type 1 and type 2 diabetes (28–31). To better understand the role of eNOS-derived NO in the pathogenesis of DN, Wang and coworkers generated C57BL/6 $eNOS^{-/-}Ins2^{C96Y/+}$ as a mouse model of type 1 diabetes with deficient eNOS activity (31). These diabetic mice, however, died by the age of 5 months before development of DN. Therefore, $eNOS^{-/-}Ins2^{C96Y/+}$ and $eNOS^{+/-}Ins2^{C96Y/+}$ mice that are F1 between C57BL/6 and 129S6/SvEvTac were created, which were as genetically uniform as inbred mice but lacked the detrimental recessive mutations that affected the survival of their parents. Compared with Akita mice having fully intact *eNOS* expression, $eNOS^{-/-}$ Akita and $eNOS^{+/-}$ Akita mice developed 2.5-fold higher urinary albumin excretion at both 3 and 7 months of age. The GFR in diabetic mice was increased by both reduction ($eNOS^{+/-}$) and absence ($eNOS^{-/-}$) of eNOS at 3 months of age. Morphometric analysis revealed that mesangial expansion, glomerulosclerosis, and GBM thickening were progressively worse in diabetic Akita mice in the order: $eNOS^{+/+}$ Akita < $eNOS^{+/-}$ Akita < $eNOS^{-/-}$ Akita, and these changes were independent from BP. Finally, along with exacerbation of DN, loss of eNOS in diabetic Akita mice increased renal fibrin deposition, and expression of inflammatory and fibrinogenic factors including tumor necrosis factor (TNF), interleukin (IL)-6, monocyte chemotactic protein 1 (MCP1), intercellular adhesion molecule 1 (ICAM1), vascular cell adhesion molecule 1 (VCAM1), and TGF-β. In summary, eNOS deficiency in Akita mice accelerated the renal injury associated with diabetes and provided insight into molecular pathways involved in the development of DN.

1.3.3. Angiotensin-Converting Enzyme 2 Deficiency in Akita Mice

Activation of renin–angiotensin system (RAS) with subsequent generation of angiotensin II (ANGII) holds an important role in the pathogenesis of kidney injury associated with diabetes (18). Blockade of the RAS has been shown to ameliorate the development of DN (18, 19). Angiotensin-converting enzyme 2 (ACE2) is a homologue of classical ACE that is also membrane-bound, but is a monocarboxypeptidase that generates ANG from the decapeptide ANGI and from the octapeptide ANGII (32, 33). As such, ACE2 represents an endogenous negative regulator of the RAS by degrading the vasoconstrictor ANGII while producing the vasodilator ANG-(1–7). In this regards, early increases in ACE2 mRNA levels, protein expression (34), and ACE2 activity have been reported in animal models of diabetes (33), whereas ACE2 mRNA and protein levels were decreased in older experimentally induced diabetic rats (32). In humans with type 2 diabetes, glomerular and tubular ACE2 expressions are reduced while ACE expression is increased (35, 36). Together, these data suggest a protective role for ACE2 in the early stage of DN. To test this hypothesis, Wong and coworkers recently studied the effect of deletion of the *Ace2* gene ($Ace2^{-/y}$) on DN in Akita mice (37). They generated $Ace2^{-/y}Ins2^{C96Y/+}$ by crossing ACE2 knockout mice with Akita mice. At 3 months of age, the absence of ACE2 led to a twofold increase in urinary albumin excretion in $Ace2^{-/y}Ins2^{C96Y/+}$ mice compared with Akita mice with *Ace2* gene intact despite similar blood glucose levels. Histomorphometric analysis of the kidneys of mice at 3 months of age revealed increased glomerular volume, mesangial matrix expansion, and GBM thickening accompanied by increased glomerular expression of fibronectin and α-smooth muscle actin as markers of glomerular injury. Although ANGII level was not increased in kidneys of diabetic $Ace2^{-/y}Ins2^{C96Y/+}$ mice, treatment with an angiotensin type 1 (AT1) receptor blocker (ARB) reduced urinary albumin excretion rate in these diabetic animals. In a study by Oudit and coworkers, treatment of Akita mice for 4 weeks with human recombinant ACE2 (hrACE2) increased plasma ACE2 activity, reduced urinary albumin excretion, and decreased glomerular volume, mesangial matrix expansion, and GBM thickness (38). Treatment with hrACE2 also lowered ANGII levels in renal cortex, and reduced ANGII-induced oxidative stress and NADPH oxidase activity (38). Taken together, these findings in diabetic Akita mice suggest that ACE2 plays a protective role in the diabetic kidney as a negative regulator of RAS and again demonstrate the utility of the Akita model.

1.3.4. Reversal of Kidney Injury by a Ketogenic Diet in Akita Mice

Increasing evidence suggests that the ketogenic diet may prevent and even reverse kidney pathologies associated with diabetes (39–41). In this regard, chronic caloric restriction and ketogenic diet reroute cellular metabolism away from glucose utilization and toward the use of alternative fuels, including the ketone

3-beta-hydroxybutyric acid (3-OHB) (39, 42). Prolonged elevation of 3-OHB, on the other hand, has been recently shown to reduce molecular response to glucose metabolism (43) and may ultimately lead to the reversal of diabetic kidney pathology (39). To address this hypothesis, Poplawski and coworkers examined if a ketogenic diet can reverse DN in C57BL/6 Akita mice (39). After the development of DN had been confirmed in the Akita mice at 20 weeks of age by the presence of tenfold increase in albuminuria, half of the Akita mice and half of the nondiabetic controls were placed on a ketogenic diet while the remaining animals were maintained on a standard high-carbohydrate diet. Ketogenic diet increased blood 3-OHB level, and after 2 months on the diet, both blood glucose level as well as urinary albumin excretion was completely normalized in diabetic Akita mice without insulin treatment. Ketogenic diet also normalized expression of kidney genes induced by oxidative and other forms of stress associated with diabetes in Akita mice. Interestingly, however, histological pathology such as glomerular sclerosis was only partially reversed by the dietary intervention in diabetic animals suggesting that reversal of functional and molecular markers of DN occur more rapidly than reversal of histological aspects of DN. These studies demonstrate that DN can potentially be altered in Akita mice by therapies such as prolonged maintenance on a ketogenic diet. The mechanism by which the simple dietary intervention reverses kidney injury associated with this model of type 1 diabetes, however, remains to be determined.

1.4. Potential for Akita Mice as a Model of DN

Significant progress has been made during the past decade toward development of better mouse models of DN, which has helped to advance our understanding of the pathogenesis of diabetic kidney injury in humans (6, 7). In this regard, the Akita model appears to be quite promising. These mice develop sustained and robust hyperglycemia as a result of a spontaneous mutation in the $Ins2$ gene accompanied by enhanced levels of albuminuria and consistent mesangial pathology (6, 8, 9). Similar to humans, these phenotypic features are significantly influenced by genetic background (8). Moreover, Akita mice also develop hypertension, cardiac hypertrophy, and echocardiographic evidence of heart failure which are complications commonly associated with diabetes mellitus in humans (44). Finally, Akita mice are commercially available, and the $Ins2^{+/C96Y}$ mutation can be easily intercrossed on other transgenic mouse lines to facilitate model development. As described in this chapter, these features of the Akita model may provide an ideal experimental platform for studying the mechanisms of diabetic kidney injury that exist in humans, and ultimately advance our progress toward a treatment for DN.

2. Materials

2.1. 24-Hour Urine Collection for Mice (see Fig. 1)

1. Cage lid: Holds disposable air filter pad. Keeps animal securely in cage, but can be removed for easy access to the animal.
2. Mouse cage: Consists of an upper and a lower chamber and is designed to house individual mice. Constructed of transparent, gas sterilizable acryl. Easy to clean with warm soapy water or detergent solution.
3. Food chamber: Constructed of transparent acryl. Located outside cage. This tunnel allows easy access to the food drawer, while its small size discourages rodents from nesting or sleeping inside. It prevents spilled food from entering the cage and contaminating the urine collection.
4. Food drawer: Constructed of transparent acryl. Slides out for easy filling with slurries, liquids or powders, without disturbing the animal.
5. Water bottle holder: Constructed of transparent acryl. Located outside cage.
6. Water bottle: Constructed of acryl.

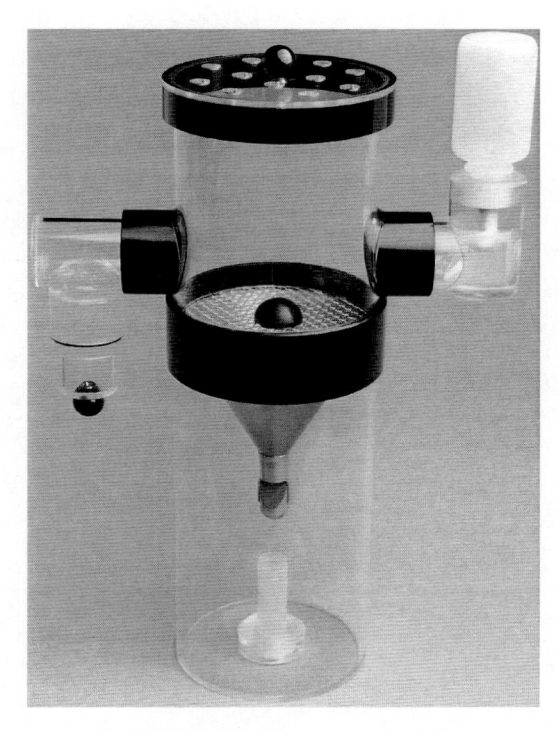

Fig. 1. Individual mouse metabolic cage (Courtesy of R. Goodman, Hatteras Instruments, NC, USA).

7. Stainless steel mesh screen floor for the cage: Lets excreta pass through the widely spaced bars.
8. Stainless steel funnel and separating cone: Urine flows along the inside surface of the collection funnel and is directed into the urine collection tube. Separates urine from feces.
9. Urine collection tube: Removable and disposable.
10. Digital scale.
11. Centrifuge capable of generating a force of $800 \times g$.
12. Pipettes (200–1,000 µL).
13. Sterile microfuge tubes (1.5 mL).

3. Methods

The intent of a metabolic cage is to collect urine and separate it from feces. There are numerous commercial rodent metabolic cages available to collect urine. Here we describe 24-h urine collection using metabolic cages purchased from Hatteras Instruments (MMC100 Metabolic Cage, Hatteras Instruments, Cary, NC, USA).

1. Determine body weight of each mouse prior to study by using a digital scale.
2. Determine weight of each urine collection tube prior to study by using a digital scale as this will be used to determine volume of urine collected (see Note 1).
3. Fill feeder drawer with rodent diet (e.g., rodent chow) (see Note 2). Slide the filled drawer cautiously into the food chamber. Food consumption can be monitored by weighing food drawer and the food inside before and after the study.
4. Fill water bottle with distilled water and attach it to the holder (see Note 3). Water consumption can be monitored by weighing the water-filled bottles before and after the study (see Note 4).
5. Place urine collection tube in the lower chamber of the cage.
6. Put stainless steel funnel in the lower chamber of the cage with the spout of the funnel positioned directly above the urine collection tube to collect the urine (see Note 5).
7. Place stainless steel mesh screen floor above the funnel (see Note 5).
8. Attach the upper chamber to the lower chamber above the stainless mesh screen (see Note 6).
9. Put single mouse into the upper chamber on the stainless steel mesh.

10. Close the upper chamber of the mouse cage with the cage lid.
11. The start time of the study is recorded.
12. After 24 h mice are removed from the cages and the body weight and the amount of water consumed and urine produced recorded (see Notes 4, 7, and 8).
13. The collected urine is centrifuged at $800 \times g$ for 15 min to remove solid contaminants and then the supernatant is aliquotted into 1.5 mL tubes (see Note 9). Store samples at $-70\,°C$.
14. Avoid repeated freeze–thaw cycles (see Note 10).

4. Notes

1. Label both urine collection tube as well as its lid for identification. Use fade and water resistant ink. This is important since spilled urine can wash away the ink.
2. Clean the food drawer each time with warm soapy water or detergent solution. Fill the drawer with fresh diet prior to each study.
3. Clean the water bottle each time with warm soapy water or detergent solution. Fill the bottle with fresh distilled water prior to each study.
4. Water consumption over a 24-h period can be calculated by using the formula: Water consumption per 24 h = Filled water bottle$^{pre\text{-}study}$ – Filled water bottle$^{post\text{-}study}$.
5. Make sure to dry the stainless steel funnel and the mesh screen floor completely after cleaning prior to each study. Remaining debris from cleaning can prevent flow of urine, and contaminate and dilute sample, causing false results.
6. Take care to attach both chambers together to avoid spilling of food and water from food chamber and water bottle, respectively.
7. Urine 24-h volume can be calculated by using the formula: Urine 24-h volume = Urine collection tube$^{post\text{-}study}$ – Urine collection tube$^{pre\text{-}study}$ (empty).
8. In diabetic animals, urine may overflow the collection tube's capacity and spill in the lower chamber of mouse cage. Larger containers can be used or the overflow urine should be collected carefully in an additional urine collection tube. Avoid transferring accidently feces into the collection tube. Determine volume of overflow urine by using above formula for urine volume.

9. Avoid disrupting the pellet since this contains feces, hair, cells, and crystals.
10. Repeated freeze–thaw cycles will damage and potentially denature most proteins in urine including albumin and should be avoided.

References

1. Reutens AT, Atkins RC (2011) Epidemiology of diabetic nephropathy. Contrib Nephrol 170:1–7
2. de Boer IH et al (2011) Temporal trends in the prevalence of diabetic kidney disease in the United States. JAMA 305:2532–2539
3. (2003) USRDS: the United States Renal Data System. Am J Kidney Dis 42:1–230
4. Chavers BM et al (1989) Glomerular lesions and urinary albumin excretion in type I diabetes without overt proteinuria. N Engl J Med 320:966–970
5. Dalla VM et al (2000) Structural involvement in type 1 and type 2 diabetic nephropathy. Diabetes Metab 26(Suppl 4):8–14
6. Breyer MD et al (2005) Mouse models of diabetic nephropathy. J Am Soc Nephrol 16:27–45
7. Brosius FC 3rd et al (2009) Mouse models of diabetic nephropathy. J Am Soc Nephrol 20:2503–2512
8. Gurley SB et al (2010) Influence of genetic background on albuminuria and kidney injury in Ins2(+/C96Y) (Akita) mice. Am J Physiol Renal Physiol 298:F788–795
9. Gurley SB et al (2006) Impact of genetic background on nephropathy in diabetic mice. Am J Physiol Renal Physiol 290:F214–222
10. Yoshioka M et al (1997) A novel locus, Mody4, distal to D7Mit189 on chromosome 7 determines early-onset NIDDM in nonobese C57BL/6 (Akita) mutant mice. Diabetes 46:887–894
11. Ron D (2002) Proteotoxicity in the endoplasmic reticulum: lessons from the Akita diabetic mouse. J Clin Invest 109:443–445
12. Cowie CC (1993) Diabetic renal disease: racial and ethnic differences from an epidemiologic perspective. Transplant Proc 25:2426–2430
13. Qi Z et al (2005) Characterization of susceptibility of inbred mouse strains to diabetic nephropathy. Diabetes 54:2628–2637
14. Kakoki M, Smithies O (2009) The kallikrein-kinin system in health and in diseases of the kidney. Kidney Int 75:1019–1030
15. Kakoki M et al (2010) Lack of both bradykinin B1 and B2 receptors enhances nephropathy, neuropathy, and bone mineral loss in Akita diabetic mice. Proc Natl Acad Sci U S A 107:10190–10195
16. Kakoki M et al (2004) Diabetic nephropathy is markedly enhanced in mice lacking the bradykinin B2 receptor. Proc Natl Acad Sci U S A 101:13302–13305
17. Rigat B et al (1990) An insertion/deletion polymorphism in the angiotensin I-converting enzyme gene accounting for half the variance of serum enzyme levels. J Clin Invest 86:1343–1346
18. Gurley SB, Coffman TM (2007) The renin-angiotensin system and diabetic nephropathy. Semin Nephrol 27:144–152
19. Lewis EJ et al (1993) The effect of angiotensin-converting-enzyme inhibition on diabetic nephropathy. The Collaborative Study Group. N Engl J Med 329:1456–1462
20. Spillmann F et al (2002) Regulation of cardiac bradykinin B1- and B2-receptor mRNA in experimental ischemic, diabetic, and pressure-overload-induced cardiomyopathy. Int Immunopharmacol 2:1823–1832
21. Schremmer-Danninger E et al (1998) B1 bradykinin receptors and carboxypeptidase M are both upregulated in the aorta of pigs after LPS infusion. Biochem Biophys Res Commun 243:246–252
22. Ahluwalia A, Perretti M (1999) B1 receptors as a new inflammatory target. Could this B the 1? Trends Pharmacol Sci 20:100–104
23. Chopra B et al (2005) Expression and function of bradykinin B1 and B2 receptors in normal and inflamed rat urinary bladder urothelium. J Physiol 562:859–871
24. Duka I et al (2001) Vasoactive potential of the b(1) bradykinin receptor in normotension and hypertension. Circ Res 88:275–281
25. Futrakul N et al (2006) Early detection of endothelial injury and dysfunction in conjunction with correction of hemodynamic maladjustment can effectively restore renal function

26. Ignarro LJ et al (1987) Endothelium-derived relaxing factor produced and released from artery and vein is nitric oxide. Proc Natl Acad Sci U S A 84:9265–9269
27. Bogdan C (2001) Nitric oxide and the immune response. Nat Immunol 2:907–916
28. Zanchi A et al (2000) Risk of advanced diabetic nephropathy in type 1 diabetes is associated with endothelial nitric oxide synthase gene polymorphism. Kidney Int 57:405–413
29. Ksiazek P et al (2003) Endothelial nitric oxide synthase gene intron 4 polymorphism in type 2 diabetes mellitus. Mol Diagn 7:119–123
30. Ezzidi I et al (2008) Association of endothelial nitric oxide synthase Glu298Asp, 4b/a, and -786 T > C gene variants with diabetic nephropathy. J Diabetes Complications 22:331–338
31. Wang CH et al (2011) A modest decrease in endothelial NOS in mice comparable to that associated with human NOS3 variants exacerbates diabetic nephropathy. Proc Natl Acad Sci U S A 108:2070–2075
32. Tikellis C et al (2003) Characterization of renal angiotensin-converting enzyme 2 in diabetic nephropathy. Hypertension 41:392–397
33. Wysocki J et al (2006) ACE and ACE2 activity in diabetic mice. Diabetes 55:2132–2139
34. Ye M et al (2004) Increased ACE 2 and decreased ACE protein in renal tubules from diabetic mice: a renoprotective combination? Hypertension 43:1120–1125
35. Mizuiri S et al (2008) Expression of ACE and ACE2 in individuals with diabetic kidney disease and healthy controls. Am J Kidney Dis 51:613–623
36. Reich HN et al (2008) Decreased glomerular and tubular expression of ACE2 in patients with type 2 diabetes and kidney disease. Kidney Int 74:1610–1616
37. Wong DW et al (2007) Loss of angiotensin-converting enzyme-2 (Ace2) accelerates diabetic kidney injury. Am J Pathol 171:438–451
38. Oudit GY et al (2010) Human recombinant ACE2 reduces the progression of diabetic nephropathy. Diabetes 59:529–538
39. Poplawski MM et al (2011) Reversal of diabetic nephropathy by a ketogenic diet. PLoS One 6:e18604
40. Al-Khalifa A et al (2009) Therapeutic role of low-carbohydrate ketogenic diet in diabetes. Nutrition 25:1177–1185
41. Badman MK et al (2009) A very low carbohydrate ketogenic diet improves glucose tolerance in ob/ob mice independent of weight loss. Am J Physiol Endocrinol Metab 297(5):E1197–204
42. Chmiel-Perzynska I et al (2011) Novel aspect of ketone action: beta-hydroxybutyrate increases brain synthesis of kynurenic acid in vitro. Neurotox Res 20:40–50
43. Ma W, Berg J, Yellen G (2007) Ketogenic diet metabolites reduce firing in central neurons by opening K(ATP) channels. J Neurosci 27:3618–3625
44. Hong EG et al (2007) Nonobese, insulin-deficient Ins2Akita mice develop type 2 diabetes phenotypes including insulin resistance and cardiac remodeling. Am J Physiol Endocrinol Metab 293:E1687–1696

Chapter 3

The BB Rat as a Model of Human Type 1 Diabetes

Rita Bortell and Chaoxing Yang

Abstract

The BB rat is an important rodent model of human type 1 diabetes (T1D) and has been used to study mechanisms of diabetes pathogenesis as well as to investigate potential intervention therapies for clinical trials. The Diabetes-Prone BB (BBDP) rat spontaneously develops autoimmune T1D between 50 and 90 days of age. The Diabetes-Resistant BB (BBDR) rat has similar diabetes-susceptible genes as the BBDP, but does not become diabetic in viral antibody-free conditions. However, the BBDR rat can be induced to develop T1D in response to certain treatments such as regulatory T cell (T_{reg}) depletion, toll-like receptor ligation, or virus infection. These diabetes-inducible rats develop hyperglycemia under well-controlled circumstances and within a short, predictable time frame (14–21 days), thus facilitating their utility for investigations of specific stages of diabetes development. Therefore, these rat strains are invaluable models for studying autoimmune diabetes and the role of environmental factors in its development, of particular importance due to the influx of studies associating virus infection and human T1D.

Key words: BB rat, Type 1 diabetes, Regulatory T cell, Toll-like receptor, Virus infection, Major histocompatibility complex, Lymphopenia, Insulitis, Kilham rat virus, Enterovirus, Innate immunity

1. Spontaneous Autoimmune Diabetes in the Rat

1.1. Generation of the Diabetes-Prone BB Rat

In the 1970s, the diabetes-prone BioBreeding (BB) rat colony was established in Canada from outbred Wistar rats by selection of animals that spontaneously developed hyperglycemia and ketoacidosis. One colony, named "BBDP/Wor," has been inbred in Worcester, Massachusetts, USA. A second colony, the outbred rat colony named "BBdp," stayed in Ottawa, Canada. Many other "BB" rat colonies have been derived from these earlier colonies; however, experimental data obtained from different rat colonies may not be transferable. When housed in a conventional environment, more than half of BBDP/Wor (hereafter designated as "BBDP") rats develop diabetes spontaneously. Interestingly, the rat colony has a higher frequency of diabetes incidence and the animals develop disease at an earlier age when they are housed in viral antibody-free (VAF) vivaria (1).

As with humans, certain major histocompatibility complex (MHC) genes of rats have been shown to be critical for autoimmune risk. The rat MHC, designated RT1, has two class I loci (*A* and *C*) and two class II loci (*B* and *D*). The *RT1 B/D* region is designated *Iddm1*, and is the most important locus for conferring susceptibility to autoimmune type 1 diabetes (T1D) (earlier referred to as insulin-dependent diabetes mellitus). Data derived from studies on many different rat strains indicate that at least one class II *RT1 B/D^u* allele is required for diabetes onset (2, 3). Mitogen-activated spleen cells from diabetic BBDP rats can transfer disease to MHC-compatible naïve recipients, confirming that the diabetes is autoimmune mediated (4).

The most striking phenotype in all BBDP rats is a profound T cell lymphopenia which results from the spontaneous apoptosis of peripheral T cells soon after their emigration from the thymus (5–7). The presence of lymphopenia is required for T1D onset in BBDP rats (8), although this is not typical of human T1D. Interestingly, however, a polyadenylation signal polymorphism in the human *GIMAP5* gene has been associated with increased levels of IA-2 autoantibodies in T1D patients (9), as well as increased risk for the multisystem autoimmune disease, systemic lupus erythematosus (10).

The cause of the T cell lymphopenia characteristic of BBDP rats was pinpointed to a frameshift mutation in the *Gimap5* (GTPase of the immune-associated protein 5) gene (11, 12). GIMAP5 is a putative small GTPase, and its cellular localization has been reported in the endoplasmic reticulum (ER), lysosomes, and related compartments (13–15). Absence of the protein encoded by *Gimap5* in T cells causes mitochondrial dysfunction, increased mitochondrial levels of stress-inducible chaperonins, and T cell specific spontaneous apoptosis (16). T cell death is initiated through disruptions in ER homeostasis mediated by the C/EBP-homologous protein (CHOP) apoptotic pathway (17).

1.2. Pathogenesis

1.2.1. Pathogenesis of Pancreatic Islets

Diabetes in BBDP rats typically develops between 50 and 90 days of age, with both sexes having a similar frequency of occurrence (1). Although increased neonatal beta cell apoptosis has been suggested to play a role in diabetes susceptibility in the BB rat (and non-obese diabetic (NOD) mouse) (18), the first histomorphological change detectable in the BBDP pancreas is the infiltration of immune cells in the islets of Langerhans (insulitis). In this regard, the morphology of insulitis observed in humans is more similar to the BB rat than to that of the NOD mouse. In NOD mice, immune cells accumulate *around* the islets (peri-insulitis), whereas this is not typically observed in diabetic rats or humans (19, 20).

In the BBDP rat, different lymphoid cells infiltrate the islets at different stages of insulitis, which usually occurs 2–3 weeks before overt diabetes. Among the first are macrophages and dendritic cells, later natural killer (NK) cells, T cells, and some B cells invade the islets (21). Beta cells are selectively destroyed, and the rat rapidly develops hyperglycemia. Alpha, delta, and pancreatic polypeptide cells are not apparently affected by infiltration of the immune cells. Without insulin treatment, diabetic rats develop ketoacidosis within several days following the onset of frank hyperglycemia.

1.2.2. Immunopathogenesis

As discussed above, the most profound immunopathology in the BBDP rat is T cell lymphopenia due to the *Gimap5* mutation (5–7). The CD4⁺ T cell number in these rats is greatly reduced, and there is almost no CD8⁺ T cell subpopulation (22–24). Not only is the low T cell number problematic, the functionality of the T cells is also poor, and this may contribute to the development of diabetes. Besides the greatly shortened life span, BBDP T cells have a much higher threshold for activation (25). The CD4⁺ART2⁺ T regulatory (T_{reg}) cells are also severely impaired (26). ART2 is a rat maturational T cell alloantigen that plays a role in Treg function and identification (27, 28). Bone marrow and thymus transplant studies suggest that BBDP rats also have abnormal intrathymic antigen-presenting cells with reduced T cell receptor (TCR) repertoire (29). Dendritic cells (DCs) of BBDP rats express much less MHC class II, with limited ability to differentiate into mature T cell-stimulatory DCs (30, 31). In addition, NK cells, NKT cells, and intraepithelial lymphocyte populations are also reduced in numbers and/or function compared to other rat strains (32, 33).

1.3. Prevention and Reversal of Diabetes in the Diabetes-Prone Rat Model

The BBDP rat model has historically been used in many studies to discover and evaluate potential treatments to prevent or reverse autoimmune human T1D. Administration of parenteral insulin and certain dietary modifications can prevent or delay diabetes onset in the BBDP rat (34, 35). Insulin gene therapy has been tested in BBDP rats using adenovirus to deliver a glucose-regulated insulin transgene (36). Diabetes in BBDP rats can also be prevented by intrathymic islets transplantation (37). Although in certain cases some of these preventative treatments would not be appropriate for humans, such studies still provide mechanistic insights that may be translatable to human therapies.

As mentioned before, the *Gimap5* mutation causes a profound lymphopenia in BBDP rats, and CD4⁺ART2⁺ Treg cells are severely deficient. Transfusion of ART2⁺ cells (38, 39) or normal MHC-compatible T cells can protect the recipient from disease, if T cell reconstitution is initiated before insulitis (40). Indeed, many immune modulatory methods can prevent or delay the disease in BBDP rats, including thymectomy, anti-lymphocyte treatment, CD8⁺ T cell depletion (33), or treatment with the immune suppressant, cyclosporine (41, 42). However, most of these therapies are either not appropriate for human studies, or have had disappointing results in clinical trials.

Pancreas and islet transplantation are also effective in curing BBDP rat diabetes, although additional treatment is needed, such as the use of immunosuppressive drugs, antibodies to anti-adhesion molecules, or costimulatory blockade (43–45). Costimulatory blockade is probably preferred over the other methods due to its specificity. Diabetes in BBDP rats can be prevented by blockade of costimulatory CD28 pathways, while blockade of the CD40-CD154 pathway has less effect (46). BBDP rats exhibit a severe imbalance between Th_{17} and regulatory T cells within the first months of age (47). Adoptive transfer of T_{reg} cells, or in vivo expansion of T_{reg} cells by treatment with a CD28 agonistic antibody, interferes with the development of diabetes in these animals, whereas treatment with conventional T helper (Th) cells does not afford protection.

2. Induced Autoimmune Diabetes

2.1. Usefulness of the Inducible BB Rat Model to Study Human T1D

There is strong evidence to suggest that the development of human T1D requires a susceptible genetic background (48). The expression of diabetes has been found to correlate more significantly with HLA class II haplotypes than HLA class I. Surprisingly, however, about 85% of T1D patients have no family history of the disease, and parents/grandparents of the patient remain free of disease. Such studies likely indicate the involvement of multiple genes, as well as a potential role for environmental factors in the development of autoimmune diabetes (49). Among identical twins T1D concordance is only 30–50%, which provides further evidence for the involvement of non-genetic environmental influences (48). Indeed, it is possible that human T1D susceptibility genes may act only in the context of certain environmental perturbations.

Clinical data show that diabetes onset is often preceded by exposure to a pathogen or other environmental factors. Although the exact identity of these environmental perturbants remains obscure, suggested candidates have included toxins, certain dietary components, and vaccination, but data to support these is not conclusive (50–53). To date, the strongest epidemiologic evidence for an environmental association with T1D is provided by virus exposure (54–56). Clinical data reveal that diabetes onset is often preceded by exposure to viral infections including mumps, rubella, rotavirus, parvovirus, and enteroviruses (57). In a recent meta-analysis of 26 cohort or case–control studies in which enterovirus RNA or viral protein was measured in blood, stool, or tissue of patients with pre-diabetes and diabetes, the authors reported a clinically significant association between enterovirus infection and T1D (58). This association between enterovirus infection and diabetes was strong, with children at diagnosis of T1D ~10 times more likely to have an enterovirus infection than the diabetes-free control group. Although correlative, these studies further confirm the importance of environmental factors in T1D development. However, the mechanism(s) by which viral infection may be involved in the development of T1D remains elusive.

The genetic complexity of human populations and the inability to control the environment are the limiting factors in mechanistic studies of human T1D development. Therefore, reliable inbred animal models that develop autoimmune diabetes upon viral infection are much needed. The NOD mouse is the most well studied animal model of spontaneous autoimmune diabetes, however, viral infections of these mice often reduce the frequency of diabetes or even prevent it entirely (59). Multiple small doses of streptozotocin (STZ) can induce diabetes in immunodeficient NOD-*scid* mice (60). However, NOD-*scid* mice have no functional lymphocytes, which raise concern about its relevance as a model of T1D (61). As described in the next sections, a major advantage of the BB rat model of T1D is its utility in studies of the role of environmental factors, such as virus infection, in the development of T1D.

2.2. Generation of the Diabetes-Resistant BBDR Rat

The diabetes-resistant BBDR/Wor (hereafter designated as "BBDR") rats were derived from BBDP/Wor rats at the fifth generation of inbreeding by selection for the *absence* of T1D. Although BBDR rats have the same $RT1^u$ MHC haplotype as the BBDP rat, these animals have a wildtype *Gimap5* allele and are consequently not lymphopenic. BBDR rats do not become diabetic in VAF conditions, in contrast to the BBDP rat (1). However, the BBDR rat can be induced to develop T1D in response to certain treatments such as Treg depletion, toll-like receptor (TLR) ligation, or infection with certain viruses (4). Perturbant-induced diabetic rats develop hyperglycemia under well-controlled circumstances and within a defined time frame. These rat strains also have enhanced susceptibility to other autoimmune diseases, as is also the case with human T1D patients. Therefore, BB rats are invaluable models for studying the effects of environmental factors in human T1D development, as well as in mapping susceptible genetic backgrounds.

Upon treatment with specific diabetes-inducing protocols (discussed in detail below), BBDR rats typically develop mild insulitis beginning at ~10 days. Once insulitis starts, however, the infiltration of immune cells is rapid and occurs throughout the pancreas, typically by ~14–18 days after induction. This pancreatic insulitis, a key signature of autoimmune diabetes, mediates the ultimate destruction of the insulin-producing beta cells. The appearance of hyperglycemia only occurs at late stages of insulitis, with ketoacidosis developing several days thereafter (62). Interestingly, there is little phenotypic evidence of any abnormality in the pancreatic islets during the first 10 days of induction, and blood glucose levels remain normal even through much of the insulitic period.

2.3. Diabetes Induction Methods

2.3.1. T_{reg} Depletion

As noted before, BBDP rats are severely deficient in CD4$^+$ART2$^+$ T_{reg} cells, but transfusion with CD4$^+$ART2$^+$ T_{reg} cells can prevent development of spontaneous diabetes in these animals. Similarly, treatment with a depleting anti-ART2 antibody can induce diabetes in BBDR rats that are housed in conventional, non-VAF conditions (63). However, depletion of ART2$^+$ T_{reg} cells in BBDR rats housed in VAF conditions is insufficient to induce diabetes without additional treatment. Taken together, these data are consistent with a role for an imbalance in T_{reg} to T effector (T_{eff}) cells in the pathogenesis of autoimmune diabetes in the BB rat. Similar deficiencies in the numbers and/or function of CD4$^+$CD25$^+$ T_{reg} cells have been reported in NOD mice and patients with T1D (64, 65).

2.3.2. TLR Ligation

BBDR rats treated with the TLR3 agonist, polyinosinic:polycytidylic acid (poly I:C), develop diabetes, and the percentage of rats which develop disease is dose-dependent. About 20% of BBDR rats develop diabetes with low dose poly I:C (5 µg/g) treatment (66), while treatment with higher doses (10 µg/g) induces disease in nearly 100% of animals (67). Interestingly, low dose poly I:C treatment protects BBDP rats from development of disease (68), while high dose poly I:C accelerates disease onset (69, 70).

As mentioned earlier, depleting ART2$^+$ T cells alone does not induce diabetes in BBDR rats housed under VAF conditions. However, diabetes can be induced if these ART2$^+$ T cell-depleted rats are additionally treated with poly I:C (1, 66). Poly I:C is a synthetic double-stranded polyribonucleotide that elicits innate immune responses similar to those observed during viral infection (67). Poly I:C binds specifically to TLR3 (71) and TLR ligation, in turn, activates antigen-presenting cells and other immune responses and therefore may play a role in pre-conditioning the immune system for autoimmunity.

2.3.3. Virus Infection

In the 1980s, an outbreak of autoimmune diabetes in the BBDR rat colony led to the discovery of Kilham rat virus (KRV) infection as a T1D induction method (72). As few as 10^3 virions can cause ~5% of BBDR rats to develop diabetes, although higher dosages (as high as 10^8 virions) are insufficient to induce 100% diabetes in KRV-infected BBDR rats. In a typical protocol, 10^7 virions are injected intraperitoneally only once when rats are at the age of 24–27 days old; this method induces diabetes in about ~30% of the rats (72, 73). Interestingly, the efficiency of KRV infection for inducing diabetes is similar to the concordance rate for human diabetes reported clinically with identical twins.

KRV infection increases serum levels of the pro-inflammatory cytokine, IL12B, and increases the mRNA expression of IL12B, CXCL10, and IFNG, particularly in the pancreatic lymph nodes of infected BBDR rats (74). The virus does not infect the pancreatic islets and exocrine tissue directly, but the rats develop insulitis, as typical of autoimmune diabetes. Although the virus infects T and B lymphocytes, it does not cause lymphopenia (75). The infected lymphocytes are apparently normal phenotypically, however, their proliferative and cytolytic functions are impaired.

Many studies have shown that other environmental perturbants, such as T_{reg} depletion or TLR ligation, can act synergistically with KRV infection to produce a higher frequency of diabetes. The combination of KRV infection and depletion of ART2$^+$ T_{reg} cells can increase diabetes incident rate to ~80% in BBDR rats (76). Besides T_{reg} depletion, treatment with TLR ligands, such as heat-killed *Escherichia coli* and *Staphylococcus aureus*, can also increase diabetes induction of KRV-infected rats by 60% and 100%, respectively (74). However, these TLR ligands are unable to induce diabetes when used alone.

The most potent protocol to induce T1D in the BBDR rat is the combination of KRV infection and low dosage of poly I:C treatment. This method induces nearly 100% diabetes within a time frame of 14–21 days after treatment. In the absence of KRV infection, poly I:C treatment at this dosage level is unable to induce diabetes (76, 77). Poly I:C, as a TLR3 agonist and viral mimetic, is well known for its ability to induce activation of the innate immune system.

2.4. Mechanisms of Virus-Induced T1D

How KRV induces diabetes is not understood. One possible mechanism is that virus infection alters the immune-regulatory system by reducing T_{reg} cell frequency (77). Activation of macrophages also appears to be important for disease induction, as BBDR rats treated with KRV and poly I:C fail to develop T1D if their macrophages have been depleted (78). Although molecular mimicry of KRV antigens to putative T1D autoantigens has been suggested, this hypothesis was not borne out in studies by Chung et al. (79), as treatment of BBDR rats with viral vectors encoding KRV proteins failed to induce diabetes. Even though both adaptive and innate immune responses were generated in infected animals, including expansion of CD8$^+$ T cells, no virus-specific CD8$^+$ T cell responses were found. Together, these data fail to support a role for molecular mimicry in KRV-induced diabetes.

As expected following virus infection, KRV itself (without co-treatment) can activate the innate immune system. Ex vivo and in vitro studies indicate that KRV upregulates pro-inflammatory cytokines and chemokines in macrophages, dendritic cells, and B lymphocytes (80–82). As KRV is a single-stranded DNA virus, it was hypothesized to act through a TLR9 signaling pathway. In support of this, BBDR rat spleen cells treated with TLR9 antagonists, such as inhibitory CpG and chloroquine, produce much lower levels of pro-inflammatory cytokines in vitro. Also, BBDR rats treated with these TLR9 inhibitors have a lower diabetes frequency (81). In addition, KRV has been shown to activate signal transducer and activator of transcription (STAT)-1 in spleen cells in vitro, and this activation can be blocked by TLR9 inhibition. In vivo upregulation of STAT-1 also occurs in pancreatic lymph nodes of BB rats early after virus infection (80).

In a recent DNA microarray-based study, >500 genes were found to be upregulated in pancreatic lymph nodes following KRV infection. The most highly activated genes included IFN-γ-induced chemokines and those associated with IL1 and interferon production and signaling. In addition, a recent study by Heinig et al. (83) utilized integrated genome-wide approaches to identify an interferon regulatory factor 7 (IRF7)-driven inflammatory network (IDIN) enriched for viral response genes. The network was regulated in multiple tissues by a locus on rat chromosome 15, whereas the orthologous human locus was located on chromosome 13. Importantly, the human IDIN genes were more strongly associated with susceptibility to T1D than randomly selected immune response genes, implicating a role for the IRF7 network in human diabetes as well as highlighting the importance of virus-induced rat models in the study of its pathogenesis.

The ability of KRV to elicit diabetes induction appears to be very specific. Parvovirus H-1, which is ~98% identical by DNA sequence to KRV, is unable to induce diabetes in BBDR rats. Although parvovirus H-1 induces cellular and humoral immune responses and activation of innate immunity in infected rats, the magnitude of activation is lower than that associated with KRV infection (74, 77). This again indicates the importance of innate immune system activation for autoimmune diabetes induction. Moreover, only KRV, not the highly similar H-1 parvovirus, causes a decrease in the population of splenic T_{reg} cells (77). KRV infection has also been reported to preferentially activate T_{eff} cells, such as CD8+ and Th1-like CD45RC+CD4+ T cells (84). Thus, as with T_{reg} depletion above, the data from this virus-induced protocol is also consistent with a role for a T_{reg}/T_{eff} imbalance in the development of T1D.

Because KRV is a rat specific parvovirus, it does not infect humans. The only significant parvovirus currently identified in humans is B19. Although there is little information on a possible association between human parvovirus B19 and T1D (85), a single case has been reported (86). Despite the viral specificity, the BBDR rat model is a valuable animal model for the study of virus-induced human T1D. Unlike some mouse models, KRV virus does not infect pancreatic cells directly, but induces autoimmune diabetes through alteration of the immune system. Therefore, this rat model can provide unique insight into how the immune system is altered upon viral infection, and what magnitude of alteration is needed to induce T1D in genetically susceptible individuals. Such insights should lead to more specific and effective clinical therapies to prevent or delay the development of diabetes in at risk humans.

2.5. A Role for the BB Rat Model in Diabetes Prediction and Intervention

Because of its predictable time course of diabetes development, the inducible BBDR rat model can be used to identify biomarkers that may be relevant to clinical diagnosis. Ideally, serum biomarkers found in the rat, once verified in human patients, may contribute to the compendium of known markers (e.g., autoantibodies) used to predict diabetes in genetically susceptible humans. Such identification would enable intervention treatments as early as possible. In a study by Kruger et al. (73), proteomic profiling of serum from KRV and poly I:C-induced BBDR rats led to the discovery of elevated levels of haptoglobin that were apparent soon after virus infection. Because multiple viruses have been implicated in the etiopathogenesis of human T1D, another rat model of virally induced diabetes was also investigated—the LEW1.WR1 rat treated with rat cytomegalovirus (RCMV) (87). Importantly, in LEW1.WR1 rats treated with RCMV alone, those animals that went on to develop diabetes exhibited sustained elevations of serum haptoglobin compared to RCMV-treated rats that remained diabetes-free (73).

In a related study by Kaldunski et al. (88), sera of both spontaneously diabetic and diabetes-inducible BB rats induced transcription of cytokines, immune receptors, and signaling molecules in the peripheral blood mononuclear cells (PBMCs) of healthy donor rats compared with control sera. These authors had previously reported a similar inflammatory "signature" of PBMCs from healthy human donors that were induced by sera of recent onset diabetics or at risk patients, but not by sera from healthy controls or long standing diabetes patients (89). Together, such studies may reveal mechanisms associated with progression to T1D. Furthermore, these studies illustrate the utility of the inducible BB rat model to test the preventative efficacy of potential anti-inflammatory therapies prior to clinical trials.

Indeed, several therapies have been found to be effective in prevention or reversal in the inducible BBDR rat model, however, the effectiveness of these therapies in humans still needs to be validated. Some examples of preventative therapies include nicotinamide, docosahexaenoic acid (DHA), high dose parenteral insulin, a diet low in essential fatty acids, and treatment with aminoguanidine, an iNOS inhibitor (90–92). Anti-CD25 and mycophenolate mofetil (MMF) treatment alone or in combination are effective in delaying and preventing diabetes induced by depleting Treg cells in the BBDR rat, especially if treatment is started early (93). The immunomodulatory drug FTY720 can prevent autoimmune diabetes in Treg depleted BBDR rats if administered before and/or during stimulation and expansion of the autoreactive T cells or in the early stages of insulitis (94). FTY720 treatment has also recently been shown to prevent diabetes in another rat model of human T1D, the LEW.1AR1-*iddm* rat (95).

As noted above, several other rat models of human T1D have emerged, including the LEW.1WR1 and the LEW.1AR1-*iddm* rat (73, 87, 95, 96). Recent genetic studies suggest that a key diabetes susceptibility locus in the BB and other diabetes-susceptible rat strains is an allele of the TCR V_{beta} chain (97), raising the possibility that specific TCR alleles in humans may one day be associated with disease susceptibility. Together, such studies may identify potential new therapies for intervention to prevent T1D, especially those which allow select targeting of limited TCRs rather than broad, "across-the-board" suppression of all TCR signaling. Indeed, a thorough understanding of the immunopathology of disease development is critical to the continued improvement of therapies for human T1D. As such, diabetes-susceptible and inducible rat models remain particularly useful for such endeavors.

As would be expected, diabetes intervention therapies investigated to date in rodent models are most effective when initiated early in the diabetogenic process. Yet human clinical trials are typically done with recent onset diabetic patients. To address this, studies investigating potential therapies to *reverse* ongoing diabetes are performed in rodent models *after* the onset of diabetes. One recent study by Kruger et al. utilized the virus-inducible BBDR rat model to evaluate the therapeutic value of the adipokine, leptin, when given at three different stages of diabetes (62). High doses of leptin (given as a pre-treatment) prevented insulitis and diabetes in >90% of rats treated with the combination of KRV and poly I:C. In new onset diabetic rats, leptin treatment prevented rapid weight loss and diabetic ketoacidosis, and temporarily restored euglycemia. In addition, leptin treatment was also found to prevent autoimmune recurrence in diabetic rats transplanted with syngeneic islets (62). Of interest, leptin regulates blood glucose and the insulin secretory function of beta cells while also modulating immune cell function, suggesting that leptin may ameliorate the autoreactive immune response as well as provide beneficial effects directly to the beta cell. These findings merit further evaluation of leptin as a potential therapeutic agent for treatment of human T1D (62).

In summary, given the inherent complexity of "outbred" human populations, this compendium of studies support the use of the BB rat, in conjunction with the NOD and other rodent models, as an invaluable resource to investigate and test potential therapies for human T1D. Although much of the research on T1D has focused on understanding its immunopathogenesis, a major question in diabetes pathogenesis relates to the role of the pancreatic beta cell. For instance, does the beta cell play an active or passive role in its own demise (98, 99)? As the sole source of insulin, beta cells of the pancreatic islets have a highly developed endoplasmic reticulum (ER) due to a heavy insulin demand and rapid changes in insulin requirement. It has been proposed that excessive or unresolved ER stress can elicit beta cell death that, in turn, may contribute to the initiation and/or progression of autoimmune diabetes (100). The answers to these and many other interesting questions await further clinical and laboratory studies.

Acknowledgments

This work was supported by NIH grants AI073871 and DK352520, and grants from the Brehm Foundation and the Juvenile Diabetes Research Foundation.

References

1. Like AA, Guberski DL, Butler L (1991) Influence of environmental viral agents on frequency and tempo of diabetes mellitus in BB/Wor rats. Diabetes 40:259–262
2. Colle E (1990) Genetic susceptibility to the development of spontaneous insulin-dependent diabetes mellitus in the rat. Clin Immunol Immunopathol 57:1–9
3. Fuks A, Ono SJ, Colle E et al (1990) A single dose of the MHC-linked susceptibility determinant associated with the RT1u haplotype is permissive for insulin-dependent diabetes mellitus in the BB rat. Exp Clin Immunogenet 7:162–169
4. Mordes JP, Bortell R, Blankenhorn EP et al (2004) Rat models of type 1 diabetes: genetics, environment, and autoimmunity. ILAR J 45:278–291
5. Elder ME, Maclaren NK (1983) Identification of profound peripheral T lymphocyte immunodeficiencies in the spontaneously diabetic BB rat. J Immunol 130:1723–1731
6. Ramanathan S, Poussier P (2001) BB rat lyp mutation and type 1 diabetes. Immunol Rev 184:161–171
7. Yale JF, Grose M, Marliss EB (1985) Time course of the lymphopenia in BB rats. Relation to the onset of diabetes. Diabetes 34:955–959
8. Awata T, Guberski DL, Like AA (1995) Genetics of the BB rat: association of autoimmune disorders (diabetes, insulitis, and thyroiditis) with lymphopenia and major histocompatibility complex class II. Endocrinology 136:5731–5735
9. Shin JH, Janer M, McNeney B et al (2007) IA-2 autoantibodies in incident type I diabetes patients are associated with a polyadenylation signal polymorphism in GIMAP5. Genes Immun 8:503–512
10. Hellquist A, Zucchelli M, Kivinen K et al (2007) The human GIMAP5 gene has a common polyadenylation polymorphism increasing risk to systemic lupus erythematosus. J Med Genet 44:314–321
11. Hornum L, Romer J, Markholst H (2002) The diabetes-prone BB rat carries a frameshift mutation in Ian4, a positional candidate of Iddm1. Diabetes 51:1972–1979
12. MacMurray AJ, Moralejo DH, Kwitek AE et al (2002) Lymphopenia in the BB rat model of type 1 diabetes is due to a mutation in a novel immune-associated nucleotide (Ian)-related gene. Genome Res 12:1029–1039
13. Wong VW, Saunders AE, Hutchings A et al (2010) The autoimmunity-related GIMAP5 GTPase is a lysosome-associated protein. Self Nonself 1:259–268
14. Keita M, Leblanc C, Andrews D et al (2007) GIMAP5 regulates mitochondrial integrity from a distinct subcellular compartment. Biochem Biophys Res Commun 361:481–486
15. Sandal T, Aumo L, Hedin L et al (2003) Irod/Ian5: an inhibitor of gamma-radiation- and okadaic acid-induced apoptosis. Mol Biol Cell 14:3292–3304
16. Pandarpurkar M, Wilson-Fritch L, Corvera S et al (2003) Ian4 is required for mitochondrial integrity and T cell survival. Proc Natl Acad Sci U S A 100:10382–10387
17. Pino SC, O'Sullivan-Murphy B, Lidstone EA et al (2009) CHOP mediates endoplasmic reticulum stress-induced apoptosis in Gimap5-deficient T cells. PLoS One 4:e5468
18. Trudeau JD, Dutz JP, Arany E et al (2000) Neonatal beta-cell apoptosis: a trigger for autoimmune diabetes? Diabetes 49:1–7
19. Kolb H, Worz-Pagenstert U, Kleemann R et al (1996) Cytokine gene expression in the BB rat pancreas: natural course and impact of bacterial vaccines. Diabetologia 39:1448–1454
20. Zipris D (1996) Evidence that Th1 lymphocytes predominate in islet inflammation and thyroiditis in the BioBreeding (BB) rat. J Autoimmun 9:315–319
21. Hanenberg H, Kolb-Bachofen V, Kantwerk-Funke G et al (1989) Macrophage infiltration precedes and is a prerequisite for lymphocytic insulitis in pancreatic islets of pre-diabetic BB rats. Diabetologia 32:126–134

22. Jackson RA, Eisenbarth GS (1983) Type I diabetes of man and the BB rat: monoclonal antibody-defined T-cell abnormalities. Diagn Immunol 1:240–244
23. Marliss EB, Nakhooda AF, Poussier P et al (1982) The diabetic syndrome of the 'BB' Wistar rat: possible relevance to type 1 (insulin-dependent) diabetes in man. Diabetologia 22:225–232
24. Woda BA, Like AA, Padden C et al (1986) Deficiency of phenotypic cytotoxic-suppressor T lymphocytes in the BB/W rat. J Immunol 136:856–859
25. Ramanathan S, Norwich K, Poussier P (1998) Antigen activation rescues recent thymic emigrants from programmed cell death in the BB rat. J Immunol 160:5757–5764
26. Greiner DL, Handler ES, Nakano K et al (1986) Absence of the RT-6 T cell subset in diabetes-prone BB/W rats. J Immunol 136: 148–151
27. Bortell R, Kanaitsuka T, Stevens LA et al (1999) The RT6 (Art2) family of ADP-ribosyltransferases in rat and mouse. Mol Cell Biochem 193:61–68
28. Bortell R, Waite DJ, Whalen BJ et al (2001) Levels of Art2+ cells but not soluble Art2 protein correlate with expression of autoimmune diabetes in the BB rat. Autoimmunity 33:199–211
29. Gold DP, Bellgrau D (1991) Identification of a limited T-cell receptor beta chain variable region repertoire associated with diabetes in the BB rat. Proc Natl Acad Sci U S A 88: 9888–9891
30. Sommandas V, Rutledge EA, Van Yserloo B et al (2005) Aberrancies in the differentiation and maturation of dendritic cells from bone-marrow precursors are linked to various genes on chromosome 4 and other chromosomes of the BB-DP rat. J Autoimmun 25:1–12
31. Sommandas V, Rutledge EA, Van Yserloo B et al (2005) Defects in differentiation of bone-marrow derived dendritic cells of the BB rat are partly associated with IDDM2 (the lyp gene) and partly associated with other genes in the BB rat background. J Autoimmun 25:46–56
32. Todd DJ, Forsberg EM, Greiner DL et al (2004) Deficiencies in gut NK cell number and function precede diabetes onset in BB rats. J Immunol 172:5356–5362
33. Whalen BJ, Mordes JP, Rossini AA (2001) The BB rat as a model of human insulin-dependent diabetes mellitus. Curr Protoc Immunol Chapter 15:Unit 15.13
34. Lefebvre DE, Powell KL, Strom A et al (2006) Dietary proteins as environmental modifiers of type 1 diabetes mellitus. Annu Rev Nutr 26:175–202
35. Wang GS, Kauri LM, Patrick C et al (2010) Enhanced islet expansion by beta-cell proliferation in young diabetes-prone rats fed a protective diet. J Cell Physiol 224:501–508
36. Olson DE, Paveglio SA, Huey PU et al (2003) Glucose-responsive hepatic insulin gene therapy of spontaneously diabetic BB/Wor rats. Hum Gene Ther 14:1401–1413
37. Posselt AM, Barker CF, Friedman AL et al (1992) Prevention of autoimmune diabetes in the BB rat by intrathymic islet transplantation at birth. Science 256:1321–1324
38. Burstein D, Mordes JP, Greiner DL et al (1989) Prevention of diabetes in BB/Wor rat by single transfusion of spleen cells. Parameters that affect degree of protection. Diabetes 38:24–30
39. Rossini AA, Mordes JP, Pelletier AM et al (1983) Transfusions of whole blood prevent spontaneous diabetes mellitus in the BB/W rat. Science 219:975–977
40. Ramanathan S, Poussier P (1999) T cell reconstitution of BB/W rats after the initiation of insulitis precipitates the onset of diabetes. J Immunol 162:5134–5142
41. Laupacis A, Stiller CR, Gardell C et al (1983) Cyclosporin prevents diabetes in BB Wistar rats. Lancet 1:10–12
42. Like AA, Anthony M, Guberski DL et al (1983) Spontaneous diabetes mellitus in the BB/W rat. Effects of glucocorticoids, cyclosporin-A, and antiserum to rat lymphocytes. Diabetes 32:326–330
43. Dugoni WE Jr, Bartlett ST (1990) Evidence that cyclosporine prevents rejection and recurrent diabetes in pancreatic transplants in the BB rat. Transplantation 49:845–848
44. Tori M, Ito T, Yumiba T et al (1999) Significant role of intragraft lymphoid tissues in preventing insulin-dependent diabetes mellitus recurrence in whole pancreaticoduodenal transplantation. Microsurgery 19:338–343
45. Kover KL, Geng Z, Hess DM et al (2000) Anti-CD154 (CD40L) prevents recurrence of diabetes in islet isografts in the DR-BB rat. Diabetes 49:1666–1670
46. Beaudette-Zlatanova BC, Whalen B, Zipris D et al (2006) Costimulation and autoimmune diabetes in BB rats. Am J Transplant 6:894–902
47. van den Brandt J, Fischer HJ, Walter L et al (2010) Type 1 diabetes in BioBreeding rats is critically linked to an imbalance between Th17 and regulatory T cells and an altered TCR repertoire. J Immunol 185: 2285–2294

48. Castano L, Eisenbarth GS (1990) Type-I diabetes: a chronic autoimmune disease of human, mouse, and rat. Annu Rev Immunol 8:647–679
49. Horn GT, Bugawan TL, Long CM et al (1988) Allelic sequence variation of the HLA-DQ loci: relationship to serology and to insulin-dependent diabetes susceptibility. Proc Natl Acad Sci U S A 85:6012–6016
50. Couper JJ, Steele C, Beresford S et al (1999) Lack of association between duration of breast-feeding or introduction of cow's milk and development of islet autoimmunity. Diabetes 48:2145–2149
51. Norris JM, Barriga K, Klingensmith G et al (2003) Timing of initial cereal exposure in infancy and risk of islet autoimmunity. JAMA 290:1713–1720
52. Hviid A, Stellfeld M, Wohlfahrt J et al (2004) Childhood vaccination and type 1 diabetes. N Engl J Med 350:1398–1404
53. Helgason T, Jonasson MR (1981) Evidence for a food additive as a cause of ketosis-prone diabetes. Lancet 2:716–720
54. Pietropaolo M, Trucco M (1996) Viral elements in autoimmunity of type I diabetes. Trends Endocrinol Metab 7:139–144
55. Yoon JW, Jun HS (2004) Viruses in type 1 diabetes: brief review. ILAR J 45:343–348
56. Laron Z (2002) Interplay between heredity and environment in the recent explosion of type 1 childhood diabetes mellitus. Am J Med Genet 115:4–7
57. Bortell R, Pino SC, Greiner DL et al (2008) Closing the circle between the bedside and the bench: toll-like receptors in models of virally induced diabetes. Ann N Y Acad Sci 1150:112–122
58. Yeung WC, Rawlinson WD, Craig ME (2011) Enterovirus infection and type 1 diabetes mellitus: systematic review and meta-analysis of observational molecular studies. BMJ 342:d35
59. Atkinson MA, Leiter EH (1999) The NOD mouse model of type 1 diabetes: as good as it gets? Nat Med 5:601–604
60. Seung E, Iwakoshi N, Woda BA et al (2000) Allogeneic hematopoietic chimerism in mice treated with sublethal myeloablation and anti-CD154 antibody: absence of graft-versus-host disease, induction of skin allograft tolerance, and prevention of recurrent autoimmunity in islet-allografted NOD/Lt mice. Blood 95:2175–2182
61. Gerling IC, Friedman H, Greiner DL et al (1994) Multiple low-dose streptozotocin-induced diabetes in NOD-scid/scid mice in the absence of functional lymphocytes. Diabetes 43:433–440
62. Kruger AJ, Yang C, Lipson KL et al (2011) Leptin treatment confers clinical benefit at multiple stages of virally induced type 1 diabetes in BB rats. Autoimmunity 44:137–148
63. Greiner DL, Mordes JP, Handler ES et al (1987) Depletion of RT6.1+ T lymphocytes induces diabetes in resistant biobreeding/Worcester (BB/W) rats. J Exp Med 166:461–475
64. Kukreja A, Cost G, Marker J et al (2002) Multiple immuno-regulatory defects in type-1 diabetes. J Clin Invest 109:131–140
65. Brusko TM, Wasserfall CH, Clare-Salzler MJ et al (2005) Functional defects and the influence of age on the frequency of CD4+ CD25+ T-cells in type 1 diabetes. Diabetes 54:1407–1414
66. Thomas VA, Woda BA, Handler ES et al (1991) Altered expression of diabetes in BB/Wor rats by exposure to viral pathogens. Diabetes 40:255–258
67. Doukas J, Cutler AH, Mordes JP (1994) Polyinosinic:polycytidylic acid is a potent activator of endothelial cells. Am J Pathol 145:137–147
68. Sobel DO, Goyal D, Ahvazi B et al (1998) Low dose poly I:C prevents diabetes in the diabetes prone BB rat. J Autoimmun 11:343–352
69. Ewel CH, Sobel DO, Zeligs BJ et al (1992) Poly I:C accelerates development of diabetes mellitus in diabetes-prone BB rat. Diabetes 41:1016–1021
70. Sobel DO, Azumi N, Creswell K et al (1995) The role of NK cell activity in the pathogenesis of poly I:C accelerated and spontaneous diabetes in the diabetes prone BB rat. J Autoimmun 8:843–857
71. Alexopoulou L, Holt AC, Medzhitov R et al (2001) Recognition of double-stranded RNA and activation of NF-kappaB by toll-like receptor 3. Nature 413:732–738
72. Guberski DL, Thomas VA, Shek WR et al (1991) Induction of type I diabetes by Kilham's rat virus in diabetes-resistant BB/Wor rats. Science 254:1010–1013
73. Kruger AJ, Yang C, Tam SW et al (2010) Haptoglobin as an early serum biomarker of virus-induced autoimmune type 1 diabetes in biobreeding diabetes resistant and LEW1.WR1 rats. Exp Biol Med (Maywood) 235:1328–1337
74. Zipris D, Lien E, Xie JX et al (2005) TLR activation synergizes with Kilham rat virus infection to induce diabetes in BBDR rats. J Immunol 174:131–142
75. McKisic MD, Paturzo FX, Gaertner DJ et al (1995) A nonlethal rat parvovirus infection suppresses rat T lymphocyte effector functions. J Immunol 155:3979–3986

76. Ellerman KE, Richards CA, Guberski DL et al (1996) Kilham rat triggers T-cell-dependent autoimmune diabetes in multiple strains of rat. Diabetes 45:557–562
77. Zipris D, Hillebrands JL, Welsh RM et al (2003) Infections that induce autoimmune diabetes in BBDR rats modulate CD4+CD25+ T cell populations. J Immunol 170:3592–3602
78. Chung YH, Jun HS, Kang Y et al (1997) Role of macrophages and macrophage-derived cytokines in the pathogenesis of Kilham rat virus-induced autoimmune diabetes in diabetes-resistant BioBreeding rats. J Immunol 159:466–471
79. Chung YH, Jun HS, Son M et al (2000) Cellular and molecular mechanism for Kilham rat virus-induced autoimmune diabetes in DR-BB rats. J Immunol 165:2866–2876
80. Nair A, Wolter TR, Meyers AJ et al (2008) Innate immune pathways in virus-induced autoimmune diabetes. Ann N Y Acad Sci 1150:139–142
81. Zipris D, Lien E, Nair A et al (2007) TLR9-signaling pathways are involved in Kilham rat virus-induced autoimmune diabetes in the biobreeding diabetes-resistant rat. J Immunol 178:693–701
82. Wolter TR, Wong R, Sarkar SA et al (2009) DNA microarray analysis for the identification of innate immune pathways implicated in virus-induced autoimmune diabetes. Clin Immunol 132:103–115
83. Heinig M, Petretto E, Wallace C et al (2010) A trans-acting locus regulates an anti-viral expression network and type 1 diabetes risk. Nature 467:460–464
84. Yoon JW, Jun HS (2006) Viruses cause type 1 diabetes in animals. Ann N Y Acad Sci 1079:138–146
85. Chen S, Howard O (2004) Images in clinical medicine. Parvovirus B19 infection. N Engl J Med 350:598
86. Munakata Y, Kodera T, Saito T et al (2005) Rheumatoid arthritis, type 1 diabetes, and Graves' disease after acute parvovirus B19 infection. Lancet 366:780
87. Mordes JP, Guberski DL, Leif JH et al (2005) LEW.1WR1 rats develop autoimmune diabetes spontaneously and in response to environmental perturbation. Diabetes 54:2727–2733
88. Kaldunski M, Jia S, Geoffrey R et al (2010) Identification of a serum-induced transcriptional signature associated with type 1 diabetes in the BioBreeding rat. Diabetes 59:2375–2385
89. Wang X, Jia S, Geoffrey R et al (2008) Identification of a molecular signature in human type 1 diabetes mellitus using serum and functional genomics. J Immunol 180:1929–1937
90. Gottlieb PA, Handler ES, Appel MC et al (1991) Insulin treatment prevents diabetes mellitus but not thyroiditis in RT6-depleted diabetes resistant BB/Wor rats. Diabetologia 34:296–300
91. Lefkowith J, Schreiner G, Cormier J et al (1990) Prevention of diabetes in the BB rat by essential fatty acid deficiency. Relationship between physiological and biochemical changes. J Exp Med 171:729–743
92. Mendez I, Chung YH, Jun HS et al (2004) Immunoregulatory role of nitric oxide in Kilham rat virus-induced autoimmune diabetes in DR-BB rats. J Immunol 173:1327–1335
93. Ugrasbul F, Moore WV, Tong PY et al (2008) Prevention of diabetes: effect of mycophenolate mofetil and anti-CD25 on onset of diabetes in the DRBB rat. Pediatr Diabetes 9:596–601
94. Popovic J, Kover KL, Moore WV (2004) The effect of immunomodulators on prevention of autoimmune diabetes is stage dependent: FTY720 prevents diabetes at three different stages in the diabetes-resistant biobreeding rat. Pediatr Diabetes 5:3–9
95. Jorns A, Rath KJ, Terbish T et al (2010) Diabetes prevention by immunomodulatory FTY720 treatment in the LEW.1AR1-iddm rat despite immune cell activation. Endocrinology 151:3555–3565
96. Peschke E, Hofmann K, Bahr I et al (2011) The insulin-melatonin antagonism: studies in the LEW.1AR1-iddm rat (an animal model of human type 1 diabetes mellitus). Diabetologia 54:1831–1840
97. Mordes JP, Cort L, Norowski E et al (2009) Analysis of the rat Iddm14 diabetes susceptibility locus in multiple rat strains: identification of a susceptibility haplotype in the Tcrb-V locus. Mamm Genome 20:162–169
98. Bottazzo GF (1986) Lawrence lecture. Death of a beta cell: homicide or suicide? Diabet Med 3:119–130
99. Atkinson MA, Bluestone JA, Eisenbarth GS et al (2011) How does type 1 diabetes develop?: the notion of homicide or beta-cell suicide revisited. Diabetes 60:1370–1379
100. Lipson KL, Fonseca SG, Urano F (2006) Endoplasmic reticulum stress-induced apoptosis and auto-immunity in diabetes. Curr Mol Med 6:71–77

Part II

Rodent Models of Type 2 Diabetes

Chapter 4

Diabetes in Mice with Monogenic Obesity: The *db/db* Mouse and Its Use in the Study of Cardiac Consequences

Darrell D. Belke and David L. Severson

Abstract

The leptin receptor deficient *db/db* mouse has served as a rodent model for obesity and type 2 diabetes for more than 40 years. Diabetic features in *db/db* mice follow an age-dependent progression, with early insulin resistance followed by an insulin secretory defect resulting in profound hyperglycemia. Diabetic *db/db* mice have been utilized to assess the cardiac consequences of diabetes, specifically evidence for a distinct diabetic cardiomyopathy. The *db/db* model is characterized by a contractile function deficit in the heart which becomes manifest 8–10 weeks after birth. Metabolic changes include an increased reliance on fatty acids and a decreased reliance on glucose as a fuel source for oxidative metabolism within the heart. As a mouse model for type 2 diabetes, both drug treatment and transgenic manipulation have proven beneficial towards improving metabolism and contractile function. The *db/db* mouse model has provided a useful resource to understand and treat the type 2 diabetic condition.

Key words: Hyperinsulinemia, Echocardiography, Magnetic resonance imaging, Cardiomyocytes, Bioenergetics, Type 2 diabetes, Obesity, Leptin

1. Diabetic *db/db* Mice: History, General Features and Genetics

Diabetic *db/db* mice were discovered at Jackson Laboratory as the consequence of a spontaneous autosomal recessive mutation (1, 2). The natural history of homozygous *db/db* mice follows a distinct pattern (3, 4). Initially, peripheral insulin resistance is accompanied by increased pancreatic beta-cell insulin secretion; thus, hyperinsulinemia is a compensatory mechanism to counteract insulin resistance, allowing normoglycemia to be maintained. Increased levels of plasma insulin are the earliest feature of *db/db* mice, evident as soon as 10–12 days of age with beta-cell hyperplasia and hypertrophy. Hyperglycemia eventually develops when enhanced beta-cell insulin secretion can no longer compensate for peripheral and hepatic insulin resistance. The maximal extent of hyperinsulinemia occurs at 2–3 months of age; insulin levels then fall rapidly as beta-cells exhibit a severe secretory defect due to beta-cell apoptosis. Body weights of *db/db* mice increase progressively and plateau at about 2 months of age (40–50 g), almost double the weight of control mice. The general features (natural history) of this age-dependent progression are shown in Fig. 1. An experimental advantage of the *db/db* mouse model system is the ability to study diabetic features at an early (6 weeks of age) or established (12 weeks) stage. Specific measurements of body weight and plasma insulin and glucose concentrations (5) are presented in Fig. 2. At 6 weeks of age, *db/db* mice exhibited hyperinsulinemia and increased body weight but plasma glucose concentration was still normal. In contrast, 12 weeks old *db/db* mice exhibit marked obesity, persistent hyperinsulinemia, and a profound degree of hyperglycemia. There is a marked influence of strain in terms of severity of diabetic features (6). The *db/db* mouse is typically maintained on the KsJ background; mice maintained on the diabetes resistant BL/6 background exhibit severe insulin resistance but no diabetic hyperglycemia. Thus, the general metabolic features of *db/db* mice (2), with initial insulin resistance followed by an insulin

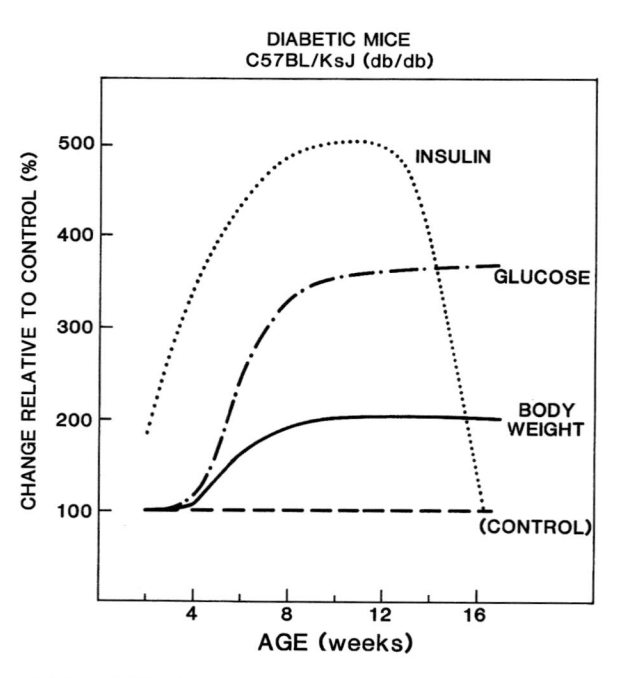

Fig. 1. Natural history of diabetic changes in *db/db* mice relative to control (100 %): plasma insulin (······), blood glucose (– · –), and body weight (—). Insulin resistance (hyperinsulinemia) precedes the development of hyperglycemia and obesity. Insulin concentration eventually falls due to a pancreatic β-cell secretory defect and the profound hyperglycemia is maintained. This figure is a composite from early publications (1–4) describing the characteristics of *db/db* mice.

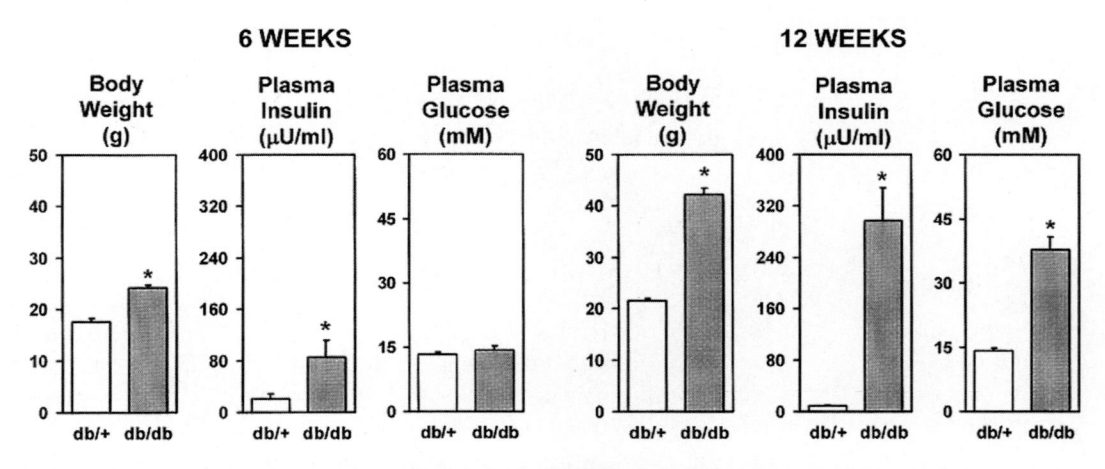

Fig. 2. Age-dependent progression of diabetes in *db/db* mice. Body weight (g), plasma insulin (μU/mL), and plasma glucose (mM) measurements were obtained from control *db/+* and *db/db* mice at 6 and 12 weeks of age, representing early and established stages in the diabetic progression. Results are from Aasum et al. (5), with permission from *Diabetes* journal.

secretion defect, are very similar to the pathogenesis of type 2 diabetes in humans (7).

The *db* mutation (*Lepr*^{db}) was subsequently identified as a G→T point mutation in the leptin receptor gene on mouse chromosome 4 that produces a frameshift which selectively eliminates the "long" isoform (Ob-Rb) of the leptin receptor, one of the five differentially spliced mRNA transcripts, resulting in defective leptin signaling (8). Thus, *db/db* mice represent a model of leptin resistance, in contrast to obese *ob/ob* mice which are a model of leptin deficiency. Interestingly, *db/+* heterozygotes with one mutant copy of the leptin receptor, as well as *ob/+* heterozygotes with one mutant copy of leptin, are phenotypically normal with respect to body weight and blood concentrations of glucose and lipids.

2. Diabetic *db/db* Mice and Diabetic Cardiomyopathy

Patients with diabetes mellitus (types 1 and 2) have an increased risk for cardiovascular disease, such that cardiovascular complications are the leading cause of diabetes-related morbidity and mortality (9–12). Diabetes-induced cardiac disease has multiple causes: (a) accelerated coronary atherosclerosis (macroangiopathy) because of associated risk factors (visceral obesity, dyslipidemia, and hypertension), resulting in ischemic heart disease progressing to myocardial infarction and heart failure; (b) microangiopathy in the coronary microvasculature; and (c) alterations in cardiac structure and function without coronary artery disease or hypertension, a condition termed diabetic cardiomyopathy (13–15). Thus, diabetic cardiomyopathy is characterized by ventricular dysfunction that is independent of coronary artery disease or hypertension; diastolic dysfunction often precedes systolic dysfunction.

Since rodents are resistant to atherosclerosis, experimental studies with rodent models of diabetes allow assessment of the deleterious effects of diabetes on cardiac function (diabetic cardiomyopathy) without any contribution of coronary artery disease (16, 17). Despite substantial dyslipidemia with elevated plasma fatty acid and triacylglycerol concentrations (18), *db/db* mice actually exhibit less atherosclerosis on a high fat diet (19) compared to lean *db/+* heterozygotes on both C57BL/6 and C57BL/Ks genetic backgrounds. Therefore, *db/db* mice provide an excellent model to examine the manifestation of a diabetic cardiomyopathy without confounding heart disease. Furthermore, some studies have observed that *db/db* mice are not hypertensive (20). An early ultrastructural study by Giacomelli and Weiner (21) provided evidence for damage to myocardial cells in *db/db* hearts without any coronary artery disease. Consequently, features of diabetic cardiomyopathy have been revealed in studies that have measured cardiac function with type 2 diabetic *db/db* mice (15, 17, 22).

3. Cardiac Phenotyping in *db/db* Mice: Contractile Dysfunction

Although the *db/db* mouse model of type 2 diabetes was discovered more than 40 years ago (1), the development of techniques to accurately assess heart function in this model was driven by the increasing availability of genetically engineered mouse models as a tool for cardiovascular research. The development of conduction catheters small enough to record pressure–volume loops in the mouse heart, along with the development of probes for echocardiography in mice and advancements in magnetic resonance imaging (MRI) have enabled researchers to track the development of cardiac dysfunction in *db/db* mice. Coupled with the development of methods to enzymatically isolate viable cardiac myocytes from mouse hearts, an improved picture of the development of cardiac dysfunction and its underlying mechanisms has emerged for the *db/db* model.

3.1. In Vivo Non-invasive Measures of Cardiac Function

Non-invasive in vivo measures of cardiac function in *db/db* mice have been obtained using echocardiography and MRI. These methods are most suitable for longitudinal studies of cardiac function in *db/db* mice to identify when alterations in contractile function begin. Echocardiography in the short axis requires sampling at a 90° angle to the papillary muscle to accurately measure changes in chamber diameter and wall thickness. M-mode analysis provides a two-dimensional image of left ventricle (LV) changes over time allowing for fractional shortening to be calculated from systolic and diastolic measurements. The earliest echo studies did not observe any difference in fractional shortening between *db/db* and *db/+* mice at 6 weeks of age but did observe a significant decrease in fractional shortening in *db/db* mice at 12 weeks of age (23). Later studies also found no difference in mice as young as 7 weeks of age but did observe a decrease in fractional shorting at 20 weeks (24). Greer et al. (25) did not observe any difference in fractional shortening measured by echo in 10 week old mice, however other studies were able to detect differences at 12 weeks (26) and 15 weeks (27) of age. Hence, analysis of fractional shortening by echocardiography suggests the development of a functional cardiomyopathy between 10 and 12 weeks of age in *db/db* mice. Some longitudinal studies from 8 to 18 weeks have indicated no change in cardiac function under normal conditions, but a blunted response to the beta 2 adrenergic receptor agonist dobutamine at later time periods, indicating a loss of contractile reserve (28). The echo measurements are most effective in estimating cardiac workload when accompanied by blood pressure measurements. Using tail cuff plethysmography, Dong and Ren (29) observed higher systolic pressure in 16–20 week old mice, however other studies suggest that an increase in adiposity prevents meaningful pressure measurements by tail cuff after 10 weeks of age in *db/db* mice (30).

Measurement of heart function by MRI requires more specialized equipment to obtain high resolution images and the capacity to gate imaging to the cardiac cycle (such as the QRS complex of the ECG) to obtain clean images. This method allows for the accumulation of multiple heart slices from apex-base permitting a reconstruction of heart volume. Yue et al. (30) performed a longitudinal study on heart function using MRI and while they observed an increase in LV mass by as early as 9 weeks, they did not observe a significant increase in LV diastolic volume or a decrease in ejection fraction in diabetic mice relative to control mice until 13 weeks. An increase in LV dilatation was also observed by MRI in *db/db* mice at 16 weeks of age (31) with a decrease in ejection fraction being observed at 8, 12, and 16 weeks of age. This contrasts with a high resolution MRI study by Stuckey et al. (32) in which they found no difference in heart mass, systolic volumes, ejection fraction, or cardiac output in 12 week old *db/db* mice relative to lean controls. By using high temporal resolution, however, they did observe a peak ejection rate of blood which was significantly slower in diabetic *db/db* mice. MRI imaging provides an additional advantage in that it can be coupled with procedures such as positron emission tomography to estimate metabolic changes in conjunction with the high resolution images obtained by MRI. Yue et al. (30) were able to observe a decrease in 18-fluorodeoxyglucose uptake at 9 weeks of age just prior to the development of LV dysfunction in *db/db* mice.

3.2. In Vivo Invasive Measures of Cardiac Function

One critique of the imaging studies described in the preceding paragraphs is the lack of blood pressure measurements required to estimate the workload of the heart. Some longitudinal studies have incorporated tail cuff plethysmography to estimate systolic and diastolic blood pressure (30), however the development of obesity in *db/db* mice may preclude an accurate assessment of blood pressure beyond 10 weeks (30). Conduction catheters small enough for mice permit the direct measurements of LV pressure and volume changes in mice over the cardiac cycle. Buchanan et al. (33) performed a longitudinal study on 4, 8, and 15 week old mice using a conduction catheter. They observed an increase in systolic pressure in *db/db* mice relative to lean controls at 8 weeks, but not 4 or 15 weeks. Consistent with the non-invasive results described above, they only observed a significant decrease in the rate of relaxation ($-dP/dt$) at the 15 week time point. Similar studies in 16 week old mice reveal a significant increase in Tau (rate constant for ventricular relaxation) in the *db/db* diabetic group, indicative of a slower rate of relaxation for the left ventricle (31). They did not observe any difference in systolic or diastolic pressures between *db/db* and *db/+* mice at 8, 12, or 16 weeks of age, suggesting the absence of a hypertensive phenotype.

3.3. Ex Vivo Measures of Cardiac Function

To complement the in vivo measurements, ex vivo perfused heart preparations were adapted to permit analysis of heart function under controlled loading conditions (preload and afterload), and substrate supply in the perfusion solution. A longitudinal study by Aasum et al. (34) examining either the product of cardiac output or heart rate times peak systolic pressure did not show any difference between diabetic and non-diabetic mice at 5 weeks, but did observe a significant decrease in both parameters by 14–15 weeks of age. This data parallels a similar study by this group (5) in which no differences in cardiac contractile function between *db/db* and *db/+* mice were observed at 6 weeks, but both measures were significantly depressed at 12 weeks. Belke et al. (35) observed a decrease in pressure development and $+/-dP/dt$ in 12 week old mice in an isovolumic Langendorff perfusion model. In this model all contractile force is registered as pressure change in the absence of volume change, rendering it a more accurate measure of cardiac function as a measure of calcium handling than the working heart. Cardiac power is a measure of the pressure generated by the heart multiplied by the volume ejected by the heart, and is the basis for increased oxygen consumption at higher workloads. Belke et al. (36) observed a decrease in cardiac power in ex vivo perfused *db/db* hearts at 10–14 weeks of age. Similarly, Buchanan et al. (33) observed a decrease in cardiac power output at 15 weeks of age. These observations suggest that the contractile dysfunction observed during in vivo studies can be replicated in ex vivo isolated perfused heart models.

With ex vivo perfused hearts, contractile function can be measured during normoxic perfusions and after a period of ischemia (reduced coronary flow) and reperfusion, to determine pre- and post-ischemic function. Perfused working *db/db* hearts exhibit increased susceptibility to ischemia–reperfusion injury, manifested as reduced functional recovery (5).

3.4. In Vitro Studies Using Isolated Cardiac Myocytes

Longitudinal studies reveal the development of a contractile defect in *db/db* mice occurring between 10 and 12 weeks of age but provide little insight into the mechanism(s) underlying the defect. Analysis of calcium handling in myocytes isolated from 12 week old *db/db* mice indicate smaller calcium transients with decreased loading of the sarcoplasmic-reticulum (SR) in comparison to *db/+* mice (35). Similar observations were obtained in 15–20 week old mice (24, 27, 29, 37). The smaller transients are associated with a slower decline of the calcium signal indicative of a reduced capacity to remove calcium from the cytosol. In type 1 diabetic models, this slow decline has been linked to a decrease in SERCA2a expression (38). In the *db/db* model a decrease in SERCA2a expression has not been uniformly associated with contractile dysfunction, with some studies reporting no change in SERCA2a expression (35, 37) and others noting a decrease in SERCA2a expression (24). Yue et al. (30) examined SERCA expression in a longitudinal study and observed a significant decrease in SERCA2a mRNA levels between 9 and 13 weeks, suggesting a decrease in SERCA2a expression contributes to the decline in contractile function at later time points. Other studies have noted a decrease in the phosphorylation of phospholamban (an inhibitory protein of SERCA2a) which would decrease SERCA2a activity in the absence of any change in SERCA2a expression (35).

In addition to the decreased SERCA2a activity, the smaller calcium transient associated with *db/db* mice has also been attributed to increased calcium removal from the myocyte through the sodium calcium exchanger (NCX) and abnormal activity of the ryanodine receptor (RyR2). Some studies have reported an increase in NCX activity in *db/db* mice contributing to the removal of calcium from the myocyte (24, 27), although not all studies have reported an increase in exchanger activity in *db/db* mice (35). The RyR2, responsible for regulating the coordinated release of calcium from the SR, is also altered in *db/db* mice. Normal RyR2a expression levels are reported for *db/db* mice (24, 35) although some studies have noted a decrease in RyR2 expression (27). An increased level of calcium leak through the RyR2 has been observed in *db/db* mice which could contribute to the decreased calcium loading of SR and the diminished calcium transient (24, 35). The increased leak has been attributed to a decrease in FKBP 12.6 (calstabin) expression (35) or an increase in calcium–calmodulin-dependent protein kinase activity (24), both of which would lead to an increased phosphorylation of RyR2, increasing leak. In addition to these observations, Pereira et al. (27) reported a decrease in L-type calcium channel expression in the *db/db* mouse which could reduce calcium current triggering calcium induced calcium release from RyR2.

In individual myocytes it is possible to observe contraction and relaxation and measure the extent and rate of change in myocyte length. The extent to which myocytes decrease in length is analogous to fractional shortening measured in echo, and changes in rate at which cells shorten and re-lengthen (dL/dt) is analogous to pressure changes (dP/dt). Dong and Ren (29) observed a smaller fractional shortening and a decreased rate of length change in the *db/db* mice at 16–20 weeks of age, consistent with a poor contractile performance. Kralik et al. (37) observed similar results in myocytes isolated from 20 week old mice. In summary, the decreased contractile performance observed in vivo or under ex vivo perfusion conditions is confirmed by measurements of the contractile performance of individual cardiac myocytes due to alterations in calcium handling reflected in decreased calcium loading of the SR and a smaller calcium transient.

4. Diabetic *db/db* Hearts: Altered Metabolic Phenotype and Reduced Cardiac Efficiency

Ex vivo heart perfusions permit control over the supply of substrates (fuels) in the perfusate. Typically, working heart perfusates contain two substrates: glucose and palmitate as a representative fatty acid (FA). Use of radiolabeled substrates allows calculation of metabolic rates based on the appearance of metabolites in the perfusate: glycolysis ((5-^{3}H)glucose → ^{3}H$_2$O); glucose oxidation ((U-^{14}C)glucose → ^{14}CO$_2$); and FA oxidation ((9,10-^{3}H)palmitate → ^{3}H$_2$O). Consequently, dual-label scintillation counting permits the simultaneous determination of glucose oxidation and FA oxidation from a single perfused heart. Perfused *db/db* hearts exhibit an altered metabolic phenotype, with decreased glycolysis and glucose oxidation and a reciprocal increase in FA oxidation (36). In fact, increased FA oxidation was the earliest metabolic change in perfused *db/db* hearts, detectable at 6 weeks of age (5). Increased esterification of FA into cellular triacylglycerols is also a feature of *db/db* hearts (22). Increased FA utilization was also evident when *db/db* hearts were perfused with high concentrations of glucose and FA to mimic diabetic conditions (39). Interestingly, although insulin-stimulated glucose uptake was reduced markedly in *db/db* cardiomyocytes (40), working perfused *db/db* hearts were insulin sensitive (increased glucose oxidation and reduced FA oxidation) (39). The complex regulation of glucose transport in a beating heart must, therefore, reduce cardiac insulin resistance.

The chronic over-utilization of FA as an energy source for diabetic hearts represents a metabolic maladaptation that can be a causative factor in the development of diabetic cardiomyopathy (15, 22, 41–43). The hypothesis that normalization of the altered metabolism of diabetic *db/db* hearts should improve contractile performance was tested using transgenic *db/db* mice with overexpression of the insulin-regulatable glucose transporter-4 (*db/db*-hGLUT4 mice) (36). Perfused *db/db*-hGLUT4 hearts exhibited increased rates of glucose utilization and reduced FA oxidation to the normal values in non-diabetic (*db/+*) perfused hearts, with a concomitant increase in contractile performance (23, 36).

The altered metabolic phenotype of *db/db* hearts also has bioenergetic implications. Cardiac efficiency is the ratio between energy output (cardiac work) and energy input (myocardial O_2 consumption, MVO_2). The cardiac work term that correlates best with MVO_2 is pressure–volume area (PVA) (44), determined by inserting a combined micromanometer (pressure)–conductance (volume) catheter into the LV lumen of ex vivo perfused working mouse hearts (45). MVO_2 measurements were obtained from fiber-optic oxygen probes. Extrapolation of the linear MVO_2-PVA relationship to zero work gives unloaded (PVA-independent) MVO_2. Increasing perfusate FA concentration produced a parallel upward shift of the MVO_2-PVA relationship; the resulting increase in unloaded MVO_2 is an indicator of reduced cardiac efficiency (45). Unloaded MVO_2 represents the O_2 costs for (1) basal metabolism (BM) and (2) excitation–contraction (EC) coupling.

Perfused *db/db* hearts showed reduced cardiac efficiency (46). Recently, Boardman et al. (47) have reported that the reduced cardiac efficiency in *db/db* hearts was due to an increase in both the BM and EC coupling components of unloaded MVO_2, reflecting increased FA utilization, and altered Ca^{2+} homeostasis, respectively.

Reduced cardiac efficiency in *db/db* hearts will likely be a causal link to the observation of increased susceptibility of *db/db* hearts to ischemia–reperfusion injury (5). Both acute perfusion with high glucose–high insulin (48) and in vivo treatment with the peroxisome proliferator-activated receptor-γ agonist rosiglitazone (49) improved cardiac efficiency and increased functional recovery after ischemia–reperfusion.

References

1. Hummel KP, Dickie MM, Coleman DL (1966) Diabetes, a new mutation in the mouse. Science 153:1127–1128
2. Coleman DL (1982) Diabetes-obesity syndromes in mice. Diabetes 31:1–6
3. Wyse BM, Dulin WE (1970) The influence of age and dietary conditions on diabetes in the *db* mouse. Diabetologia 6:268–273
4. Coleman DL, Hummel KP (1974) Hyperinsulinemia in pre-weaning diabetes (*db*) mice. Diabetologia 10:607–610
5. Aasum E, Hafstad AD, Severson DL et al (2003) Age-dependent changes in metabolism, contractile function, and ischemic sensitivity in hearts from *db/db* mice. Diabetes 52:434–441

6. Hummel KP, Coleman DL, Lane PW (1972) The influence of genetic background on expression of mutations at the diabetes locus in the mouse. I. C57BL/KsJ and C57BL/6J strains. Biochem Genet 7:1–13
7. Cavaghan MK, Ehrmann DA, Polonsky KS (2000) Interactions between insulin resistance and insulin secretion in the development of glucose intolerance. J Clin Invest 106:329–333
8. Leibel RL, Chung WK, Chua SC Jr (1997) The molecular genetics of rodent single gene obesities. J Biol Chem 272:31937–31940
9. Garcia MJ, McNamara PM, Gordon T et al (1974) Morbidity and mortality in diabetics in the Framingham population: sixteen year follow-up study. Diabetes 23:105–111
10. Grundy SM, Benjamin IJ, Burke GL et al (1999) Diabetes and cardiovascular disease. A statement for healthcare professionals from the American Heart Association. Circulation 100:1134–1146
11. Haffner SM, Lehto S, Ronnemaa T et al (1998) Mortality from coronary heart disease in subjects with type 2 diabetes and in nondiabetic subjects with and without prior myocardial infarction. N Engl J Med 339:229–234
12. Lee C, Folsom A, Pankow J et al (2004) Cardiovascular events in diabetic and nondiabetic adults with or without history of myocardial infarction. Circulation 109:855–860
13. Rubler S, Dlugash J, Yuceoglu YZ et al (1972) New type of cardiomyopathy associated with diabetic glomerulosclerosis. Am J Cardiol 30:595–602
14. Regan TJ, Lyons MM, Ahmed SS et al (1977) Evidence for cardiomyopathy in familial diabetes mellitus. J Clin Invest 60:885–899
15. Boudina S, Abel ED (2007) Diabetic cardiomyopathy revisited. Circulation 115:3213–3223
16. Tomlinson KC, Gardiner SM, Hebden RA et al (1992) Functional consequences of streptozotocin-induced diabetes mellitus, with particular reference to the cardiovascular system. Pharmacol Rev 44:103–179
17. Severson DL (2004) Diabetic cardiomyopathy: recent evidence from mouse models of type 1 and type 2 diabetes. Can J Physiol Pharmacol 82:813–823
18. Kobayashi Y, Fortre TM, Taniguchi S et al (2000) The *db/db* mouse, a model for diabetic dyslipidemia: molecular characterization and effects of Western diet feeding. Metabolism 49:22–31
19. Nishina PM, Naggert JK, Verstuyft J et al (1994) Atherosclerosis in genetically obese mice: the mutants obese, diabetes, fat, tubby, and lethal yellow. Metabolism 43:554–558
20. Jones SP, Girod WG, Granger DN et al (1999) Reperfusion injury is not affected by blockade of P-selectin in the diabetic mouse heart. Am J Physiol Heart Circ Physiol 277:H763–H769
21. Giacomelli F, Wiener J (1979) Primary myocardial disease in the diabetic mouse. An ultrastructural study. Lab Invest 40:460–473
22. Carley AN, Severson DL (2005) Review. Fatty acid metabolism is enhanced in type 2 diabetic hearts. Biochim Biophys Acta 1734:112–126
23. Semeniuk LM, Kryski AJ, Severson DL (2000) Echocardiographic assessment of cardiac function in diabetic *db/db* and transgenic *db/db*-hGLUT4 mice. Am J Physiol Heart Circ Physiol 283:H976–H982
24. Stolen TO, Høydal MA, Kemi OJ et al (2009) Interval training normalizes cardiomyocyte function, diastolic Ca^{2+} control, and SR Ca^{2+} release synchronicity in a mouse model of diabetic cardiomyopathy. Circ Res 105:527–536
25. Greer JJ, Ware DP, Lefer DJ (2006) Myocardial infarction and heart failure in the *db/db* diabetic mouse. Am J Physiol Heart Circ Physiol 290:H146–H153
26. Carley AN, Semeniuk LM, Shimoni Y et al (2004) Treatment of type 2 diabetic *db/db* mice with a novel PPARgamma agonist improves cardiac metabolism but not contractile function. Am J Physiol Endocrinol Metab 286:E449–E455
27. Pereira L, Matthes J, Schuster I et al (2006) Mechanisms of $(Ca^{2+})i$ transient decrease in cardiomyopathy of *db/db* type 2 diabetic mice. Diabetes 55:608–615
28. Daniels A, van Bilsen M, Janssen BJ et al (2010) Impaired cardiac functional reserve in type 2 diabetic *db/db* mice is associated with metabolic, but not structural, remodeling. Acta Physiol (Oxf) 200:11–22
29. Dong F, Ren J (2009) Adiponectin improves cardiomyocyte contractile function in *db/db* diabetic obese mice. Obesity (Silver Spring) 17:262–268
30. Yue P, Arai T, Terashima M et al (2007) Magnetic resonance imaging of progressive cardiomyopathic changes in the *db/db* mouse. Am J Physiol Heart Circ Physiol 292:H2106–H2118
31. Nielsen JM, Kristiansen SB, Nørregaard R et al (2009) Blockage of receptor for advanced glycation end products prevents development of cardiac dysfunction in *db/db* type 2 diabetic mice. Eur J Heart Fail 11:638–647
32. Stuckey DJ, Carr CA, Tyler DJ et al (2008) Novel MRI method to detect altered left

ventricular ejection and filling patterns in rodent models of disease. Magn Reson Med 60:582–587
33. Buchanan J, Mazumder PK, Hu P et al (2005) Reduced cardiac efficiency and altered substrate metabolism precedes the onset of hyperglycemia and contractile dysfunction in two mouse models of insulin resistance and obesity. Endocrinology 146:5341–5349
34. Aasum E, Cooper M, Severson DL et al (2005) Effect of BM 17.0744, a PPARalpha ligand, on the metabolism of perfused hearts from control and diabetic mice. Can J Physiol Pharmacol 83:183–190
35. Belke DD, Swanson EA, Dillmann WH (2004) Decreased sarcoplasmic reticulum activity and contractility in diabetic *db/db* mouse heart. Diabetes 53:3201–3208
36. Belke DD, Larsen TS, Gibbs EM et al (2000) Altered metabolism causes cardiac dysfunction in perfused hearts from diabetic (*db/db*) mice. Am J Physiol Endocrinol Metab 279: E1104–E1113
37. Kralik PM, Ye G, Metreveli NS et al (2005) Cardiomyocyte dysfunction in models of type 1 and type 2 diabetes. Cardiovasc Toxicol 5:285–292
38. Trost SU, Belke DD, Bluhm WF et al (2002) Overexpression of the sarcoplasmic reticulum Ca(2+)-ATPase improves myocardial contractility in diabetic cardiomyopathy. Diabetes 51:1166–1171
39. Hafstad AD, Solevåg GH, Severson DL et al (2006) Perfused hearts from Type 2 diabetic (*db/db*) mice show metabolic responsiveness to insulin. Am J Physiol Heart Circ Physiol 290:H1763–H1769
40. Carroll R, Carley AN, Dyck JRB et al (2005) Metabolic effects of insulin on cardiomyocytes from control and diabetic *db/db* mouse hearts. Am J Physiol Endocrinol Metab 288: E900–E906
41. An D, Rodrigues B (2006) Role of changes in cardiac metabolism in development of diabetic cardiomyopathy. Am J Physiol Heart Circ Physiol 291:H1489–H1506
42. Taegtmeyer H, McNulty P, Young ME (2002) Adaptation and maladaptation of the heart in diabetes. Part I: general concepts. Circulation 105:1727–1733
43. Young ME, McNulty P, Taegtmeyer H (2002) Adaptation and maladaptation of the heart in diabetes. Part II: potential mechanisms. Circulation 105:1861–1870
44. Suga H (1990) Ventricular energetics. Physiol Rev 70:247–277
45. How O-J, Aasum E, Kunnathu S et al (2005) Influence of substrate supply on cardiac efficiency, as measured by pressure-volume analysis in *ex vivo* mouse hearts. Am J Physiol Heart Circ Physiol 288:H2979–H2985
46. How O-J, Aasum E, Severson DL et al (2006) Increased myocardial oxygen consumption reduces cardiac efficiency in diabetic mice. Diabetes 55:466–473
47. Boardman N, Hafstad AD, Larsen TS et al (2009) Increased O_2 cost of basal metabolism and excitation-contraction coupling in hearts from type 2 diabetic mice. Am J Physiol Heart Circ Physiol 296:H1373–H1379
48. Hafstad AD, Khalid AM, How O-J et al (2007) Glucose and insulin improve cardiac efficiency and postischemic functional recovery in perfused hearts from type 2 diabetic (*db/db*) mice. Am J Physiol Endocrinol Metab 292:E1288–E1294
49. How O-J, Larsen TS, Hafstad AD et al (2007) Rosiglitazone treatment improves cardiac efficiency in hearts from diabetic mice. Arch Physiol Biochem 113:211–220

Chapter 5

Pathophysiology and Genetics of Obesity and Diabetes in the New Zealand Obese Mouse: A Model of the Human Metabolic Syndrome

Reinhart Kluge, Stephan Scherneck, Annette Schürmann, and Hans-Georg Joost

Abstract

The New Zealand Obese (NZO) mouse is one of the most thoroughly investigated polygenic models for the human metabolic syndrome and type 2 diabetes. It presents the main characteristics of the disease complex, including early-onset obesity, insulin resistance, dyslipidemia, and hypertension. As a consequence of this syndrome, a combination of lipotoxicity and glucotoxicity produces beta-cell failure and apoptosis resulting in hypoinsulinemia and diabetic hyperglycemia. With NZO as a breeding partner, several adipogenic and diabetogenic gene variants have been identified by hypothesis-free positional cloning (*Tbc1d1*, *Zfp69*) or by combining genetic screens and candidate gene approaches (*Pctp*, *Abcg1*, *Nmur2*, *Lepr*). This chapter summarizes the present knowledge of the NZO strain and describes its pathophysiology as well as the known underlying genetic defects.

Key words: Metabolic syndrome, Insulin resistance, Type 2 diabetes, Obesity, New Zealand Obese mouse, Leptin receptor, High-fat diet, Glucotoxicity, Lipotoxicity, Positional cloning, QTL (quantitative trait locus), Neuromedin U, Neuromedin U receptor

1. Introduction: Mouse Models of Human Type 2 Diabetes: Potential and Limitations

Human type 2 diabetes is a complex, polygenic disease characterized by chronic hyperglycemia and hypoinsulinemia. Its main pathogenetic factor is visceral obesity leading to ectopic fat deposition, insulin resistance, and to failure of the insulin-producing cells by incompletely understood processes. Previous research has shown that several inbred mouse strains such as the New Zealand Obese (NZO) mouse, the C57KS/J-*db/db* mouse, and the TALLYHO mouse present a similar obesity-associated diabetes mellitus. Thus, it is reasonable to assume that many, if not all, pathogenetic mechanisms leading to hyperglycemia are similar in mice and humans. Furthermore, direct genetic evidence for the involvement of a particular protein or pathway can be obtained in mice but very rarely in humans. Thus, inbred mouse models are ideally suited for the investigation of human type 2 diabetes. However, the genetic homogeneity of the inbred strains is not only an advantage, it also limits their potential. Individuals of an inbred mouse line are genetically identical, and it is therefore unlikely that a single strain presents all pathogenetic mechanisms of a complex disease. Selecting the "right" mouse model for the metabolic syndrome and type 2 diabetes is therefore of crucial importance, and more than one model is required for a complete analysis of complex traits (1). In addition, previous and ongoing research supports the view that the combination of individual genomes—by intercross of inbred strains and by the generation of congenic lines—will reveal effects of many more genes and gene interactions than can be observed in a single inbred strain. Because of its metabolic phenotype, the NZO mouse appears to be a well-suited breeding partner for such an experimental approach.

2. Origin and Breeding of the NZO Mouse Model

2.1. Origin

The original NZO strain was developed by Dr. Franz Bielschowsky at the New Zealand Otago Medical School from a colony of randomly bred mice which were brought to New Zealand from the Imperial Cancer Research Fund Laboratories in London by W.H. Hall in 1930 (2, 3). Bielschowsky started inbreeding and selection for different coat colors in 1948, and generated the NZB, NZO, NZC, and NZW lines. The NZO strain was derived from offspring of agouti-colored mice which were inbred by brother × sister mating, leading to homozygosity at the agouti locus. From F10 on, an obese phenotype was observed in the progeny, and was used for further selection between F12 and F17 (3, 4). This selection resulted in the present NZO strain which presents an early onsetting adiposity associated with metabolic consequences such as impaired glucose tolerance and reduced insulin sensitivity (4). In addition, the strain presents characteristics of the human metabolic syndrome such as dyslipidemia, hypertension, and beta-cell failure leading to overt type 2 diabetes (5).

From the New Zealand Otago Medical School, NZO mice (NZO/Bl) started their tour around the world. Breeding colonies from NZO/Bl were established at the Walter and Eliza Hall Institute in Melbourne, Australia (NZO/Wehi) (6) and at the German Diabetes Centre Düsseldorf (Lieselotte Herberg, NZO/Hl). Subsequently, the Düsseldorf NZO mice were distributed further. The Hl substrain was used by Edward Leiter to found the

HlLtJ colony at the Jackson Laboratory (Bar Harbor, Maine), derived from a single brother/sister pair by in vitro fertilization (7). It is available as the defined inbred strain NZO/HlLtJ (Jax Mice Database 002105). In 1988, the commercial breeder Bomholtgard (Ry, Denmark) obtained a breeding nucleus from Düsseldorf in F92 (Bomholtgard Breeder Information, 1994).

In 1996, NZO mice were transferred from Bomholtgard to the Institute of Laboratory Animals at the Technical University of Aachen, and were maintained as an inbred colony. In 2002, breeding pairs were transferred from Aachen to the German Institute of Human Nutrition (DIfE) in Potsdam-Rehbrücke; the resulting colony is registered at the Jackson Laboratory as the substrain NZO/HlBomDife.

In addition to the registered substrains, several colonies of NZO exist at other laboratories all over the world, and are maintained as inbred or randomly bred populations. These lines may harbor genetic differences fixed in the background genome, and these differences may be the reason for variable and contrasting metabolic subphenotypes among the single colonies (8). So far, no systematic genetic or phenotypic comparison of the existing substrains has been made.

2.2. Breeding

At the DIfE, the NZO/HlBomDife substrain is maintained as an inbred strain by consequent brother × sister mating of a small breeding nucleus. In addition, we keep an experimental colony mated by chance which is continuously restocked with mice from the inbreeding nucleus. As consistently described (2, 9, 10), fertility and reproduction of the NZO strain is generally rather poor. On the average, about one third of the mated females do not produce a single litter. This reduced fertility appears to be due to decreased ovulation and increased number of primordial and atretic follicles (10). Those becoming pregnant often do not raise their first litter, presumably due to a poor and/or blocked lactation with consequent starvation of the pups. However, the second and additional litters are usually normal. Having successfully raised one litter, most females subsequently produce 6–8 litters with a mean of 4–6 pups per litter. Fortnight weights of the offspring (as an indication of the maternal lactation) were found to be almost independent of litter number and offspring sex. They vary between 7.0 and 9.6 g (mean: 8.9 g) and exceed the weight of other strains already at this age. There is also no close relationship between litter size and individual pup weight. Body weights at weaning (3 weeks of age) reach 17–19 g showing no sex difference. The poor reproduction appears to be a consequence of the early development of obesity in females. In addition, the fertility of NZO males can also be reduced; they display large seminal vesicles and a clotted seminal fluid (4).

In order to maintain the strain by continuous brother × sister mating, the breeder animals have to be mated at an early age of about 6 weeks, when the degree of adiposity—especially in the females—is still moderate. In addition, adiposity of the breeder mice can be reduced by the composition of the diet: A fiber-enriched diet will slow down the development of adiposity but will also influence lactation and milk composition. Such a dietary intervention may affect the development of body weight, adiposity, and insulin resistance of the offspring, altering the target characteristics of the model. These potential alterations have to be considered when modifications of breeding or maintenance conditions are planned.

3. Physiological Characteristics of the NZO Mouse

3.1. Body Weight and Growth Characteristics

The most striking characteristic of NZO mice is its marked obesity (2). The body weight of the animals can vary in the first month of life, but most males exceed a body weight of 45 g at the age of approximately 3 months (4). At this age, males are heavier than females; the latter exhibit a higher body fat content. Adult females display a comparable body weight and fat content as males (11). At the age of 22 weeks, male mice fed with a high-fat diet have lower body weights than females because of their diabetes leading to growth arrest and ultimately weight loss (5). Females continue to gain weight and can reach weights of >100 g. In addition to its higher fat mass, NZO mice exhibit a larger body size (length) than most other inbred strains (12).

The diet of the animals has an important influence to the development of the obese phenotype. Based on a comparison of a low-fat chow diet with a semisynthetic diet containing 40% of calories as fat, NZO mice were considered markedly sensitive to the dietary fat content (13). However, a subsequent study comparing semisynthetic diets indicated that the development of obesity was identical under dietary fat contents of 40 and 15%. In contrast, chow diet with a high fiber content significantly inhibited the development of obesity and diabetes in NZO mice (14).

Several physiological and genetic approaches were performed to investigate the primary causes of the obese phenotype of NZO mice. In the first publications on the NZO strain, Bielschowsky and Bielschowsky found no correlation between body length and weight of the mice, suggesting that the obese phenotype does not depend on excessive growth, but on increased deposition of fat in the abdominal and retroperitoneal regions (2, 4). Gonadectomy of 4–6-weeks-old mice had no distinctive effect on body weight of the castrates. Interestingly, the treatment with the synthetic nonsteroidal estrogen diethylstilbestrol led to a distinct decrease in body weight in both males and females (4). In a comprehensive study, early characteristics of the NZO strain were compared to lean C57BL/6J (B6), NZB, and obese controls B6.V-$Lep^{ob/ob}$ (ob/ob) (15). As early as at 8 weeks of age, NZO mice exhibited hyperphagia compared to NZB and B6, but had a comparable food intake compared to the *ob/ob* strain. Analysis of the meal pattern revealed that NZO mice consumed larger portions, ate more frequently than NZB mice, and showed extended meal duration. It has been suggested that the hyperphagia of NZO reflects impaired leptin signaling. Like in other obese animals, leptin levels of NZO mice are elevated. The strain shows resistance to subcutaneously (16) but not to intracerebroventricularly administered leptin (17, 18), suggesting a defect in leptin transport from the periphery to the central nervous system, possibly due to a leptin receptor variant (16).

Similar to *ob/ob* mice, NZO mice exhibited a lower core body temperature than the lean NZB mice, but were in contrast to *ob/ob* mice resistant to cold stress (15). Interestingly, GLUT4 expression as compared with muscle and white adipose tissue is reduced in brown adipose tissue at an early stage of the obesity (19). These data suggest a potential mechanism for the lower body temperature of NZO. In addition, NZO mice exhibited lower voluntary running wheel activity but no differences in spontaneous locomotor activity compared to NZB. Total energy expenditure in NZO mice is reduced compared to NZB (15). Interestingly, in the post-absorptive state NZO mice has greater oxygen consumption and carbon dioxide production compared to the lean NZC strain (20).

Larkins checked the possible influence of the pituitary growth hormone (GH) on the metabolic disorders of NZO mice (21). GH was measured in different age groups of NZO animals both under basal conditions and after glucose administration compared to B6 mice. The results showed a greater variability in NZO mice under basal conditions but did not reveal significant differences. Both strains responded to a glucose load by a rapid decline of plasma GH. According to these results, the author considered it unlikely that GH plays a major role in the development of the metabolic syndrome of NZO mice (21).

3.2. Insulin Resistance

Because of their obesity, NZO mice develop severe insulin resistance: 8-months-old mice tolerate very high doses of insulin without any signs of convulsions (2, 11, 22). Insulin resistance in NZO is dependent on the extent of their obesity as has been shown by glucose clamp experiments: highest doses of insulin are required to maintain the desired glucose levels in mice that are rendered extremely obese by a high-fat, carbohydrate-free diet (23).

Compared to the lean NZC strain, 1-month-old NZO mice exhibit elevated hepatic glucose production and insulin insensitivity of brown adipose tissue, soleus, diaphragm, red quadriceps, and red gastrocnemius, whereas white quadriceps, white gastrocnemius, and heart were not affected (24). In perfused liver from NZO mice, gluconeogenesis and glucose output were markedly elevated and were resistant to insulin (22, 25). NZO mice exhibit lower levels of liver glycogen, and tracer glucose injected into NZO mice is not incorporated into liver as glycogen. Thus, the liver and also most muscles appear to be the primary sites of insulin resistance of NZO. In later studies, this conclusion was confirmed by glucose clamp experiments (23). In addition, insulin insensitivity of white adipose tissue was observed in some, but not all, experimental studies (22, 26, 27), but was proven by hyperinsulinemic clamp studies in 20-weeks-old mice (24).

In experiments designed to study the role of adiponectin as a humoral vasodilator, Fesus et al. determined the effects of the peptide hormone in connection with the anti-contractile effects of perivascular fat in mesenteric arteries of the NZO model. The results show no association between adiponectin levels and the anti-contractile effects of the perivascular fat. The adiponectin levels remain nearly constant in mouse groups of 20-, 25-, and 34-weeks of age. In addition, the mesenteric fat of NZO showed a normal response to recombinant mouse adiponectin (28).

3.3. Type 2 Diabetes

NZO mice develop type-2-like hyperglycemia, comparable with the human disease (8, 29–31). However, the degree and the severity of the syndrome differ between the published studies. Bielschowsky and Bielschowsky observed 176 NZO mice over a maximum period of 20 months. No animal developed a manifest type 2 diabetes characterized by blood glucose levels >300 mg/dL; males and females showed comparable values (4). Crofford and Davis measured significantly higher blood glucose levels in male NZO mice compared to females, but no severe hyperglycemia was observed (11). Bray and York summarized the hyperglycemic phenotype of the NZO mouse as "minimal" compared to *ob/ob* and *db/db* mice (32). However, the majority of studies on the NZO strain reported a manifest type 2 diabetes with plasma glucose levels >300 mg/dL in male mice on both standard chow and high-fat diet (5, 16, 23, 30, 33). An explanation for the discrepant metabolic phenotypes could be due to the used substrains of NZO mice (34). In addition, the energy and fat content of the used diets play an important role in the disease progression (14, 23, 35). In our colony, approximately 50% of males raised on a low-fat chow diet exhibit type 2 diabetes (plasma glucose levels >300 mg/dL = >16.6 mM) at the age of 23 weeks. A semisynthetic high-fat diet accelerates and enhances the development of diabetes: 80–100% of males become diabetic during a time span of 14–23 weeks of age under these conditions. Furthermore, for the high-fat diet a threshold body weight of 45 g at week 7 predicts diabetes at week 14, whereas for the chow diet a threshold body weight of 50 g at week 12 predicts diabetes at week 23. Thus, the development of diabetes in NZO is mainly determined by the increment of adipose tissue stores, and the variability of the latter may cause a reduction in the diabetes prevalence. It should be noted that the numbers given above can vary depending on the season and on other unknown factors.

It is generally accepted that the diabetic hyperglycemia in NZO reflects a failure of the pancreatic beta-cell to compensate insulin resistance (30, 31, 35). The mechanism of this beta-cell failure is insufficiently understood. In prediabetic mice, basal insulin levels are increased, but the response to an acute insulinotropic stimulus is impaired (36); this effect is comparable to that seen in human type 2 diabetics. In diabetic NZO mice, beta-cells undergo apoptosis, and beta-cell mass as well as pancreatic insulin content are markedly reduced (35). Thus, diabetes in NZO is similar to that observed in other obese mouse models with a genetic diabetes-sensitive background such as C57KS/J-*db/db*. It differs from the models on a diabetes-resistant background such as the C57BL/6-*ob/ob* and C57BL/6-*db/db*, where a marked proliferation of beta-cells compensates insulin resistance. This heterogeneity of the diabetes-sensitive or resistant background indicates that obesity and diabetes can be dissociated. Consequently, in all likelihood diabetes in NZO depends on the presence of diabetogenic alleles that are not adipogenic. The identification of these alleles will help to understand the mechanism of the obesity-induced beta-cell failure and apoptosis.

Interestingly, restriction of carbohydrates protects the animals from hyperglycemia, but re-exposure to carbohydrates causes rapid development of hyperglycemia and beta-cell apoptosis within a few days (23). Thus, glucose toxicity is a major factor in the development of diabetes in NZO. On the molecular level, early events of this pathogenesis are decreased levels of glucose transporter 2, decreased phosphorylation of the transcription factor FoxO1, and decreased Akt signaling in the islets of Langerhans (23, 35). Furthermore, β-cell expansion in diabetic NZO mice in response to a glucose stimulus is limited (37). A possible role of autoimmunity, e.g., by autoantibodies to the insulin receptor, and a contribution of B lymphocyte function were discussed (34, 38). However, lymphocytic infiltrations like those observed in type 1 diabetes were observed at the late stages of the diabetes only, and could be a consequence, not the cause of the beta-cell degeneration. Interestingly, transplantation of islets from lean mice improved the blood glucose levels of NZO mice (39, 40). This effect seems not to be dependent exclusively on β-cell function, because implantation of streptozotocin-treated islets also improved the diabetic metabolic state (41).

It should be noted that the onset of type 2 diabetes is limited to males in all available NZO substrains (1, 5). Gender dichotomy of diabetes has previously been shown to depend on a slow inactivation of estrogen by sulfation (42), emphasizing the critical role of estrogen as an anti-diabetic factor. Furthermore, preliminary data indicate that ovarectomy leads to type 2 diabetes in NZO females and suggest that estrogen exerts a beta-cell protecting effect (Taugner, Liehl and Kluge, unpublished data).

3.4. Other Characteristics of the NZO Mouse

In addition to obesity and insulin resistance, NZO mice develop other features of the human metabolic syndrome such as hypertension (elevated systolic and diastolic blood pressure, higher heart rates) and elevated triglyceride and cholesterol levels (5, 29). Hypertension does not appear to be an obligatory consequence of obesity in mice, since the obese TALLYHO mouse presents a normal blood pressure (see Chap. 2, Subheading 3). Also, data from an outcross of NZO with C3H indicate that obesity and hypertension are associated with distinct susceptibility loci (43). An atypical form of diabetic nephropathy occurs after crossing of NZO with NON mice, assuming the NON genome to be responsible for the susceptibility to nephropathy (44, 45). Additional remarkable characteristics of the NZO strain are a small airway caliber with greater parapharyngeal fat pad volumes, a greater volume of other upper airway soft tissue structures (46), and the susceptibility to develop malignant lymphomas, duodenal, and lung tumors (47).

4. The NZO Mouse as a Model for the Identification of Obesity and Diabetes Genes

The NZO strain has successfully been used for identification of adipogenic or diabetogenic gene variants (Table 1). Three different strategies were employed: First, susceptibility loci (QTL, quantitative trait loci) were identified by conventional crossbreeding of NZO with a lean strain and linkage analysis in an F2 or backcross

Table 1
Adipogenic and/or diabetogenic gene variants identified in NZO or NZO-derived outcross populations

Gene symbol	Gene name/function	Variant	Trait associated with variant	Variant strain	References
Tbc1d1	Rab-GTPase activating protein	Deletion/frameshift	Accumulation of body fat	SJL	(61)
Zfp69	Zinc finger domain transcription factor	Gene trap by retrotransposon	Plasma glucose and insulin	B6, NZO	(65)
Pctp	Phosphatidylcholine transfer protein	1 Amino acid substitution	Serum insulin	NZO	(52)
Abcg1	ATP-binding cassette transporter G1	201 bp insertion in intron 2	Accumulation of body fat	NZO	(54)
Nmur2	Neuromedin U receptor 2	2 Amino acid substitutions	Feeding behavior	NZO	(53)
Lepr	Leptin receptor	3 Amino acid substitutions	Feeding behavior	NZO	(16)

progeny (see also Subheading 5). Subsequently, by generation of congenic lines carrying different chromosomal segments, the QTL were narrowed down to a critical region comprising 10–50 genes. Detailed hypothesis-free analysis of these critical regions by expression profiling and sequencing led to the identification of *Tbc1d1* and *Zfp69* (a more detailed description of these genes is given below), and will allow identification of the gene(s) underlying the effects of the QTL *Nob3*. This strategy was successful with outcross populations of NZO with NON, Swiss Jim Lambert (SJL), and C57BL/6J. It was also successfully employed by other groups that identified diabetogenic variants of *Sorcs1* and *Lisch-like* in crosses of obese (*ob/ob*, *db/db*) mice with a lean, diabetes-sensitive background strain (48, 49). However, it is applicable only to major QTL, since the effects of minor QTL seem to require the NZO background and are usually lost after transfer to a lean strain. Other crosses of NZO with the strains small (SM) and C3H detected new QTL, but so far not the responsible gene variants (43, 50). Furthermore, in addition to the QTL associated with obesity and hyperglycemia, other metabolic phenotypes were investigated such as elevated plasma cholesterol levels associated with a NZO-derived QTL on distal Chr 5 (51).

A second strategy for identification of diabetogenic or adipogenic genes is the analysis of selected candidates within a whole QTL. This strategy led to the identification of variants of *Pctp* (52) and *NmuR2* (53). In addition, candidates located in minor mouse QTL such as *Abcg1* and *Hdh* were obtained from mutagenesis screens in other species (*Drosophila*, *Caenorhabditis*), and their involvement in adipogenesis was shown by generation of knockout mice (54, 55). Thirdly, a candidate gene approach without any prior genetic evidence led to identification of a leptin receptor variant in NZO (16).

An important, general conclusion from the crossbreeding experiments is that not only NZO but also the lean, non-diabetic breeding partners can contribute diabetogenic or adipogenic alleles to the phenotype of the progeny. This was expected when NZO was crossed with the leaner NON strain (30), since NON mice develop a late onsetting, moderate glucose intolerance. Two major QTL for decompensated hyperglycemia (>300 mg/dL) in the F2 progeny, *Nidd1* on chromosome Chr 4, and *Nidd2* on Chr 18, were contributed by the NON genome, and only *Nidd3* on Chr 11 was found to be NZO-derived (30). Subsequently, the contribution of a diabetogenic allele (*Nidd/SJL*) by the lean breeding partner was unexpectedly observed in a backcross of NZO with the high-fat diet resistant SJL strain (31).

The outcross of NZO with NON was also used to combine the different diabetogenic alleles on the NON background. By this strategy, recombinant-congenic mouse lines were generated that exhibit various phenotypes with different degree of obesity as well as different onset and severity of hyperglycemia (56). These lines exhibit differential sensitivity to the effects of thiazolidinediones and represent useful tools for pharmacogenetic analysis (44, 57–59).

4.1. Tbc1d1

Tbc1d1 was identified as the causal gene of the obesity QTL *Nob1*, which was found in an outcross of NZO mice with the lean and high-fat diet resistant SJL strain (60). A combination of expression profiling and sequencing of genes in a critical region defined by congenic lines led to a 7 bp deletion causing a frame shift and truncation of a functional domain of the protein (61). The mutation leads to a suppression of obesity and diabetes in the intercross progeny under high-fat diet conditions (61). *Tbc1d1* is member of the TBC1 domain family, and encodes a Rab-GTPase activating protein (RabGAP). Its overexpression in skeletal muscle cells causes a reduction in fatty acid oxidation and an increase in glucose oxidation, knockdown produces the opposite effect (61). Mice carrying the loss-of-function mutant exhibit a reduced RQ, enhanced palmitate, and reduced glucose oxidation in skeletal muscle *ex-vivo*. Thus, *Tbc1d1* appears to be an important regulator of substrate utilization in muscle, and could be a novel target for an anti-adipogenic and anti-diabetogenic intervention. Since a rare mutant was associated with morbid obesity in two unrelated families (62, 63), the gene is likely to play a role in the development of the human disease.

4.2. Zfp69

Zfp69 was identified as the presumably causal gene in the susceptibility locus *Nidd/SJL* on Chr 4 found in an intercross of NZO with the lean SJL strain. Interestingly, this QTL was contributed by the lean SJL strain (31), and maps to the same region as the QTL *Niddm1* identified in the NZO × NON cross (30), and *Tanidd4* identified in a TALLYHO × B6 cross (64). The phenotype associated with *Nidd/SJL* is severe hyperglycemia, hypoinsulinemia, and beta-cell degeneration. This effect was dependent on a body weight threshold of 45 g at week 12; the QTL itself produced no alteration of the weight development (13, 31). By introgression of various segments of SJL chromosome 4 into the C57BL/6J strain and subsequent "reporter" cross of the resulting congenic lines with NZO, a critical region harboring ten genes was identified. Expression profiling and sequencing identified a retrotransposon in the third intron of *Zfp69* from NZO and B6 which caused premature polyadenylation of the mRNA, thereby disrupting the synthesis of a functional protein (65).

Zfp69 encodes a zinc-finger domain transcription factor that harbors an additional, inhibitory KRAB domain. A possible mechanism of the diabetogenic effect of *Zfp69* could be reduced storage of triglycerides in white adipose tissue leading to hepatosteatosis and hyperglycemia, as was suggested by a characterization of *ob/ob* mice carrying the QTL on the B6 background (65, 66). Previous data indicating a strong interaction with the adipogenic allele of the QTL *Nob1* (*Tbc1d1*, see above) (13) are consistent with this conclusion and emphasize the crucial role of fat storage and oxidation in the pathogenesis of diabetes. Furthermore, the human orthologue of *Zfp69* appears to be involved in the pathogenesis of human diabetes, since its expression in adipose tissue from human patients with type 2 diabetes was significantly increased (65).

4.3. Pctp

The gene-encoding phosphatidylcholine transfer protein (*Pctp*) is located in the QTL *Nidd3* identified in the NZO × NON intercross. Since NZO mice exhibit alterations in phosphatidyl choline metabolism, the gene was sequenced, and a non-synonymous point mutation resulting in the R120H substitution was identified. Functional studies indicated that the R120H variant is inactive. Thus, it was concluded that the loss-of-function mutation causes the deficiencies in phosphatidyl choline metabolism in the NZO strain and contributes to the development of diabetes (52).

4.4. Abcg1

The ATP-binding cassette transporter gene *Abcg1* maps to a minor, suggestive adiposity QTL on Chr 17 contributed by the NZO genome. Since its Drosophila ortholog had previously been identified as an adipogenic gene in a random mutagenesis screen, the gene was sequenced, its expression in NZO was determined, and a knockout mouse was generated. As was expected, disruption of *Abcg1* caused resistance to an adipogenic diet. Furthermore, NZO mice exhibited an increased expression of *Abcg1* in white adipose tissue which could be caused by a 210 base pair insertion in intron 2 of the gene. Thus, it was concluded that the NZO variant of *Abcg1* contributes to the obese phenotype of the strain (54).

4.5. Nmur2

The neuromedin U receptor 2 gene (*Nmur2*) maps to a minor QTL for obesity on chromosome 11, and is a candidate obesity gene because of the anorexigenic effect of neuromedin U. Sequencing of the *Nmur2* cDNA identified two non-synonymous nucleotide exchanges causing amino acid exchanges in an extracellular loop of the receptor (I202M and V190M). The anorexigenic effect of an intracerebroventricular injection of neuromedin U was markedly reduced in NZO compared with B6 mice. In addition, the potency of neuromedin U was threefold lower in HEK293 cells expressing the variant receptor than in cells transfected with cDNA of wild-type receptor (53).

4.6. Nob3

In an outcross F2 population of NZO with the diabetes-resistant B6 strain, a major QTL on Chr 1 (*Nob3*) responsible for obesity and hyperglycemia was identified (67). By introgression of the chromosomal segment into B6, several congenic lines were generated that presented the phenotype, and a critical region harboring approximately 30 genes was defined. Efforts to identify the causal gene(s) are ongoing. The QTL is particularly important, since it interacted with the diabetogenic *Zfp69* allele; the two loci accounted for almost all of the diabetes in the cross experiments NZO×B6.Cg-*Nidd/SJL* designed to identify the diabetogenic gene in *Nidd/SJL* (68).

5. Epigenetic Modification of Obesity and Diabetes in NZO

A strong factor modifying obesity and diabetes in NZO-derived outcross populations is the body weight of the mothers. In a backcross population NON×NZO, adipogenic and diabetogenic QTL were identified on Chr 1, 5, 12, and 15. The effects of these QTL were modified by the maternal postparturitional environment. By cross-fostering experiments, the authors could demonstrate that this presumably epigenetic effect is at least in part due to obesity-inducing factors in the milk of obese F1 dams (69). So far, neither these factors nor the epigenetic mechanisms have been identified.

6. Concluding Remarks

The NZO mouse represents an excellent model for the study of the pathophysiology and genetics of an obesity-associated diabetes mellitus that is caused by beta-cell failure and degeneration, and thereby resembles the human type 2 diabetes. It is therefore ideally suited for the identification of the underlying genes as well as for elucidation of the pathogenetic mechanisms. Previous research has shown that these genes and the involved pathways may not only be relevant for the mouse but also for the human disease. In the case of the adipogenic and diabetogenic genes *Tbc1d1* and *Zfp69* it was shown that the human orthologues may be involved in the progression of human obesity and type 2 diabetes (62, 63, 65, 66). Thus, NZO mice will remain an important tool in future experimental diabetes research.

References

1. Leiter EH (2009) Selecting the "right" mouse model for metabolic syndrome and type 2 diabetes research. Methods Mol Biol 560:1–17
2. Bielschowsky M, Bielschowsky F (1953) A new strain of mice with hereditary obesity. Proc Univ Otago Med School 31:29–31
3. Bielschowsky M, Goodall CM (1970) Origin of inbred NZ mouse strains. Cancer Res 30:834–836
4. Bielschowsky F, Bielschowsky M (1956) The New Zealand strain of obese mice; their response to stilboestrol and to insulin. Aust J Exp Biol Med Sci 34:181–198
5. Ortlepp JR et al (2000) A metabolic syndrome of hypertension, hyperinsulinaemia and hypercholesterolaemia in the New Zealand obese mouse. Eur J Clin Invest 30:195–202

6. Festing M (1997) Inbred strains of mice. Mouse Genome 95:519–686
7. Koza RA et al (2004) Contributions of dysregulated energy metabolism to type 2 diabetes development in NZO/H1Lt mice with polygenic obesity. Metabolism 53:799–808
8. Herberg L, Coleman DL (1977) Laboratory animals exhibiting obesity and diabetes syndromes. Metabolism 26:59–99
9. Chankiewitz E (2005) Beiträge zur Charakterisierung eines diabetischen Tiermodells: die New Zealand obese-Maus (NZO). In: Medizinische Fakultät. Martin-Luther-Universität, Halle-Wittenberg, p 79
10. Radavelli-Bagatini S et al (2011) The New Zealand obese mouse model of obesity insulin resistance and poor breeding performance: evaluation of ovarian structure and function. J Endocrinol 209(3):307–315
11. Crofford OB, Davis CK Jr (1965) Growth characteristics, glucose tolerance and insulin sensitivity of New Zealand obese mice. Metabolism 14:271–280
12. Ackert-Bicknell C et al (2011) Aging study: bone mineral density and body composition of 32 inbred strains of mice. Mouse Phenome Database web site, The Jackson Laboratory, Bar Harbor, ME. http://phenome.jax.org
13. Plum L et al (2002) Characterisation of the mouse diabetes susceptibility locus Nidd/SJL: islet cell destruction, interaction with the obesity QTL Nob1, and effect of dietary fat. Diabetologia 45:823–830
14. Mirhashemi F et al (2011) Diet dependence of diabetes in the New Zealand obese (NZO) mouse: total fat, but not fat quality or sucrose accelerates and aggravates diabetes. Exp Clin Endocrinol Diabetes 119:167–171
15. Jürgens HS et al (2006) Hyperphagia, lower body temperature, and reduced running wheel activity precede development of morbid obesity in New Zealand obese mice. Physiol Genomics 25:234–241
16. Igel M et al (1997) Hyperleptinemia, leptin resistance, and polymorphic leptin receptor in the New Zealand obese mouse. Endocrinology 138:4234–4239
17. Friedman JM, Halaas JL (1998) Leptin and the regulation of body weight in mammals. Nature 395:763–770
18. Halaas JL et al (1997) Physiological response to long-term peripheral and central leptin infusion in lean and obese mice. Proc Natl Acad Sci U S A 94:8878–8883
19. Ferreras L et al (1994) Early decrease in GLUT4 protein levels in brown adipose tissue of New Zealand obese mice. Int J Obes Relat Metab Disord 18:760–765
20. Subrahmanyam K (1960) Metabolism in the New Zealand strain of obese mice. Biochem J 76:548–556
21. Larkins RG (1971) Plasma growth hormone in the New Zealand obese mouse. Diabetologia 7:302–307
22. Huchzermeyer H, Rudorff KH, Staib W (1973) (Experimental studies on the problem of insulin resistance in adipositas and diabetes mellitus, with the aid of New Zealand obese mice. Pathogenesis of the obese-hyperglycaemic syndrome (author's transl)). Z Klin Chem Klin Biochem 11:249–256
23. Jürgens HS et al (2007) Development of diabetes in obese, insulin-resistant mice: essential role of dietary carbohydrate in beta cell destruction. Diabetologia 50:1481–1489
24. Veroni MC, Proietto J, Larkins RG (1991) Evolution of insulin resistance in New Zealand obese mice. Diabetes 40:1480–1487
25. Rudorff KH et al (1970) The influence of insulin on the alanine gluconeogenesis in isolated perfused livers of New Zealand obese mice. Eur J Biochem 16:481–486
26. Sneyd JG (1964) Pancreatic and serum insulin in the New Zealand strain of obese mice. J Endocrinol 28:163–172
27. Stauffacher W, Renold AE (1969) Effect of insulin in vivo on diaphragm and adipose tissue of obese mice. Am J Physiol 216:98–105
28. Fesus G et al (2007) Adiponectin is a novel humoral vasodilator. Cardiovasc Res 75:719–727
29. Joost HG (2010) The genetic basis of obesity and type 2 diabetes: lessons from the New Zealand obese mouse, a polygenic model of the metabolic syndrome. Results Probl Cell Differ 52:1–11
30. Leiter EH et al (1998) NIDDM genes in mice: deleterious synergism by both parental genomes contributes to diabetogenic thresholds. Diabetes 47:1287–1295
31. Plum L et al (2000) Type 2 diabetes-like hyperglycemia in a backcross model of NZO and SJL mice: characterization of a susceptibility locus on chromosome 4 and its relation with obesity. Diabetes 49:1590–1596
32. Bray GA, York DA (1971) Genetically transmitted obesity in rodents. Physiol Rev 51:598–646
33. Stauffacher W et al (1967) Measurements of insulin activities in pancreas and serum of mice with spontaneous ("Obese" and "New Zealand Obese") and induced (Goldthioglucose) obe-

sity and hyperglycemia, with considerations on the pathogenesis of the spontaneous syndrome. Diabetologia 3:230–237
34. Haskell BD et al (2002) The diabetes-prone NZO/HlLt strain. I. Immunophenotypic comparison to the related NZB/BlNJ and NZW/LacJ strains. Lab Invest 82:833–842
35. Kluth O et al (2011) Dissociation of lipotoxicity and glucotoxicity in a mouse model of obesity associated diabetes: role of forkhead box O1 (FOXO1) in glucose-induced beta cell failure. Diabetologia 54:605–616
36. Cameron DP, Opat F, Insch S (1974) Studies of immunoreactive insulin secretion in NZO mice in vivo. Diabetologia 10(suppl):649–654
37. Lange C et al (2006) The diabetes-prone NZO/Hl strain. Proliferation capacity of beta cells in hyperinsulinemia and hyperglycemia. Arch Physiol Biochem 112:49–58
38. Junger E et al (2002) The diabetes-prone NZO/Hl strain. II. Pancreatic immunopathology. Lab Invest 82:843–853
39. Gates RJ et al (1972) Return to normal of blood-glucose, plasma-insulin, and weight gain in New Zealand obese mice after implantation of islets of Langerhans. Lancet 2:567–570
40. Gates RJ et al (1972) Studies on implanted islets of Langerhans: normalization of blood glucose concentration, blood insulin concentration and weight gain in New Zealand obese mice. Biochem J 130:26P–27P
41. Gates RJ, Hunt MI, Lazarus NR (1974) Further studies on the amelioration of the characteristics of New Zealand obese (NZO) mice following implantation of islets of Langerhans. Diabetologia 10:401–406
42. Leiter EH, Chapman HD, Falany CN (1991) Synergism of obesity genes with hepatic steroid sulfotransferases to mediate diabetes in mice. Diabetes 40:1360–1363
43. Tsukahara C et al (2004) Blood pressure in 15 inbred mouse strains and its lack of relation with obesity and insulin resistance in the progeny of an NZO/HILtJ x C3H/HeJ intercross. Mamm Genome 15:943–950
44. Leiter EH, Reifsnyder PC (2004) Differential levels of diabetogenic stress in two new mouse models of obesity and type 2 diabetes. Diabetes 53(suppl 1):S4–S11
45. Brosius FC III et al (2009) Mouse models of diabetic nephropathy. J Am Soc Nephrol 20:2503–2512
46. Brennick MJ et al (2009) Altered upper airway and soft tissue structures in the New Zealand obese mouse. Am J Respir Crit Care Med 179:158–169
47. Goodall CM et al (1973) Oncological and survival reference data for NZO-B1 inbred mice. Lab Anim 7:65–71
48. Clee SM et al (2006) Positional cloning of Sorcs1, a type 2 diabetes quantitative trait locus. Nat Genet 38:688–693
49. Dokmanovic-Chouinard M et al (2008) Positional cloning of "Lisch-Like", a candidate modifier of susceptibility to type 2 diabetes in mice. PLoS Genet 4:e1000137
50. Taylor BA et al (2001) Multiple obesity QTLs identified in an intercross between the NZO (New Zealand obese) and the SM (small) mouse strains. Mamm Genome 12:95–103
51. Giesen K et al (2003) Diet-dependent obesity and hypercholesterolemia in the New Zealand obese mouse: identification of a quantitative trait locus for elevated serum cholesterol on the distal mouse chromosome 5. Biochem Biophys Res Commun 304:812–817
52. Pan HJ et al (2006) A polymorphism in New Zealand inbred mouse strains that inactivates phosphatidylcholine transfer protein. FEBS Lett 580:5953–5958
53. Schmolz K et al (2007) Role of neuromedin-U in the central control of feeding behavior: a variant of the neuromedin-U receptor 2 contributes to hyperphagia in the New Zealand obese mouse. Obes Metab Milan 3:28–37
54. Buchmann J et al (2007) Ablation of the cholesterol transporter adenosine triphosphate-binding cassette transporter G1 reduces adipose cell size and protects against diet-induced obesity. Endocrinology 148:1561–1573
55. Schulz N et al (2011) Role of medium- and short-chain L-3-hydroxyacyl-CoA dehydrogenase in the regulation of body weight and thermogenesis. Endocrinology 152:4641–4651
56. Reifsnyder PC, Leiter EH (2002) Deconstructing and reconstructing obesity-induced diabetes (diabesity) in mice. Diabetes 51:825–832
57. Pan HJ et al (2005) Pharmacogenetic analysis of rosiglitazone-induced hepatosteatosis in new mouse models of type 2 diabetes. Diabetes 54:1854–1862
58. Leiter EH et al (2006) Differential endocrine responses to rosiglitazone therapy in new mouse models of type 2 diabetes. Endocrinology 147:919–926
59. Pan HJ et al (2006) Adverse hepatic and cardiac responses to rosiglitazone in a new mouse model of type 2 diabetes: relation to dysregulated phosphatidylcholine metabolism. Vascul Pharmacol 45:65–71
60. Kluge R et al (2000) Quantitative trait loci for obesity and insulin resistance (Nob1,

Nob2) and their interaction with the leptin receptor allele (LeprA720T/T1044I) in New Zealand obese mice. Diabetologia 43: 1565–1572
61. Chadt A et al (2008) Tbc1d1 mutation in lean mouse strain confers leanness and protects from diet-induced obesity. Nat Genet 40: 1354–1359
62. Meyre D et al (2008) R125W coding variant in TBC1D1 confers risk for familial obesity and contributes to linkage on chromosome 4p14 in the French population. Hum Mol Genet 17: 1798–1802
63. Stone S et al (2006) TBC1D1 is a candidate for a severe obesity gene and evidence for a gene/gene interaction in obesity predisposition. Hum Mol Genet 15:2709–2720
64. Stewart TP, Kim HY, Saxton AM et al (2010) Genetic and genomic analysis of hyperlipidemia, obesity and diabetes using (C57BL/6J×TALLYHO/JngJ) F2 mice. BMC Genomics 11:713
65. Scherneck S et al (2009) Positional cloning of zinc finger domain transcription factor Zfp69, a candidate gene for obesity-associated diabetes contributed by mouse locus Nidd/SJL. PLoS Genet 5:e1000541
66. Scherneck S et al (2010) Role of zinc finger transcription factor zfp69 in body fat storage and diabetes susceptibility of mice. Results Probl Cell Differ 52:57–68
67. Vogel H et al (2009) Characterization of Nob3, a major quantitative trait locus for obesity and hyperglycemia on mouse chromosome 1. Physiol Genomics 38:226–232
68. Scherneck S (2007) Identifizierung eines diabetogenen Allels im Suszeptibilitätslocus Nidd/SJL der Maus. Department of Pharmacology (German Institute of Human Nutrition), Universität Potsdam, Potsdam, p 85
69. Reifsnyder PC, Churchill G, Leiter EH (2000) Maternal environment and genotype interact to establish diabesity in mice. Genome Res 10: 1568–1578

Chapter 6

The TALLYHO Mouse as a Model of Human Type 2 Diabetes

Jung Han Kim and Arnold M. Saxton

Abstract

The TALLYHO/Jng (TH) mouse is an inbred polygenic model for type 2 diabetes (T2D) with moderate obesity. Both male and female TH mice are characterized by increased body and fat pad weights, hyperleptinemia, hyperinsulinemia, and hyperlipidemia. Glucose intolerance and hyperglycemia are exhibited only in males. Reduced 2-deoxy-glucose uptake occurs in adipose tissue and skeletal muscle of male TH mice. While both sexes of TH mice exhibit enlarged pancreatic islets, only males have degranulation and abnormal architecture in islets. Endothelial dysfunction and considerably decreased bone density are also observed in male TH mice. The blood pressure of male TH mice is normal. Genetic outcross experiments with non-diabetic strains revealed multiple susceptibility loci (quantitative trait loci) for obesity, hypertriglyceridemia, hypercholesterolemia, and hyperglycemia. In conclusion, TH mice encompass many aspects of polygenic human diabetes and are a very useful model for T2D.

Key words: TALLYHO, Mice, Insulin resistance, Glucose intolerance, Obesity, Hyperlipidemia, Hyperglycemia, Islet degranulation, QTL, Congenics

1. Introduction

Type 2 diabetes (T2D) is the most common form of human diabetes, accounting for over 90% of diagnosed patients, and often coexists with obesity (1, 2). The etiology of T2D involves multiple factors, including multiple susceptibility genes and environmental factors (e.g., obesity, age, diet, life style, etc.) (3, 4). The pathophysiological mechanism of T2D is characterized by a combination of peripheral insulin resistance and β-cell dysfunction (5). Often, T2D is associated with secondary complications, such as cardiovascular disease, vision loss, kidney disease, and degeneration of peripheral nerves (6).

The TALLYHO/Jng (TH) mice spontaneously develop T2D as in humans. The development of T2D in TH mice follows a complex mode of inheritance, which accurately reflects the common T2D in humans. TH mice manifest many phenotypic traits that are consistent with those in T2D patients. To demonstrate that TH mice are an appropriate model for human T2D, this chapter discusses the current information on metabolic and genetic characteristics of TH mice.

1.1. TALLYHO Mice

The TALLYHO/Jng (TH) mouse strain was developed by Dr. Jürgen Naggert's research group at The Jackson Laboratory (TJL) (Bar Harbor, ME) (7). This strain originally derived from two deviant male mice that spontaneously became polyuric, glucosuric, hyperinsulinemic, and hyperglycemic at 5–7 months of age, identified in a colony of outbred Theiler Original mice (Harrow, UK) in 1992. Some diabetic mice produced from the deviants were imported into TJL in 1994 and subjected to brother–sister mating in combination with backcrossing with phenotypic selection for male hyperglycemia (non-fasting plasma glucose levels >300 mg/dL). The resultant diabetes prone inbred strain was named TALLYHO.

Until September of 2001, TH mice were bred only in Dr. Naggert's laboratory. A sub-colony was then initiated in our laboratory with breeding pairs from Dr. Naggert's research colony. Since 2004, TH mice are also available commercially from TJL (http://jaxmice.jax.org). Other sub-colonies exist in Calgary, Canada (8) and Daejon, Korea (9, 10). Hyperglycemia in male TH mice is consistent across the locations although the onset of hyperglycemia varies. There are some discrepancies in metabolic phenotypes across the locations, and presently it is unknown whether the observed differences are environmental or reflect genetic change. Fertility is very well maintained in the TH mouse strain with a large litter size of around 8–12.

Due to polygenic inheritance of T2D in TH mice, there is no precise genetic control strain for TH mice, which is the case for all polygenic models (11). TH mice appear to be a Swiss-derived strain and therefore strains including SWR, SJL, and FVB are more genetically related to TH mice than others (11). Nonetheless, the C57BL/6 (B6) mice, one of the most widely used strains in obesity and diabetes research, have been used as a comparison strain for TH mice in publications to date.

2. Metabolic Characteristics of TALLYHO Mice

2.1. Obesity

Obesity in TH mice is characterized by increased body weight as well as fat pad weight including subcutaneous and visceral fat. The obesity in TH mice is moderate compared to some other polygenic T2D models, showing mean 4-week body weight of 16 g (female) and 19 g (male) (12) (vs. 26 g of male NZO/H1Lt mice (13)). At 12 weeks of age, the mean body weight becomes 32 g (female) and

35 g (male) (vs. 21 g (female) and 27 g (male) for B6 mice) (12). The higher body weight in TH mice persists throughout life. However, weight loss is occasionally observed in males with long-term severe hyperglycemia (10) (unpublished observations).

Mean adiposity index (sum of five fat pad weights (inguinal, epididymal, mesenteric, retroperitoneal, and subscapular)/body weight without the fat pads) was about 2.3 fold (males) and 7.8 fold (females) higher in TH mice than age- and sex-matched B6 mice (26 weeks of age) (7).

Rhee et al. reported that food intake, determined as food consumed/day/body weight, was significantly higher in male TH mice than male B6 mice (but not in females), without differences in food efficiency (body weight gain/food consumed) (10). There appears to be differences in food intake across the TH sub-colonies. In our colony maintained since 2001, food intake (food consumed/day/body weight) was comparable among TH (0.19 ± 0.01 g/day/g, $n=4$), SWR (0.21 ± 0.01 g/day/g, $n=7$), and B6 (0.20 ± 0.01 g/day/g, $n=4$) strains under normal rodent chow feeding (mean ± SE; males; 7 weeks of age) (unpublished data).

2.2. Glucose Intolerance and Hyperglycemia

T2D is a progressive disease, preceded by a period of insulin resistance and impaired glucose tolerance (14). At 4 weeks of age, both male and female TH mice were tolerant to glucose loading, but after puberty male TH mice, not females, developed impaired tolerance to glucose loading (12). This impaired glucose tolerance was accompanied by hyper-secretion of insulin during the intraperitoneal glucose tolerance test (IPGTT) (1 mg glucose/g body weight) (12). With age the glucose intolerance increased, and insulin secretion during the IPGTT became less profound in male TH mice (12). However, Sung et al. reported mild glucose intolerance and reduced insulin secretion during oral GTT (2 mg glucose/g body weight) in male TH mice at 4 weeks of age (9). Currently, it is unknown what causes this discrepancy across the studies.

The glucose intolerance progresses to hyperglycemia in male TH mice (12). In post-puberty, plasma glucose levels in male TH mice continuously increased with age and reached full-blown diabetes levels (300–400 mg/dL, non-fasting) around 14 weeks of age (Fig. 1). However, the extent and onset of hyperglycemia varies from litter to litter; a plausible speculation is that the susceptibility to T2D in TH mice might be influenced by experiences in early life or environmental factors.

2.3. Hyperinsulinemia and Insulin Resistance

Hyperinsulinemia in TH mice was detectable as early as 4 weeks of age and persistently increased with age in both males and females (12). The mean plasma insulin levels (non-fasting) were 6 ± 1 ng/mL for female and 8 ± 1 ng/mL for male TH mice (vs. 0.4 ± 0.1 ng/mL for female and 0.6 ± 0.2 ng/mL for male B6 mice) (6 weeks of age) (12). While the degree of hyperinsulinemia remained stable in female

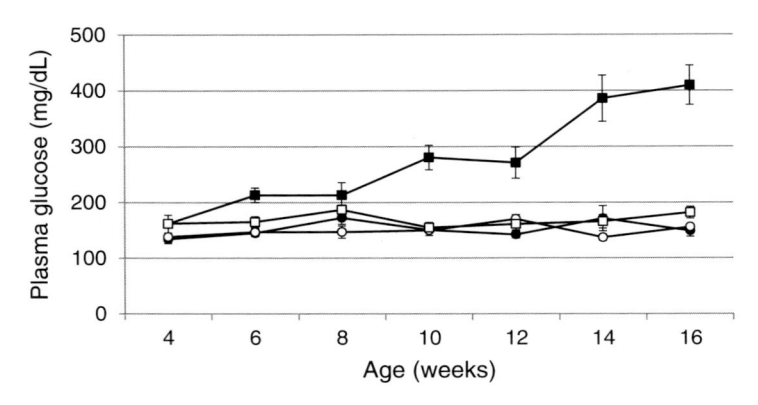

Fig. 1. Changes in plasma glucose levels in TALLYHO/Jng (*filled symbols*) and C57BL/6 (*open symbols*) mice from 4 to 16 weeks of age (non-fasting). *Squares* and *circles* represent male and female, respectively. The original data were presented as a part of Fig. 2 in (12). Data are means ± SE.

TH mice, it further increased in males reaching mean maximal levels of 12±0.7 ng/mL (non-fasting) around 12 weeks of age and remained high throughout the period of study (16 weeks of age) (12). The Langerhans islets were hypertrophied in both sexes of TH mice compared to B6 mice at 4 weeks through adult ages, suggesting the presence of sustained potent stimuli for insulin secretion (12). However, degranulation of β-cell and abnormal architecture in islets were evident only in male TH mice (7, 12). Plasma insulin levels varied across colony locations, and hyperinsulinemia was absent in the Calgary-based TH colony at 16 weeks of age (8). Study of β-cells in this sub-colony might explain this discrepancy.

Glucose uptake stimulated by insulin was impaired in soleus muscle and adipocytes isolated from male TH mice compared to B6 mice (12, 15). This impaired glucose uptake was associated with altered translocation and redistribution of the glucose transporter-4 (GLUT-4) from internal membrane to the plasma membrane (15). Reduced GLUT-4 translocation in TH mice appears to be preceded by alterations in insulin-signaling cascade, involving reduced tyrosine phosphorylation of the insulin receptor substrate 1 (IRS1) protein and reduced activation of the phosphatidylinositol (PI) 3-kinase (15). Hyper-serine phosphorylation of IRS1 on Ser307 was shown in adipose tissue of TH mice, which possibly occurs in response to elevated intracellular serine kinase JNK (15). Serine phosphorylation of the IRS1 protein may prime proteasomal degradation of IRS1 in TH mice, which then impairs downstream effectors of insulin (15).

In addition to adipose tissue and skeletal muscle, liver is one of the major sites of insulin action. Hepatic insulin resistance confers increased glucose production after fasting and reduced suppression of postprandial glucose production (16). Male TH mice, not females, exhibit overnight fasting hyperglycemia (7). However, thus far, hepatic insulin resistance has not been well characterized in TH mice.

2.4. Hyperleptinemia and Leptin Resistance

Leptin is produced by adipocytes and is known to decrease food intake and increase energy expenditure (17). Leptin is also known to have an anti-adipogenic effect (18).

Circulating leptin levels are proportion to fat mass as adaptive responses to energy stores. At 4 weeks of age, both male and female TH mice exhibited about threefold higher plasma leptin levels than age- and sex-matched B6 mice (12). Won et al. also observed hyperleptinemia in male TH mice at 8 weeks of age (19). On the other hand, Cheng et al. reported the absence of hyperleptinemia and obesity in male TH mice at 16 weeks of age (8). It is speculated that variation in fat mass associated with severity of diabetes and environmental factors may cause the differences in hyperleptinemia. It may also reflect genetic drift from further selective inbreeding of the local TH colony by Cheng et al. (8).

Rhee et al. reported blunted food intake response to intravenous leptin injection in TH mice at 4 weeks of age (10). This blunted response was accompanied by reduced mRNA levels in hypothalamic neuropeptides, including NPY, AgRP, and POMC, without changes in leptin signaling protein levels (10). Unlike the leptin resistance shown in the hypothalamus of TH mice in vivo, Kim et al. reported that leptin treatment effectively inhibited adipogenesis of preadipocytes isolated from TH mice (20).

2.5. Dyslipidemia

Many T2D patients display dyslipidemia characterized by increased triglycerides, increased small dense LDL cholesterol, and decreased HDL cholesterol (21). This atherogenic lipid profile contributes to cardiovascular disease in T2D patients, a prominent cause of death associated with T2D (22). Notably, hypertriglyceridemia occurs years before diabetes in T2D patients and is known to be a strong predictor of diabetes (23).

Similar to the pattern of hyperinsulinemia, hypertriglyceridemia in TH mice was detectable at 4 weeks of age (12). While the degree of hypertriglyceridemia remains stable in females (282 ± 23 mg/dL vs. 109 ± 9 mg/dL in B6 females, non-fasting, 6 weeks of age), it further increases in male TH mice with age, reaching mean levels of 632 ± 36 mg/dL (vs. 148 ± 24 mg/dL in male B6 mice, 10 weeks of age). Both male and female TH mice exhibited approximately twofold higher levels of plasma cholesterol and free fatty acids (26 weeks of age) (7). Hyperlipidemia in male TH mice compared to B6 males was also observed by Cheng et al. (8).

2.6. Diabetes-Associated complications

Diabetes-associated complications are not yet well characterized in TH mice, but certain degrees of abnormalities in vasculature and skeleton have been reported to date and are summarized here.

A large body of evidence indicates that dysfunction of the endothelium plays a key role in the pathogenesis of vascular disease in T2D patients, such as retinopathy, nephropathy, and atherosclerosis (24). Endothelial dysfunction, demonstrated as impaired relaxation in response to acetylcholine and augmented contraction in response to phenylephrine, was evident in aorta, small mesenteric arteries, carotid arteries, and cerebral arterioles from male TH mice (8, 25). Potential mechanisms underlying the endothelial dysfunction may include oxidative stress and enhanced Rho kinase activity (25), prostaglandin H_2/thromboxane A_2 receptor activity and cytochrome p450 products (8). Despite the endothelial dysfunction, male TH mice were not hypertensive based on systolic blood pressure determined by tail-cuff plethysmography (25). Hypertension and diabetes are well known to be concomitant frequently, with a 75% prevalence of hypertension in patients with diabetes (26). Accordingly, the normotensive phenotype of TH mice is rather unique, especially when compared to other obese and diabetic models such as NZO mice discussed extensively in a separate chapter of this volume.

Substantial evidence from health care databases and experimental and clinical studies indicates bone fragility in T2D (27). Bone fragility in T2D involves decreased bone mineral density (BMD) and bone quality (28). Male TH mice, but not females, exhibited significantly lower BMD compared to age- and sex-matched B6 mice at 4, 8, and 12 weeks of age (19). These mice also showed lower bone mineral content. The lower BMD was associated with the imbalance of osteoblasts and osteoclasts, demonstrated as reduced osteoblastic gene expression (osteoprotegerin and osteocalcin) and increased osteoclastic gene expression (receptor activator of NF-κB ligand (RANKL) and interleukin 6 (IL-6)), in bone marrow of male TH mice. Reduced serum levels of osteocalcin and increased serum levels of IL-6 and IFN-γ (both induce RANKL) were also shown in male TH mice (19). The bone abnormalities observed in male TH mice were associated with enhanced activity of IL-17-producing CD4+ T cell (T_H17), stimulating synthesis of RANKL (19). The authors speculated that hyperleptinemia in TH mice may be responsible for the enhanced pro-osteoclastogenic activity of T_H17 (19). Administration of alendronate, a bisphosphonate drug used for osteoporosis, restored decreased BMD in male TH mice (19).

3. Genetic Characteristics of TALLYHO Mice

3.1. Genetic Crossing of TALLYHO Mice and Phenotypes

Because of male sex bias in hyperglycemia, all genetic crosses were carried out using male diabetic TH mice and normal female inbred strains, and the genetic analysis was performed using only male progeny (7, 29). In these crossbreeding experiments, hyperglycemia and all other metabolic phenotypes including body weight, fat pad weight, hypertriglyceridemia, and hypercholesterolemia showed continuous values, reflecting contributions from multiple quantitative trait loci (QTLs). All significant QTLs identified in crosses of TH with non-diabetic inbred strains are depicted in Table 1.

3.2. QTLs for Hyperglycemia

A genome-wide linkage analysis of the male backcross (BC) progeny from TH mice crossed with B6 mice identified two TH-derived QTLs for hyperglycemia (non-fasting) on chromosomes 19 (TALLYHO-associated-non-insulin-dependent-diabetes-1, *Tanidd1*) and 13 (*Tanidd2*) (7). The *Tanidd1* locus was also identified for hyperglycemia in the male BC mice from F1(CAST×TH)×TH. In this CAST cross, a third TH-derived QTL for hyperglycemia (non-fasting), *Tanidd3*, was identified on chromosome 16 (7).

Recent meta-analysis of numerous crossbreeding studies revealed mouse chromosome 19 as one of the prominent consensus regions linked to the traits of glucose levels, insulin levels, and glucose tolerance (30). Multiple diabetes candidate genes, including *Sorcs1*, *Hhex*, *Ide*, and *Tcf7l2*, are mapped to the *Tanidd1* locus on mouse chromosome 19 (31, 32). Studies suggest that risk variants of these candidate genes are associated with impaired insulin secretion and β-cell dysfunction (31, 33).

We also conducted a genome-wide QTL analysis using male F2 mice from a cross between TH and B6 mice and identified a fourth TH-derived QTL for hyperglycemia (4-h fasting), *Tanidd4*, on chromosome 4 (29). Multiple QTLs linked to hyperglycemia coincide with the *Tanidd4* locus and include the *Nidd1* locus in NZO×NON, a QTL near *D4Mit203* in C57BL/KsJ×DBA/2, and the *Nidd/SJL* locus in F1(NZO×SJL)×NZO (30). The causative gene for the *Nidd/SJL* locus is known to be zinc finger protein 69 (*Zfp69*) that plays a role in regulating fat storage in adipose tissue (34, 35).

The molecular bases for the *Tanidd* loci (1–4) have not yet been identified.

3.3. QTLs for Hyperlipidemia

Using the (B6×TH) F2 cross, a very significant QTL for hypercholesterolemia (TALLYHO-associated-cholesterol-1, *Tachol1*) was identified on chromosome 1 near *D1Mit113* (4-h fasting total cholesterol) (29). Previously, this chromosomal location has been

Table 1
Genome-wide significant QTLs identified from genome-wide linkage analysis of TALLYHO/Jng crosses with non-diabetic inbred strains

Chr[a]	Locus	Best location, cM (CI[b])	Closest marker	Trait[c]	Susceptible allele[d]	Human ortholog	Candidate genes and QTLs in mice and humans (references)
F1(B6×TH)×TH							
19	Tanidd1	50 (20, 60)	D19Mit103	Glu	TH	10q24-25	Sorcs1, Hhex, Ide, Tcf7l2 (31, 32)
13	Tanidd2	60 (5, 70)	D13Mit148	Glu	TH	5q12	D13Mit144, D13Mit262, Gluchos1, Cdkal1, Zbed3 (30, 31)
7	Tabw	30 (18, 44)	D7Mit231	BW	Het	15q26	Igf1r, Bw14, Afw9, Epfq5, Mtgq3, D7Mit122 (40, 41)
4	Tafat	80 (68, 90)	D4Mit312	FPW	Het	1p36	Afw2, Bw8q2, Pbwg2 (39)
6	Tabw2	43	D6Mit230	BW	TH	3p14	Pfat2, Bwtq3, Adip2, Obq14, D6Mit287 (40)
F1(CAST×TH)×TH							
19	Tanidd1	55 (16, 60)	D19Mit108	Glu	TH	10q26	Sorcs1, Hhex, Ide, Tcf7l2 (31, 32)
16	Tanidd3	5 (0, 34)	D16Mit129	Glu	TH	16p13	D16Mit103, T2dm1, Igf2bp2, Adcy5 (30, 31)
7	Tabw	5 (0, 18)	D7Mit191	BW	Het	19q13	Kctd15 (41)
F2(B6×TH)							
4	Tanidd4	67.3 (66.3, 70.3)	D4Mit312	Glu	TH	1p36	Nidd1, Zfp69, Insq1, D4Mit203, D4Mit42 (30)
1	Tabw3	35.7 (33.7, 44.7)	D1Mit215	BW FPW	TH	2q35-36	Wt10q1, Wt6q1, Bw5, Obq7, Mtgq1, D1Mit251 (40)
11	Tabw4	41 (32, 43)	D11Mit41	BW CRW	TH	17q21-23	Wt6q3, Bw4, Skl5, Cara2, Q11ucd1, D11Nds16 (40)
14	Tacrw	72.5 (65.5, 76.1)	D14Mit107	CRW	B6	13q33	
1	Tachol1 Tatg1	86.7 (84.7, 87.7)	D1Mit113	Chol TG	TH	1q21-24	Apoa2, D1Mit36, D1Mit206, D1S305, D1S518, D1S1660 (36, 39)
3	Tachol2	10.6 (5.6, 11.6)	D3Mit304	Chol	B6		D3Mit46, D3Mit241 (36)
11	Tatg2	65 (20, 79)	D11Mit132	TG	TH	17q12-21	D11Mit54, D11Mit14, D17S1291 (39)
4	Tatg3	31.3 (21.3, 41.3)	D4Mit178	TG	TH	9q32-33	Ifna, D4Mit17, D4Mit143 (39)
8	Tatg4	55.75 (50, 55.7)	D8Mit242	TG	TH	16q22	D8Mit66 (39)

The QTL names of *Tanidd4, Tabw3-4, Tacrw, Tachol1-2,* and *Tatg1-4* were not assigned in the original report
[a] *Chr* chromosome
[b] *CI* confidence interval
[c] Traits: *Glu* plasma glucose; *BW* body weight; *FPW* fat pad weight; *CRW* carcass weight; *TG* plasma triglyceride; *Chol* plasma total cholesterol
[d] Susceptible allele: *TH* TALLYHO/Jng; *Het* Heterozygote; *B6* C57BL/6

reported for hypercholesterolemia in 19 different mouse crosses (36). Three different population studies also reported QTLs linked to HDL-cholesterol in the human orthologous region of this locus (36). Apolipoprotein A-II (*Apoa2*) gene maps to the *Tachol1* locus, and our sequence analysis revealed that TH mice carry the $Apoa2^b$ allele (vs. $Apoa2^a$ allele in B6 mice). The $Apoa2^b$ allele (Ala61-to-Val61) is known to be hypermorphic in increasing plasma cholesterol levels in multiple mouse strains including BALB, CBA, C3H, DDD, KK, MRL, NFS, NZB, 129/Sv, SAMP6, SAMR1, SAMR4, FVB, LP, NON, NZW, and RF (37, 38). We therefore proposed that *Apoa2* is the causative gene for the *Tachol1* locus on chromosome 1. A B6-derived QTL for hypercholesterolemia, *Tachol2* was also identified on chromosome 3 in the F2 mice (29). In mice and humans, multiple QTLs linked to HDL-cholesterol were previously reported in this chromosomal region (36).

In the F2 mice, four significant QTLs (age-specific) were detected for hypertriglyceridemia on chromosomes 1 (TALLYHO-associated-triglyceride-1, *Tatg1*), 11 (*Tatg2*), 4 (*Tatg3*), and 8 (*Tatg4*) (29). For all four loci, TH-derived alleles conferred susceptibility (29). The *Tatg1* locus overlaps the *Tachol1* locus, and presumably they are the same gene. Concordance QTLs for each *Tatg* locus (39) are listed in Table 1.

3.4. QTLs for Obesity

Genomic regions associated with subphenotypic elements of obesity, including body weight and fat pad weight, were tested by genome-wide QTL analysis. Using the BC population of TH with B6 mice, a significant QTL for body weight was identified on chromosome 7 (TALLYHO-associated-body weight, *Tabw*) and a significant QTL for fat pad weight on chromosome 4 (TALLYHO-associated-fat, *Tafat*) (7). For both loci, the heterozygotes of B6 and TH alleles showed higher phenotypic values than mice homozygous for the TH allele. Near the *Tabw* locus, a QTL for body weight was also detected in the BC mice of TH with CAST mice (7). Again, the heterozygotes of CAST and TH alleles showed higher phenotypic values than mice homozygous for the TH allele. We therefore assumed that they are the same QTL. Multiple candidate genes and QTLs are physically mapped to the *Tabw* locus (40, 41).

In the BC population of TH with B6 mice, a second body weight QTL, *Tabw2*, was identified on chromosome 6, and the TH allele was associated with higher body weight (42). The *Tabw2* locus has been confirmed by congenic line breeding (42), and the associated studies are discussed later in this chapter.

Using the F2 population of TH and B6 mice, two TH-derived obesity QTLs were detected on chromosomes 1 (*Tabw3*) and 11 (*Tabw4*), respectively (29). The *Tabw3* locus was linked to body weight as well as fat pad weight. Multiple obesity QTLs were previously reported in the region of *Tabw3* (40), and positional candidate genes include *Irs1*, *Mogat1*, and *Igfbp2*. The *Tabw4* locus on chromosome 11 was linked to body weight and carcass weight (body weight without fat pads), suggesting that the *Tabw4* locus has a major effect on lean mass. An obesity QTL (called *Wg4* or *Q11Ucd1*) identified in *hg/hg* F2 population from B6-*hg/hg* × CAST maps to the *Tabw4* location and exhibits effects similar to *Tabw4* (43).

In the F2 population, a B6-derived QTL linked to carcass weight (TALLYHO-associated carcass weight, *Tacrw*) was also detected on chromosome 14 (29), where obesity QTLs are sparse in both mice and humans.

3.5. Dissecting Quantitative Traits by Microarrays

To pursue QTL analysis at the molecular level, we applied a genetical genomics approach and identified genomic regions that are associated with variation in gene expression in the F2 population of TH and B6 mice (29). We used a subset of the F2 mice selected from the upper and lower tails of the frequency distribution of the plasma triglyceride levels without severe hyperglycemia. This sample selection strategy was chosen to focus on identifying genes responsible for early stage of T2D in TH mice, in a cost-effective manner. Using a genome-wide microarray, we analyzed gene expression levels in four critical tissues associated with diabetes, including liver, adipose tissue, skeletal muscle, and pancreas. ANOVA revealed 8,764 gene expression traits in liver, 1,410 in adipose tissue, 1,832 in skeletal muscle, and 4,130 in pancreas associated with the markers tested. Among these, coiled-coil domain containing 46 (*Ccdc46*) and chymotrypsin C (caldecrin) (*Ctrc*) genes were identified as putative *cis*-acting transcripts for the *Tatg2* locus and the *Tanidd4* locus, respectively (29).

3.6. Obesity in Congenic B6.TH-*tabw2/tabw2* Mice

Congenic strains are produced by backcross breeding along with genomic selection, so that they carry a specific chromosomal segment of interest derived from a donor strain in their genetic background (44). Congenic strains are a powerful tool to confirm QTLs and allow much more precise localizations of QTLs. They have been successfully used for identification of susceptibility genes for diabetes and obesity (34, 45–47).

We developed a congenic strain, bred by introgressing the *Tabw2* obesity QTL on chromosome 6 from the TH strain into the B6 strain, B6.TH-*tabw2/tabw2* mice (42). The B6.TH-*tabw2/tabw2* congenic mice exhibited slight, but significant increase in body weight compared to controls (27.2 ± 0.5 g (n=22) vs. 25.4 ± 0.4 g (n=17), males, 14 weeks of age), confirming the *Tabw2* locus. When fed a high-fat and high-sucrose (HFS) diet, the obesity in B6.TH-*tabw2/tabw2* congenic mice became exacerbated (32.3 ± 0.9 g vs. 27.5 ± 1.5 g in controls, males, 4 weeks of age), followed by insulin resistance of adipose tissue. This suggests that gene-diet interactions play a role in the *tabw2*-mediated obesity. The body weight differences were mainly accounted for by an increase in fat depots both on chow and HFS diet feeding (Fig. 2). The obesity in B6.TH-*tabw2/tabw2* congenic mice was accompanied by hyperleptinemia (42).

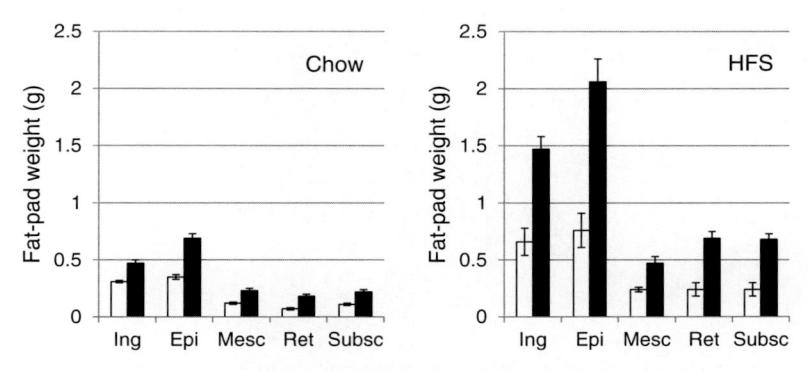

Fig. 2. Fat pad weights in male B6.TH-*tabw2/tabw2* congenic (*filled bars*) and B6-homozygous control (*open bars*) mice under chow or fed high-fat and high-sucrose (HFS) diets. Mice were weaned onto standard rodent chow. At 4 weeks of age, mice were either fed chow or HFS diets for 10 weeks. *Ing* inguinal fat pad; *Epi* epididymal fat pad; *Mesc* mesenteric fat pad; *Ret* retroperitoneal (including perirenal) fat pad; *Subsc* subscapular fat pad. The original data were presented as a part of Table 3 in (42). Data are means ± SE.

Analyzing B6.TH-*tabw2*/+ intercross mice fed HFS diets further refined the *Tabw2* interval to 15 cM (42). Gene expression profiling in adipose tissue and liver from B6.TH-*tabw2/tabw2* congenic mice vs. B6-homozygous control mice fed HFS diets revealed multiple biological pathways that may be perturbed, and included Wnt signaling pathway and intermediary metabolism pathways (48). Identifying the molecular basis and pathophysiological mechanism underlying the obesity mediated by *tabw2* will therefore allow understanding the mechanisms of gene-by-diet interactions in the development of obesity.

4. Concluding Remarks

T2D in humans is a complex polygenic disease. Animal models with a similar genetic basis, such as TH mice, are ideal resources for understanding the genetic architecture of T2D. TH mice have a profile of physiological anomalies very similar to those that are present in the majority of T2D patients. Therefore, information obtained from TH mice will provide important insights regarding diabetes genes and pathology that can be tested in humans. Furthermore, the current ever-escalating pace of modern molecular techniques will accelerate the discovery of genes underlying common complex diseases, and TH mice can serve as a valuable model for functional tests in seeking new therapeutic targets for T2D.

Acknowledgements

The preparation of this review was supported by American Heart Association Grant 0855300E and NIH/National Institute of Diabetes and Digestive and Kidney Disease Grant R01DK077202.

References

1. Gavin JR 3rd, Stolar MW, Freeman JS et al (2010) Improving outcomes in patients with type 2 diabetes mellitus: practical solutions for clinical challenges. J Am Osteopath Assoc 110:S2–S14
2. Belkina AC, Denis GV (2010) Obesity genes and insulin resistance. Curr Opin Endocrinol Diabetes Obes 17:472–477
3. Elbein SC (2009) Genetics factors contributing to type 2 diabetes across ethnicities. J Diabetes Sci Technol 3:685–689
4. Freeman H, Cox RD (2006) Type-2 diabetes: a cocktail of genetic discovery. Hum Mol Genet 15:R202–R209
5. Surampudi PN, John-Kalarickal J, Fonseca VA (2009) Emerging concepts in the pathophysiology of type 2 diabetes mellitus. Mt Sinai J Med 76:216–226
6. Israili ZH (2011) Advances in the treatment of type 2 diabetes mellitus. Am J Ther 18:117–152
7. Kim JH, Sen S, Avery CS et al (2001) Genetic analysis of a new mouse model for non-insulin-dependent diabetes. Genomics 74:273–286
8. Cheng ZJ, Jiang YF, Ding H et al (2007) Vascular dysfunction in type 2 diabetic TallyHo mice: role for an increase in the contribution of PGH2/TxA2 receptor activation and cytochrome p450 products. Can J Physiol Pharmacol 85:404–412
9. Sung YY, Lee YS, Jung WH et al (2005) Glucose intolerance in young TallyHo mice is induced by leptin-mediated inhibition of insulin secretion. Biochem Biophys Res Commun 338:1779–1787
10. Rhee SD, Sung YY, Lee YS et al (2011) Obesity of TallyHO/JngJ mouse is due to increased food intake with early development of leptin resistance. Exp Clin Endocrinol Diabetes 119:243–251
11. Leiter EH (2009) Selecting the "right" mouse model for metabolic syndrome and type 2 diabetes research. Methods Mol Biol 560:1–17
12. Kim JH, Stewart TP, Soltani-Bejnood M et al (2006) Phenotypic characterization of polygenic type 2 diabetes in TALLYHO/JngJ mice. J Endocrinol 191:437–446
13. Leiter EH, Reifsnyder PC (2004) Differential levels of diabetogenic stress in two new mouse models of obesity and type 2 diabetes. Diabetes 53:S4–S11
14. Abdul-Ghani MA, DeFronzo RA (2009) Plasma glucose concentration and prediction of future risk of type 2 diabetes. Diabetes Care 32:S194–S198
15. Wang Y, Nishina PM, Naggert JK (2009) Degradation of IRS1 leads to impaired glucose uptake in adipose tissue of the type 2 diabetes mouse model TALLYHO/Jng. J Endocrinol 203:65–74
16. Ostenson CG (2001) The pathophysiology of type 2 diabetes mellitus: an overview. Acta Physiol Scand 171:241–247
17. Myers MG Jr, Leibel RL, Seeley RJ et al (2010) Obesity and leptin resistance: distinguishing cause from effect. Trends Endocrinol Metab 21:643–651
18. Ambati S, Kim HK, Yang JY et al (2007) Effects of leptin on apoptosis and adipogenesis in 3T3-L1 adipocytes. Biochem Pharmacol 73:378–384
19. Won HY, Lee JA, Park ZS et al (2011) Prominent Bone Loss Mediated by RANKL and IL-17 Produced by CD4+T Cells in TallyHo/JngJ Mice. PLoS One 6:e18168
20. Kim KY, Kim JY, Sung YY et al (2011) Inhibitory effect of leptin on rosiglitazone-induced differentiation of primary adipocytes prepared from TallyHO/Jng mice. Biochem Biophys Res Commun 406:584–589
21. von Eckardstein A, Sibler RA (2011) Possible contributions of lipoproteins and cholesterol to the pathogenesis of diabetes mellitus type 2. Curr Opin Lipidol 22:26–32
22. Singh S, Dhingra S, Ramdath DD et al (2010) Risk factors preceding type 2 diabetes and cardiomyopathy. J Cardiovasc Transl Res 3:580–596
23. Tomkin GH (2008) Targets for intervention in dyslipidemia in diabetes. Diabetes Care 31:S241–S248

24. Schalkwijk CG, Stehouwer CD (2005) Vascular complications in diabetes mellitus: the role of endothelial dysfunction. Clin Sci (Lond) 109:143–159
25. Didion SP, Lynch CM, Faraci FM (2007) Cerebral vascular dysfunction in TallyHo mice: a new model of Type II diabetes. Am J Physiol Heart Circ Physiol 292:H1579–H1583
26. Glandt M, Bloomgarden ZT (2011) Hypertension in diabetes: treatment considerations. J Clin Hypertens (Greenwich) 13:314–318
27. Merlotti D, Gennari L, Dotta F et al (2010) Mechanisms of impaired bone strength in type 1 and 2 diabetes. Nutr Metab Cardiovasc Dis 20:683–690
28. Yaturu S (2009) Diabetes and skeletal health. J Diabetes 1:246–254
29. Stewart TP, Kim HY, Saxton AM et al (2010) Genetic and genomic analysis of hyperlipidemia, obesity and diabetes using (C57BL/6 J×TALLYHO/JngJ) F2 mice. BMC Genomics 11:713
30. Schmidt C, Gonzaludo NP, Strunk S et al (2008) A meta-analysis of QTL for diabetes-related traits in rodents. Physiol Genomics 34:42–53
31. Grarup N, Sparsø T, Hansen T (2010) Physiologic characterization of type 2 diabetes-related loci. Curr Diab Rep 10:485–497
32. Clee SM, Attie AD (2007) The genetic landscape of type 2 diabetes in mice. Endocr Rev 28:48–83
33. Goodarzi MO, Lehman DM, Taylor KD et al (2007) SORCS1: a novel human type 2 diabetes susceptibility gene suggested by the mouse. Diabetes 56:1922–1929
34. Scherneck S, Nestler M, Vogel H et al (2009) Positional cloning of zinc finger domain transcription factor Zfp69, a candidate gene for obesity-associated diabetes contributed by mouse locus Nidd/SJL. PLoS Genet 5:e1000541
35. Joost HG (2010) The genetic basis of obesity and type 2 diabetes: lessons from the New Zealand obese mouse, a polygenic model of the metabolic syndrome. Results Probl Cell Differ 52:1–11
36. Rollins J, Chen Y, Paigen B et al (2006) In search of new targets for plasma high-density lipoprotein cholesterol levels: promise of human-mouse comparative genomics. Trends Cardiovasc Med 16:220–234
37. Wang X, Korstanje R, Higgins D et al (2004) Haplotype analysis in multiple crosses to identify a QTL gene. Genome Res 14:1767–1772
38. Kitagawa K, Wang J, Mastushita T et al (2003) Polymorphisms of mouse apolipoprotein A-II: seven alleles found among 41 inbred strains of mice. Amyloid 10:207–214
39. Wang X, Paigen B (2005) Genome-wide search for new genes controlling plasma lipid concentrations in mice and humans. Curr Opin Lipidol 16:127–137
40. Wuschke S, Dahm S, Schmidt C et al (2007) A meta-analysis of quantitative trait loci associated with body weight and adiposity in mice. Int J Obes (Lond) 31(5):829–841
41. Herrera BM, Lindgren CM (2010) The genetics of obesity. Curr Diab Rep 10:498–505
42. Kim JH, Stewart TP, Zhang W et al (2005) Type 2 diabetes mouse model TallyHo carries an obesity gene on chromosome 6 that exaggerates dietary obesity. Physiol Genomics 22:171–181
43. Corva PM, Horvat S, Medrano JF (2001) Quantitative trait loci affecting growth in high growth (hg) mice. Mamm Genome 12:284–290
44. Todd JA (1999) From genome to aetiology in a multifactorial disease, type 1 diabetes. Bioessays 21:164–174
45. Clee SM, Yandell BS, Schueler KM et al (2006) Positional cloning of Sorcs1, a type 2 diabetes quantitative trait locus. Nat Genet 38:688–693
46. Chiu S, Kim K, Haus KA et al (2007) Identification of positional candidate genes for body weight and adiposity in subcongenic mice. Physiol Genomics 31:75–85
47. Dokmanovic-Chouinard M, Chung WK, Chevre JC et al (2008) Positional cloning of "Lisch-Like", a candidate modifier of susceptibility to type 2 diabetes in mice. PLoS Genet 4:e1000137
48. Kim HY, Stewart TP, Wyatt BN et al (2010) Gene expression profiles of a mouse congenic strain carrying an obesity susceptibility QTL under obesigenic diets. Genes Nutr 5:237–250

Chapter 7

Diet-Induced Diabetes in the Sand Rat (*Psammomys obesus*)

Nurit Kaiser, Erol Cerasi, and Gil Leibowitz

Abstract

Insulin deficiency is the underlying cause of hyperglycemia in type 2 diabetes. The gerbil *Psammomys obesus* (*P. obesus*) is a naturally insulin resistant rodent with tendency to develop diet-induced hyperglycemia associated with obesity. *P. obesus* does not exhibit hyperglycemia in its natural desert habitat, feeding on low caloric vegetation. However, when fed regular laboratory chow containing higher caloric density, the animals develop moderate obesity and hyperglycemia. Diabetes development and progression is very fast in *P. obesus*. The animals reach the irreversible hypoinsulinemic stage of the disease, in which a marked reduction of β-cell mass is apparent, within 4–6 weeks of high caloric diet. The present review describes the *P. obesus* of the Hebrew University colony, with emphasis on its use for the study of β-cell dysfunction in type 2 diabetes.

Key words: Type 2 diabetes, *Psammomys obesus*, β-Cell dysfunction, Sand rat, Insulin deficiency, Insulin secretion, Proinsulin, Proinsulin conversion intermediates, Insulin content, Proinsulin biosynthesis, Gerbils, Oxidative stress

1. Introduction

Type 2 diabetes mellitus (T2DM) is increasing worldwide in association with the global obesity epidemic (1). This trend is related to the exposure of a growing number of populations to food abundance and sedentary life-style that together promote insulin resistance. To normalize blood glucose in the face of augmented nutrient intake and insulin resistance, the pancreatic β-cell must adapt its secretory capacity to the increasing insulin demand; failure to do so results in hyperglycemia (2). Indeed, β-cell dysfunction is believed to play a determining role throughout the development of T2DM, and was shown to deteriorate further during disease progression, irrespective of the type of treatment used to reduce the hyperglycemia (reviewed recently in ref. (3)). The β-cell adapts to an increase in insulin demand by augmenting insulin biosynthesis and secretion and by the expansion of β-cell mass (functional as well as physical). Performance of longitudinal studies aimed to assess the β-cell response to insulin resistance in man is extremely difficult and appraisal of β-cell mass in vivo is currently not feasible. Moreover, the cellular pathways mediating the β-cell response are complex, making it difficult to decipher the critical pathways involved. Thus, animal models are required for comprehensive studies on insulin resistance and on the regulation of β-cell function and mass in T2DM.

In the present review we describe a diabetes model extensively used by our group, the *Psammomys obesus* (*P. obesus*), trivially nicknamed "sand rat," with emphasis on its utility for the study of β-cell dysfunctions in T2DM. The use of this animal model to study insulin resistance was described in a number of comprehensive reviews by Shafrir and colleagues (4–8).

2. General Description of the Model

P. obesus is a diurnal rodent that lives in the arid regions of North Africa and Eastern Mediterranean. In its natural habitat it feeds mainly on succulent leaves relatively low in energy and high in water and electrolytes. The trivial name "sand rat" was given to these rodents when first trapped on the sandy beaches of the Nile Delta by the US Naval Medical Research Unit in Egypt in the 1960s because they were thought to be rats. However, *Psammomys* is a gerbil, not a murine, belonging to the subfamily Gerbillinea. Animals living in their natural habitat are lean and normoglycemic; diabetes was discovered in *P. obesus* by chance when animals transferred from Egypt to Duke University and fed on regular laboratory chow developed hyperglycemia (9, 10). On this relatively high caloric diet, a large proportion of the animals gained weight and exhibited insulin resistance. The early investigations in the United States were performed mostly on the first generations of animals shipped from Egypt, because of difficulty to establish a multi-generation colony in captivity due to the low reproductive capacity of animals fed the regular rodent chow.

The Hebrew University *P. obesus* colony was established in the early 1970s from animals captured in the area of the Dead Sea where they feed mostly on the low calorie, high fiber salt bush (*Atriplex halimus*) (11). Feeding on a mixture of salt bush leaves with a few pellets of regular rodent chow enabled the maintenance of the colony. During the initial 20 years, no systematic longitudinal study was planned, and animals were removed at random from the colony; it was then observed that several phenotypes had developed: 32% of the animals were normoglycemic and normoinsulinemic, 26% were moderately obese with normoglycemia–hyperinsulinemia, 36%

were hyperglycemic–hyperinsulinemic, and about 6% developed hypoinsulinemia and hyperglycemia with weight loss and ketosis (12).

The digestible caloric density of the regular rodent chow is about 3 kcal/g, which for *P. obesus* represents a high-energy (HE) diet, compared to salt bush nutrition that contains only 2.3 kcal/g. To preserve normoglycemia in the *P. obesus* colony, a special low-energy (LE) pellet diet was formulated by Koffolk (Petach Tikva, Israel), containing a digestible caloric density of about 2.3 kcal/g (8). Assorted breeding using HE diet and postprandial blood glucose measurements enabled Kalman et al. to select two outbred lines of animals: diabetes-prone (DP) and diabetes-resistant (DR) *P. obesus* (13). This indicates that the natural population of *P. obesus* is composed of at least two genetically defined lines that differ in their susceptibility to diet-induced hyperglycemia. Further studies suggested that diabetes tendency in the two selected lines results from differences in energy expenditure: whereas the energy cost for a 1 g gain in body weight is 6–6.3 kcal in the DP animals, irrespective of the diet, the DR animals consumed 9.3 kcal per each 1 g increase in body weight when fed the HE diet (13). This difference in metabolic efficiency, coupled with the higher caloric HE diet, resulted in increased weight gain and progression to hyperglycemia in animals of the DP line, in the absence of hyperphagia. However, the selection procedure was incomplete. Indeed, while in the DP line 90–95% of the animals developed non-fasting hyperglycemia within 1 week of HE diet feeding, only about 55% of the animals in the DR line remained normoglycemic. The remaining animals of the DR line exhibited an extended time-course of diabetes development under HE diet, with hyperinsulinemia preceding development of hyperglycemia by several weeks. Thus, the DR line apparently consists of a mixed population, which as yet has not been sufficiently clarified. At present, the DP line of the Hebrew University *P. obesus* is available on a regular basis for animal studies (Harlan, Jerusalem, Israel).

Additional studies by Ziv et al. showed that susceptibility to diet-induced diabetes increased from weaning up to 5 months of age and decreased thereafter (14). A greater reproductive efficiency is exhibited by females of the DP line (3.3 vs. 1.3 births per female in the DP vs. the DR line, respectively) with no difference in the number of newborns per birth (~3) (8); the reason for this unexpected reproductive advantage of diabetes-prone animals is not clear. It is important to note that when challenged by increased calories, the development of non-fasting hyperglycemia in DP *P. obesus* is very rapid. We have observed that when HE pellets are placed inside the cage, instead of on top of the cage, to reduce the physical activity of the animals, non-fasting hyperglycemia (blood glucose >8.3 mmol/L) was usually observed by the fourth day of HE diet. Once established, diabetes progression is also fast, with animals reaching the hypoinsulinemic end stage of the disease between 4 and 6 weeks of feeding on the HE diet (15). Thus, unlike the evolution of diabetes in other rodent models of T2DM (16, 17), the onset and progression of diet-induced diabetes is quite rapid in the DP line of *P. obesus* (18–20).

An important characteristic of *P. obesus* in the context of diet-induced diabetes is the innate insulin resistance of these animals, detectable on the LE maintenance diet soon after weaning, while the animals are normoglycemic; as expected, the insulin resistance is exacerbated by the diabetic state. This inherent trait has been the subject of numerous studies, reviewed by Shafrir and colleagues (4–8).

We have been using the *P. obesus* model of diet-induced hyperglycemia, associated with moderate obesity and insulin resistance, to study the role of β-cell dysfunction in the development and progression of T2DM and decipher the mechanisms involved. This experimental approach is based on the contention that, notwithstanding the important role of insulin resistance in T2DM, hyperglycemia is the result of insulin deficiency (21). Furthermore, the progressive nature of T2DM is the expression of deteriorating β-cell function (3). It is important to note that in humans, many more gene variants predisposing to T2DM were found to act through perturbation of β-cell function than by affecting insulin resistance (22, 23).

Longitudinal studies using DP animals, changed from their normoglycemic maintenance LE diet to the calorie-rich HE diet, elucidated the important metabolic parameters and islet morphological changes that occur during diet-induced diabetes (15). Thus, with the initiation of high caloric intake, the animals go through a phase of partial adaptation, followed by rapid and progressive deterioration of both metabolic and β-cell-related parameters, culminating in a marked reduction of β-cell mass (Fig. 1). At this "end stage" of diabetes, the animals become ketotic and die unless exogenous insulin is administered. During the partial adaptation phase, there is increased insulin secretion. However, this is done at the expense of depleting the pancreatic insulin stores, and due to the high turnover of pancreatic insulin, there is an increase in circulating precursors of insulin (proinsulin and proinsulin conversion intermediates) which are less bioactive than insulin (24). In fact, what is determined as increased levels of circulating "immunoreactive insulin" using insulin RIA and commonly referred to as "insulin", was found by high performance liquid chromatography (HPLC) analysis to consist of 60% proinsulin and its conversion intermediates, rendering the diabetic animals insulin-deficient even during the apparent hyperinsulinemia which characterizes the adaptation phase (24). The marked pancreatic insulin depletion was not correlated with a decrease in β-cell mass: whereas the reduction of pancreatic insulin occurred already at the initial phase

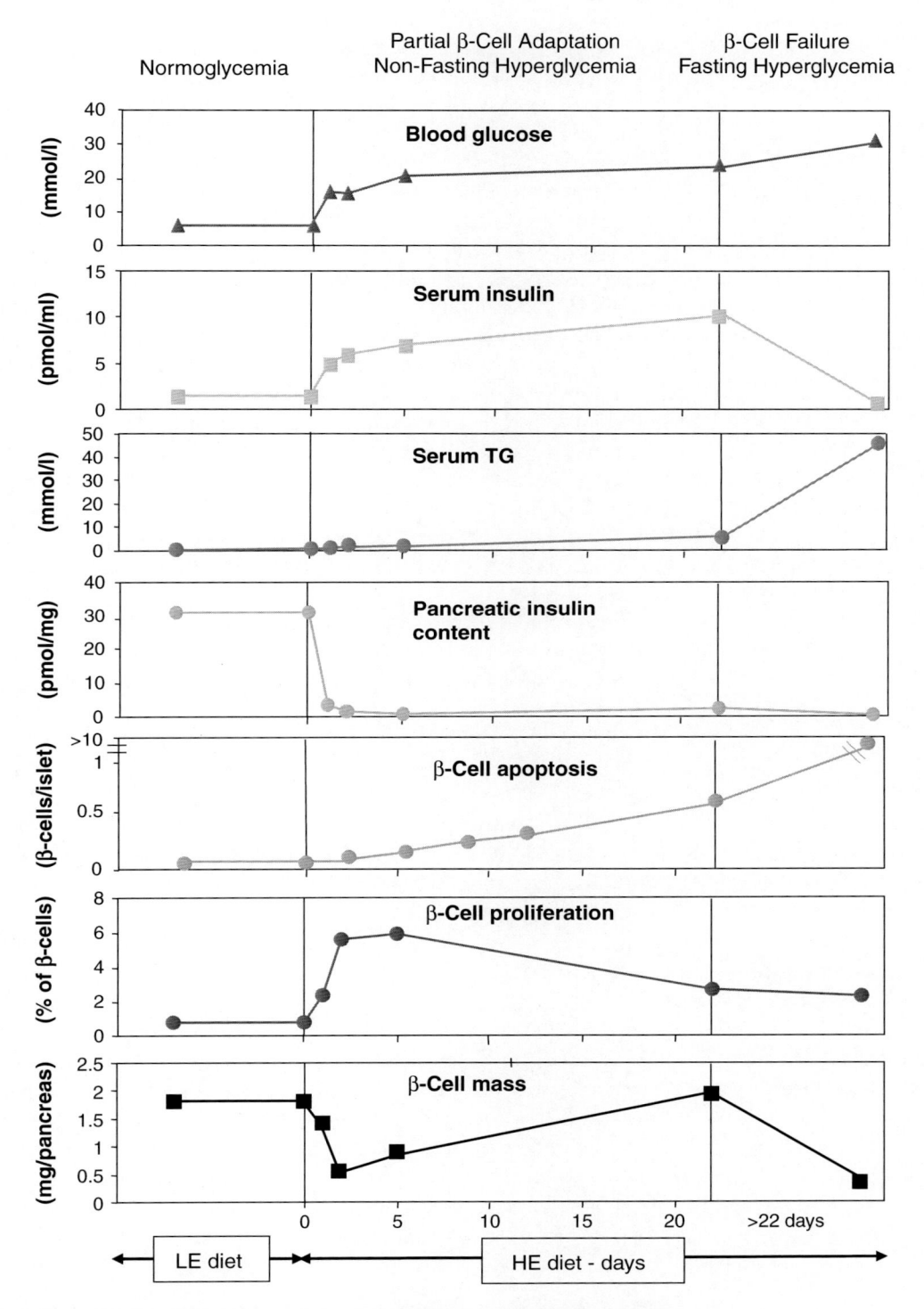

Fig. 1. Characteristics of *Psammomys obesus* during diabetes initiation and progression.

of post-prandial hyperglycemia and did not change throughout disease progression, β-cell mass showed only small variations during the adaptive phase and was reduced markedly only at the end stage of the disease, when there was a massive destruction of the β-cells by apoptosis and necrosis (15, 19, 20, 25).

During the adaptive phase, blood glucose may be normalized and diabetes progression halted in *P. obesus* by food restriction, overnight fast, or change to LE diet (6, 18, 26); increased physical activity using daily treadmill exercise also reduced the hyperglycemia in HE-fed animals (27). Pharmacologic agents, some of which are related to drugs used to treat T2DM in man, were shown to be effective in halting diabetes progression in HE diet-fed *P. obesus* when administered at the early stages of the disease, before hypoinsulinemia and β-cell destruction occur. Among these are: GLP-1 analogues (28, 29), phlorizin that promotes normoglycemia by inducing glucosuria (15), vanadyl sulfate which affects the insulin receptor signaling (30), and the PPARγ agonist rosiglitazone (31, 32). These studies suggest that *P. obesus* may be a suitable model for testing new pharmacological agents for their potential activity in T2DM.

Dealing with β-cell function in *P. obesus*, it is important to note that there is a striking similarity between the fully processed *P. obesus* insulin and human insulin, which differ by only two amino acids, none of which residing in the antigenic or active sites of the molecule (33). Therefore, human insulin RIA, using human insulin standards, is suitable for determination of *P. obesus* insulin. However, *P. obesus* proinsulin cannot be determined by a human proinsulin RIA due to a considerable variation in the C-peptide, hence, the use of HPLC for determining *P. obesus* proinsulin-like peptides.

3. β-Cell Failure in *P. obesus*

3.1. Insulin Secretion and Biosynthesis

The role of the β-cell in diet-induced diabetes was evaluated in *P. obesus* by combining in vivo and in vitro studies on insulin secretion and biosynthesis. In DP animals, HE diet-induced diabetes is characterized by high levels of immunoreactive insulin in the circulation, shown by HPLC analysis to contain increased proportions of proinsulin and proinsulin conversion intermediates (~60% vs. <10% in DP animals on LE diet). This increase in immunoreactive insulin was at the expense of a marked reduction in pancreatic insulin stores, which also contained a higher proportion of insulin precursor molecules (24, 34). The DR animals were able to adapt to HE diet-induced increase in insulin demand by doubling their serum insulin levels, while preserving their islet insulin content (18). In vitro studies in islets isolated from DP and DR animals fed

LE or HE diet revealed a leftward shift in the glucose–insulin concentration–response curves in both lines of animals compared to adult rat islets, suggesting that the increased glucose sensitivity of the islets was genetically determined. Yet, induction of diabetes in the DP line resulted in further reduction of the threshold for insulin release and a 55% decrease in the maximal insulin response (18). The biochemical basis for the increased sensitivity to glucose in *P. obesus* islets and the lower glucose threshold of insulin secretion in diabetic *P. obesus* were evaluated by investigating cellular pathways involved in stimulus-secretion coupling. Total glucose phosphorylation capacity was elevated in islets of DP *P. obesus* irrespective of their diet compared to DR animals on the HE diet. This was the result of increased activity of glucokinase with an additional increase in hexokinase activity in the hyperglycemic DP animals fed the HE diet (18). The increased glucose sensitivity of hyperglycemic *P. obesus* was accompanied by a rise in cytosolic calcium and NAD(P)H concentration observed at lower glucose levels (35). Islets from hyperglycemic *P. obesus* increased the rate of glycolysis twofold compared to islets from DR animals on either diet or DP animals on LE diet. On the other hand, all islets exhibited the same rate of mitochondrial glucose oxidation whether they originated from hyperglycemic or normoglycemic animals. Therefore, islets from DP *P. obesus* on HE diet exhibited a 50% decline in fractional glucose oxidation upon increase in glucose exposure from 1.7 to 11.1 mmol/L, suggesting an inadequate adaptation of the mitochondrial metabolism to the increased secretory demand imposed by the HE diet (36).

The rapid depletion of β-cell insulin content which coincides with increased insulin demand is the most prominent characteristic of *P. obesus* upon a change from LE to HE diet (Fig. 1). Importantly, the depletion of pancreatic insulin stores was not associated with a marked decrease in β-cell mass (15), suggesting that the relative insulin deficiency and the increase in circulating and islet insulin precursor molecules resulted from inappropriate coupling between insulin secretion and insulin production (34). Indeed, reduction in secretory demand in vivo by changing the diet from HE to LE diet or an overnight fast, as well as normalization of blood glucose by administration of the glucosuric agent phlorizin resulted in a rapid restoration of islet insulin content (15, 26, 34). Similarly, exposure of islets from prediabetic *P. obesus* to elevated glucose levels in vitro caused depletion of islet insulin stores, its extent depending on the glucose concentration, and duration of exposure (37, 38).

Our studies suggest that inadequate insulin biosynthesis plays an important role in diabetes initiation and progression under conditions of diet-induced increase in insulin demand. However, it should be emphasized that the β-cell response to elevated glucose in vitro is similar in islets derived from LE diet-fed DP and DR animals, both showing reduced glucose-stimulated proinsulin biosynthesis and depletion of pancreatic insulin content (25).

Glucose is the prime stimulus for insulin production. It has a rapid effect on preproinsulin mRNA translation and a slower effect on preproinsulin gene transcription which is responsible for maintaining the islet insulin stores under conditions of chronic increased demand. *P. obesus* fails to increase preproinsulin gene transcription in response to long-term exposure to high glucose, which contributes to the depletion of islet insulin content under conditions of hyperglycemia (39). The conserved form of the β-cell transcription factor pancreatic duodenal homeobox-1 (PDX-1) was undetectable in islets of DP or DR *P. obesus*; its forced expression using adenoviral vectors increased preproinsulin gene expression and partially prevented the depletion of insulin content during high glucose exposure (40). Thus, the poor adaptation of the β-cell biosynthetic activity to prolonged secretory drive with depletion of pancreatic insulin stores during diet-induced diabetes initiation and progression could be the result of a missing key transcription factor. Yet, the failure of the biosynthetic machinery to adapt to increased secretory demand could not account by itself for the higher incidence of diet-induced diabetes in the DP vs. the DR line in vivo, since islets from both lines exhibit insulin depletion after high glucose exposure in vitro and both lack the conserved form of PDX-1. The lack of PDX-1 is not unique to *P. obesus* and was also found in other members of the Gerbillinae subfamily (41). This was in marked contrast to other pancreatic transcription factors that are highly conserved in gerbils (40, 42). Interestingly, the spiny mouse (*Acomys cahirinus*), which is the closest relative to the gerbils, expresses PDX-1 (41). This suggests that during the evolution, PDX-1 was lost in gerbils at the time of separation of spiny mice and gerbils. PDX-1 has a critical role in pancreas development, however the pancreatic and islet morphology of gerbils is intact; thus a PDX-1 equivalent protein must be present in gerbils, including *P. obesus*. Cloning of the PDX-1-like gene of *P. obesus* was not successful, which may suggest that the gerbil PDX-1 is considerably different from the conserved gene of most species. Modern techniques of whole genome sequencing will hopefully enable to identify and characterize the gerbil PDX-1. This will allow studying the functional differences between the gerbil and the conserved PDX-1 protein and testing the hypothesis that the lack of the conserved form of PDX-1 accounts for the limited capacity of *P. obesus* to replace insulin stores under conditions of increased demand. Since the conserved form of PDX-1 is not expressed in either DP or DR *P. obesus*, the difference in the incidence of diabetes between the lines cannot be explained by this finding. Possibly, a progressive increase in insulin resistance resulting from HE diet-induced obesity, as a result of the lower energy expenditure of the DP line, coupled with a low capacity to increase preproinsulin mRNA expression, drives diabetes initiation and progression in DP *P. obesus* fed the HE diet.

3.2. β-Cell Survival and Mass

During the evolution of HE diet-induced diabetes we observed progressive changes in islet morphology, culminating in destruction of the islet architecture but without the involvement of autoimmunity (15, 25). These changes affect mostly the β-cells, whereas other islet endocrine cells are present even at the most advanced stages of the disease (15). Diet-induced hyperglycemia resulted in a short-lasting increase in β-cell proliferative activity, assessed by immunostaining for the KI-67 or PCNA nuclear antigens (15, 19). On the other hand, a progressive increase in the incidence of β-cell death, initially by apoptosis, but later on also by necrosis, was evident throughout the course of the disease (19, 25). In vitro studies implied that β-cell apoptosis was induced by exposure to the high glucose concentrations and was more pronounced in islets from DP compared to DR animals (19). Yet, β-cell mass showed little change throughout the adaptive phase of diabetes (Fig. 1), suggesting that in this animal model β-cell dysfunction rather than reduced β-cell mass drives diabetes progression (15, 25). At the end stage of the disease there was a marked decrease in β-cell mass with destruction of islet architecture.

4. Possible Mechanisms Involved in β-Cell Dysfunction in *P. obesus*

4.1. Oxidative Stress

Oxidative stress has been suggested to be involved in the development and/or progression of T2DM, either as an independent variable or in association with chronic hyperglycemia (43–46). In line with this, increased circulating levels of the lipid peroxidating product 4-hydroxy-2E-nonenal was found in diabetic *P. obesus*; it was furthermore shown to increase by elevated glucose concentrations in INS-1E β-cells (47). Moreover, thioredoxin interacting protein (TXNIP), the endogenous inhibitor of the major antioxidant system in the β-cell, was found to be increased in islets of *P. obesus* on HE diet, and by elevated glucose in vitro in *P. obesus* islets and in INS-1E β-cells (48). Notably, we found that GLP-1 analogs decreased the expression of TXNIP in β-cells (48), probably explaining their protective effect against β-cell apoptosis in vivo (28). These observations suggest that oxidative stress may be involved in HE diet-induced diabetes and in the anti-diabetic effect of GLP-1 in *P. obesus*.

4.2. Proinflammatory Cytokines

Activation of the innate immune system, with chronic increase in inflammatory mediators that may impair β-cell function, has been reported in obesity-associated T2DM (49, 50). As in islets from T2DM patients, increased IL-1β expression was documented in islets of diabetic *P. obesus* (51). Normalization of glycemia with phlorizin reduced IL-1β expression in *P. obesus* islets, suggesting that stimulation of IL-1β in this animal is mediated by glucose.

The IL-1 receptor antagonist (IL-1Ra) showed the opposite response to changes in blood glucose: its expression was reduced in islets from hyperglycemic *P. obesus* and elevated under conditions of normoglycemia (LE-diet or phlorizin). These observations complemented comprehensive studies by Donath and colleagues in human islets (reviewed in ref. (49)) and suggested that *P. obesus* may also serve to study modulation of inflammatory stress in T2DM and its effect on β-cell functional mass. It should be noted, however, that despite substantial experimental data supporting the involvement of the innate immune system in β-cell dysfunction in T2DM, this is not accepted by all investigators in the field (52, 53).

5. Concluding Remarks

P. obesus is well adapted to its natural desert habitat where the available high-fiber, low-calorie nutrition and the scarcity of rich food spare the animal hyperglycemic excursions, which would necessitate major fluctuations in insulin output to maintain normoglycemia. The reduced physical activity in captivity accentuates the innate insulin resistance of *P. obesus*, yet the animal is able to maintain normoglycemia as long as its caloric intake is limited, e.g., by the special LE diet. The increased secretory demand imposed by transition to the HE diet reduces pancreatic insulin stores, leading to increased relative levels of insulin precursor molecules in the pancreas and the blood. The decline in bioavailability of the active hormone leads to postprandial hyperglycemia that further aggravates the innate peripheral resistance. Moreover, the hyperglycemia may affect the β-cell at multiple sites, some of which involve stimulus-secretion coupling, whereas others involve insulin biosynthesis; all result in further attenuation of insulin release and depletion of pancreatic insulin content (Fig. 2). As the animal progresses to the end stage of the disease it exhibits severe fasting hyperglycemia and marked hypoinsulinemia (Fig. 2), which results in hyperlipidemia. At this stage, secondary changes related to increased serum lipids may cause further deterioration of β-cell function. An additional arm of the glucotoxicity-related processes involves the β-cells mass, with increased β-cell apoptosis not compensated for by β-cell proliferation. This arm is also aggravated by the hyperlipidemia. The hyperglycemia-related vicious cycle, causing deterioration of β-cell function and later on also reduced β-cell mass, may be interrupted during the adaptive phase of the disease by several strategies, among which are limiting caloric intake, increased physical activity, reduction of the hyperglycemia, and the administration of various pharmacologic agents that act on the β-cell (e.g., GLP-1 analogues) or reduce insulin resistance. Antioxidants and immune modulating compounds may also affect the course of

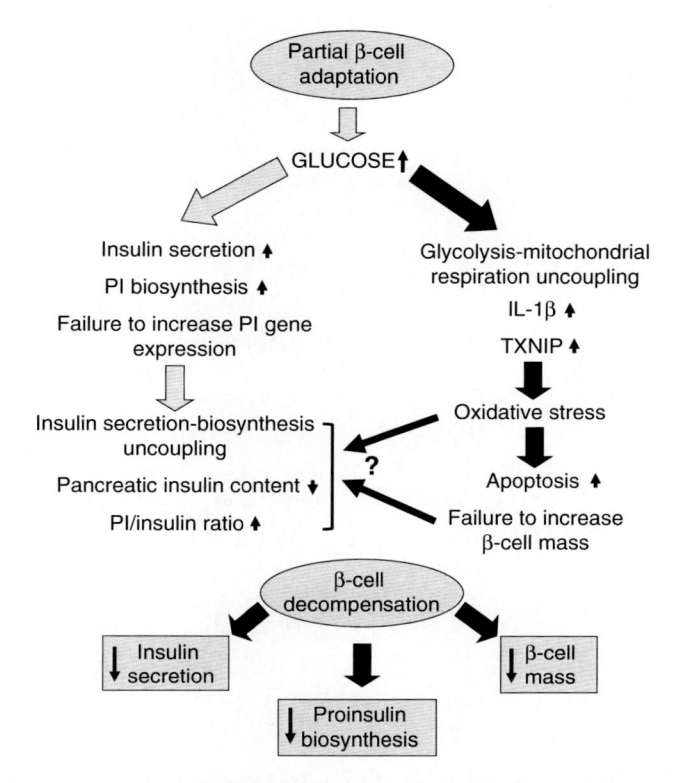

Fig. 2. β-Cell adaptation and failure in different stages of diabetes in *P. obesus*.

diabetes in *P. obesus*. Despite the demonstration of the reversible nature of diabetes at the initial adaptive phase of the disease, the different strategies may have variable efficiencies; neither are all the mechanisms involved fully understood. The fast initiation and progression to overt diabetes in this model, which culminates in insulin deficiency and β-cell destruction within 4–6 weeks of HE diet, may be advantageous for studies on the biochemical mechanisms of diabetes initiation and progression. For example, the rapid progression of diabetes in this model enabled us to capture and analyze β-cell death in situ and identify apoptosis as the main process of glucotoxicity-induced β-cell death (19), at a time that programmed β-cell death was conceived to be associated with lipotoxicity in T2DM (54). Moreover, the rapid diet-induced hyperglycemia enabled us to perform longitudinal studies and show that depletion of pancreatic insulin stores is an early β-cell pathology in *P. obesus*, preceding the decrease in β-cell mass. Hence, diabetes in this model is a result of β-cell dysfunction, with β-cell mass reduction playing a role only in the very advanced stages of the disease (15). The relative roles of β-cell dysfunction and reduced β-cell mass are still under debate in human T2DM (3). On the other hand, the fast progression of diabetes in *P. obesus* can pose a disadvantage, in particular when compounds having moderate antihypeglycemic activity and slow onset of action are tested; e.g., we were unable to demonstrate a beneficial effect of IL-1Ra administration on diet-induced diabetes in *P. obesus* (unpublished observation), unlike its effect in humans. Another limitation of this model is related to the fact that the gerbil DNA has yet to be sequenced to enable more sophisticated mechanistic and molecular studies. Nevertheless, we are convinced that *P. obesus* is at present one of the best available animal models for testing new treatment modalities that affect β-cell function in nutrition-induced obesity-associated type 2 diabetes.

References

1. Psaltopoulou T, Ilias I, Alevizaki M (2010) The role of diet and lifestyle in primary, secondary, and tertiary diabetes prevention: a review of meta-analyses. Rev Diabet Stud 7:26–35
2. Cerasi E (1995) Insulin deficiency and insulin resistance in the pathogenesis of type 2 diabetes: is a divorce possible. Diabetologia 38:992–997
3. Leibowitz G, Kaiser N, Cerasi E (2011) Beta-cell failure in type 2 diabetes. J Diabetes Invest 2:82–91
4. Shafrir E, Gutman A (1993) *Psammomys obesus* of the Jerusalem colony: a model for nutritionally induced, non-insulin-dependent diabetes. J Basic Clin Physiol Pharmacol 4:83–99
5. Shafrir E, Ziv E (1998) Cellular mechanism of nutritionally induced insulin resistance: the desert rodent *Psammomys obesus* and other animals in which insulin resistance leads to detrimental outcome. J Basic Clin Physiol Pharmacol 9:347–385
6. Shafrir E, Ziv E, Mosthaf L (1999) Nutritionally induced insulin resistance and receptor defect leading to beta-cell failure in animal models. Ann N Y Acad Sci 892:223–246
7. Shafrir E (2001) Albert Renold memorial lecture: molecular background of nutritionally induced insulin resistance leading to type 2 diabetes—from animal models to humans. Int J Exp Diabetes Res 2:299–319
8. Shafrir E, Ziv E, Kalman R (2006) Nutritionally induced diabetes in desert rodents as models of type 2 diabetes: *Acomys cahirinus* (spiny mice) and *Psammomys obesus* (desert gerbil). ILAR J 47:212–224
9. Schmidt-Nielsen K, Haines HB, Hackel DB (1964) Diabetes mellitus in the sand rat induced by standard laboratory diets. Science 143:689–690
10. Hackel DB, Mikat E, Lebovitz H et al (1967) The sand rat (*Psammomys obesus*) as an experimental animal in studies of diabetes mellitus. Diabetologia 3:130–134
11. Adler JH, Lazarovici G, Marton M et al (1986) The diabetic response of weanling sand rats (*Psammomys obesus*) to diets containing different concentrations of salt bush (*Atriplex halimus*). Diabetes Res 3:169–171
12. Kalderon B, Gutman A, Levy E et al (1986) Characterization of stages in development of obesity-diabetes syndrome in sand rat (*Psammomys obesus*). Diabetes 35:717–724
13. Kalman R, Adler JH, Lazarovici G et al (1993) The efficiency of sand rat metabolism is responsible for development of obesity and diabetes. J Basic Clin Physiol Pharmacol 4:57–68
14. Ziv E, Shafrir E, Kalman R et al (1999) Changing pattern of prevalence of insulin resistance in *Psammomys obesus*, a model of nutritionally induced type 2 diabetes. Metabolism 48:1549–1554
15. Kaiser N, Yuli M, Uckaya G et al (2005) Dynamic changes in beta-cell mass and pancreatic insulin during the evolution of nutrition-dependent diabetes in *Psammomys obesus*: impact of glycemic control. Diabetes 54:138–145
16. Peterson RG, Shaw WN, Neel MA et al (1990) Zucker diabetic fatty rat as a model of non-insulin-dependent diabetes mellitus. ILAR News 32:16–19
17. Kawano K, Hirashuma T, Mori S et al (1992) Spontaneous long-term hyperglycemic rat with diabetic complications: Otsuka Long-Evans Tokushima Fatty (OLEFT) strain. Diabetes 41:1422–1428

18. Nesher R, Gross DJ, Donath MY et al (1999) Interaction between genetic and dietary factors determines beta-cell function in *Psammomys obesus*, an animal model of type 2 diabetes. Diabetes 48:731–737
19. Donath MY, Gross DJ, Cerasi E et al (1999) Hyperglycemia-induced beta-cell apoptosis in pancreatic islets of *Psammomys obesus* during development of diabetes. Diabetes 48:738–744
20. Leibowitz G, Yuli M, Donath MY et al (2001) Beta-cell glucotoxicity in the *Psammomys obesus* model of type 2 diabetes. Diabetes 50(suppl 1):S113–S117
21. Cerasi E, Kaiser N, Gross DJ (1997) From sand rats to diabetic patients: is non-insulin-dependent diabetes mellitus a disease of the beta cell? Diabetes Metab 23(suppl 2):47–51
22. McCarthy MI (2010) Genomics, type 2 diabetes, and obesity. N Engl J Med 363:2339–2350
23. Hivert MF, Jablonski KA, Perreault L et al (2011) Updated genetic score based on 34 confirmed type 2 diabetes loci is associated with diabetes incidence and regression to normoglycemia in the diabetes prevention program. Diabetes 60:119–124
24. Gadot M, Leibowitz G, Shafrir E et al (1994) Hyperproinsulinemia and insulin deficiency in the diabetic *Psammomys obesus*. Endocrinology 135:610–616
25. Kaiser N, Nesher R, Donath MY et al (2005) *Psammomys obesus*, a model for environment-gene interactions in type 2 diabetes. Diabetes 54(suppl 2):S137–S144
26. Fraenkel M, Weiss R, Leizerman I et al (2008) Scanning electron microscopic analysis of intramyocellular lipid droplets in an animal model of type 2 diabetes. Obesity (Silver Spring) 16:695–699
27. Heled Y, Shapiro Y, Shani Y et al (2002) Physical exercise prevents the development of type 2 diabetes mellitus in *Psammomys obesus*. Am J Physiol Endocrinol Metab 282:E370–E375
28. Uckaya G, Delagrange P, Chavanieu A et al (2005) Improvement of metabolic state in an animal model of nutrition-dependent type 2 diabetes following treatment with S 23521, a new glucagon-like peptide 1 (GLP-1) analogue. J Endocrinol 184:505–513
29. Vedtofte L, Bodvarsdottir TB, Gotfredsen CF et al (2010) Liraglutide, but not vildagliptin, restores normoglycaemia and insulin content in the animal model of type 2 diabetes, *Psammomys obesus*. Regul Pept 160:106–114
30. Shafrir E, Spielman S, Nachliel I et al (2001) Treatment of diabetes with vanadium salts: general overview and amelioration of nutritionally induced diabetes in the *Psammomys obesus* gerbil. Diabetes Metab Res Rev 17:55–66
31. Hefetz S, Ziv E, Jorns A et al (2006) Prevention of nutritionally induced diabetes by rosiglitazone in the gerbil *Psammomys obesus*. Diabetes Metab Res Rev 22:139–145
32. Molero JC, Lee S, Leizerman I et al (2010) Effects of rosiglitazone on intramyocellular lipid accumulation in *Psammomys obesus*. Biochim Biophys Acta 1802:235–239
33. Kaiser N, Bailyes EM, Schneider BS et al (1997) Characterization of the unusual insulin of *Psammomys obesus*, a rodent with nutrition-induced NIDDM-like syndrome. Diabetes 46:953–957
34. Gadot M, Ariav Y, Cerasi E et al (1995) Hyperproinsulinemia in the diabetic *Psammomys obesus* is a result of increased secretory demand on the beta-cell. Endocrinology 136:4218–4223
35. Pertusa JA, Nesher R, Kaiser N et al (2002) Increased glucose sensitivity of stimulus-secretion coupling in islets from *Psammomys obesus* after diet induction of diabetes. Diabetes 51:2552–2560
36. Nesher R, Warwar N, Khan A et al (2001) Defective stimulus-secretion coupling in islets of *Psammomys obesus*, an animal model for type 2 diabetes. Diabetes 50:308–314
37. Gross DJ, Leibowitz G, Cerasi E et al (1996) Increased susceptibility of islets from diabetes-prone *Psammomys obesus* to the deleterious effects of chronic glucose exposure. Endocrinology 137:5610–5615
38. Bachar E, Ariav Y, Cerasi E et al (2010) Neuronal nitric oxide synthase protects the pancreatic beta cell from glucolipotoxicity-induced endoplasmic reticulum stress and apoptosis. Diabetologia 53:2177–2187
39. Leibowitz G, Uckaya G, Oprescu AI et al (2002) Glucose-regulated proinsulin gene expression is required for adequate insulin production during chronic glucose exposure. Endocrinology 143:3214–3220
40. Leibowitz G, Ferber S, Apelqvist A et al (2001) IPF1/PDX1 deficiency and beta-cell dysfunction in *Psammomys obesus*, an animal with type 2 diabetes. Diabetes 50:1799–1806
41. Gustavsen CR, Chevret P, Krasnov B et al (2008) The morphology of islets of Langerhans is only mildly affected by the lack of Pdx-1 in the pancreas of adult Meriones jirds. Gen Comp Endocrinol 159:241–249
42. Vedtofte L, Bodvarsdottir TB, Karlsen AE et al (2007) Developmental biology of the *Psammomys obesus* pancreas: cloning and

43. Kaneto H, Fujii J, Myint T et al (1996) Reducing sugars trigger oxidative modification and apoptosis in pancreatic beta-cells by provoking oxidative stress through the glycation reaction. Biochem J 320:855–863
44. Kaneto H, Kajimoto Y, Miyagawa J et al (1999) Beneficial effects of antioxidants in diabetes. Possible protection of pancreatic beta-cells against glucose toxicity. Diabetes 48:2398–2406
45. Tanaka Y, Gleason CE, Tran PO et al (1999) Prevention of glucose toxicity in HIT-T15 cells and Zucker diabetic fatty rats by antioxidants. Proc Natl Acad Sci U S A 96:10857–10862
46. Ihara Y, Toyokuni S, Uchida K et al (1999) Hyperglycemia causes oxidative stress in pancreatic beta-cells of GK rats, a model of type 2 diabetes. Diabetes 48:927–932
47. Cohen G, Riahi Y, Shamni O et al (2011) The role of lipid peroxidation and PPAR-delta in amplifying glucose-stimulated insulin secretion. Diabetes 60:2830–2842
48. Shaked M, Ketzinel-Gilad M, Ariav Y et al (2009) Insulin counteracts glucotoxic effects by suppressing thioredoxin-interacting protein production in INS-1E beta cells and in *Psammomys obesus* pancreatic islets. Diabetologia 52:636–644
49. Donath MY, Shoelson SE (2011) Type 2 diabetes as an inflammatory disease. Nat Rev Immunol 11:98–107
50. Böni-Schnetzler M, Donath MY (2011) Increased IL-1beta activation, the culprit not only for defective insulin secretion but also for insulin resistance? Cell Res 21:995–997
51. Maedler K, Sergeev P, Ris F et al (2002) Glucose-induced beta cell production of IL-1beta contributes to glucotoxicity in human pancreatic islets. J Clin Invest 110:851–860
52. Jorns A, Rath KJ, Bock O et al (2006) Beta cell death in hyperglycaemic *Psammomys obesus* is not cytokine-mediated. Diabetologia 49:2704–2712
53. Cnop M, Welsh N, Jonas JC et al (2005) Mechanisms of pancreatic beta-cell death in type 1 and type 2 diabetes: many differences, few similarities. Diabetes 54(suppl 2):S97–S107
54. Shimabukuro M, Zhou Y-T, Levi M et al (1998) Fatty acid-induced beta-cell apoptosis: a link between obesity and diabetes. Proc Natl Acad Sci U S A 95:2498–2502

Chapter 8

Diabetes in Zucker Diabetic Fatty Rat

Masakazu Shiota and Richard L. Printz

Abstract

Male Zucker diabetic fatty *fa/fa* (ZDF) rats develop obesity and insulin resistance at a young age, and then with aging, progressively develop hyperglycemia. This hyperglycemia is associated with impaired pancreatic β-cell function, loss of pancreatic β-cell mass, and decreased responsiveness of liver and extrahepatic tissues to the actions of insulin and glucose. Of particular interest are the insights provided by studies of these animals into the mechanism behind the progressive impairment of carbohydrate metabolism. This feature among others, including the development of obesity- and hyperglycemia-related complications, is common between male ZDF rats and humans with type 2 diabetes associated with obesity. We discuss the diabetic features and complications found in ZDF rats and why these animals are widely used as a genetic model for obese type 2 diabetes.

Key words: Zucker diabetic fatty, Zucker fatty, fa Gene mutation, Obesity, Type 2 diabetes, Hyperglycemia, Hyperlipidemia, Hyperinsulinemia, Insulin resistance, Glucotoxicity, Skeletal muscle, Liver, Pancreatic β-cell, Glucose transport, Glucose phosphorylation, Glucose production, Gluconeogenesis, Glucokinase, Leptin, Complications

1. Introduction

Hyperphagia and obesity develop in a partially outbred rat strain, Zucker fatty *fa/fa* (ZF) rats, that carry a spontaneous mutation of the leptin receptor gene (*fa* gene) (1, 2). Although ZF rats are obese and insulin-resistant, through increased insulin production and secretion, they maintain normal blood glucose levels. Occasionally, ZF rats will spontaneously acquire high blood sugars. It is these animals that were selectively inbreed to derive the Zucker diabetic fatty *fa/fa* (ZDF) strain of rats (3).

Animals of the ZDF line that are heterozygous for the *fa* gene mutation do not become obese, and hence, do not develop insulin resistance and diabetes. Female ZDF rats, homozygous for the *fa* gene mutation, rarely exhibit hyperglycemia; even though they have levels of obesity and insulin resistance comparable to males

(3, 4). Nevertheless, hyperglycemia can be consistently induced in female ZDF rats by increasing the fat content of their diet (5, 6). In contrast, male ZDF rats, homozygous for the *fa* gene mutation, develop with age a progressively greater level of insulin resistance, glucose intolerance, and impaired pancreatic β-cell function leading to frank diabetes (7). Since these features are common with human type 2 diabetes associated with obesity (3, 4), male ZDF rats are widely used as a genetic model for this disease. We focus most of our discussion of this model on the feature of impaired carbohydrate metabolism and how it resembles that of human obese type 2 diabetes.

Development of severe hyperglycemia and concomitant necrosis of β-cells in male ZDF rats appear not to be a direct consequence of the obesity syndrome associated with the fa gene, since ZF rats do not exhibit these characteristics (8, 9). Likewise, the Wister diabetic fatty rat (WDF *fa/fa*), which is a congenic strain of the Wister Kyoto rat and was established by transferring the fa gene of the ZF rat to a somewhat carbohydrate-intolerant lean Wister Kyoto rat, exhibits severe hyperglycemia that appears not to be associated with the *fa* gene (10). The rat *fa* gene is homologues with the mouse *db* gene (2). Similar to the rat *fa* gene (2), the mouse db gene mutation occurred spontaneously in the C57BL/KsJ inbred strain (11). The *db* mutation in the C57BL/KsJ stain arose through a genetic contamination of a black mouse strain with the majority (84%) of alleles being derived from C57BL/6J and the minority (16%) from DBA/2J (12). The C57BL/KsJ homozygotes for the db gene become obese after weaning and develop transient hyperinsulinemia with progressively more severe insulin resistance, followed by β-cell necrosis and establishment of chronic severe hyperglycemia in both sexes (11). When the db mutation was transferred from C57BL/KsJ into a closely related inbred C57BL/6J, however, the males develop a transient hyperglycemia, followed by remission to normoglycemia and females are completely resistant to the hyperglycemic stress (13). Therefore, the induction of severe diabetes in homozygotes of *fa* or *db* mutation depends upon interaction between the mutation and the inbred strain genetic background.

2. Progression from Obesity to Diabetes in Male ZDF Rats

2.1. Obesity

In male ZDF rats, compared with lean (ZCL) rats, body weights are greater by ~7 weeks of age, while individual growth rate and body mass index continue to increase until ~10 weeks (Fig. 1a, b). Thereafter, growth rate decreases, while the body mass index difference between ZDF and ZCL rats becomes less. Then after

~15 weeks of age, these differences in body weight and body mass index disappear between ZDF and ZCL rats (14, 15). However, body fat mass relative to body weight, adiposity, is not decreased in ZDF rats and remains nearly double to that of aged-matched ZCL rats at 15–20 weeks of age (unpublished data).

2.2. Glycemia

In ad lib-fed male ZDF rats compared with age-matched ZCL rats, mild hyperglycemia develops by 7–8 weeks of age with plasma glucose levels progressively rising and reaching 25–30 mM by 9–10 weeks (Fig. 1e) (3, 4, 16–20). In contrast, fasting plasma glucose levels after a short fast are only mildly hyperglycemic at 9–10 weeks of age, but reach ~25 mM by 14–15 weeks (Fig. 1e) (15, 16). Along with rising blood glucose levels, glucose excretion into urine and urine output increases markedly from ~7 weeks of age (19).

2.3. Lipidemia

Hyperlipidemia develops in ZDF rats (~1 mM of plasma free fatty acids and ~200 mg/dL of plasma triglyceride) compared to age-matched ZCL rats (~0.5 mM of plasma Fatty acids and ~40 mg/dL of plasma triglyceride) by 6–7 weeks of age (16, 19, 21). After which, further elevation of plasma triglyceride continues (19, 21) and reaches approximately tenfold higher levels (~500 mg/dL) than that of ZCL rats by 20 weeks of age (15, 22, 23).

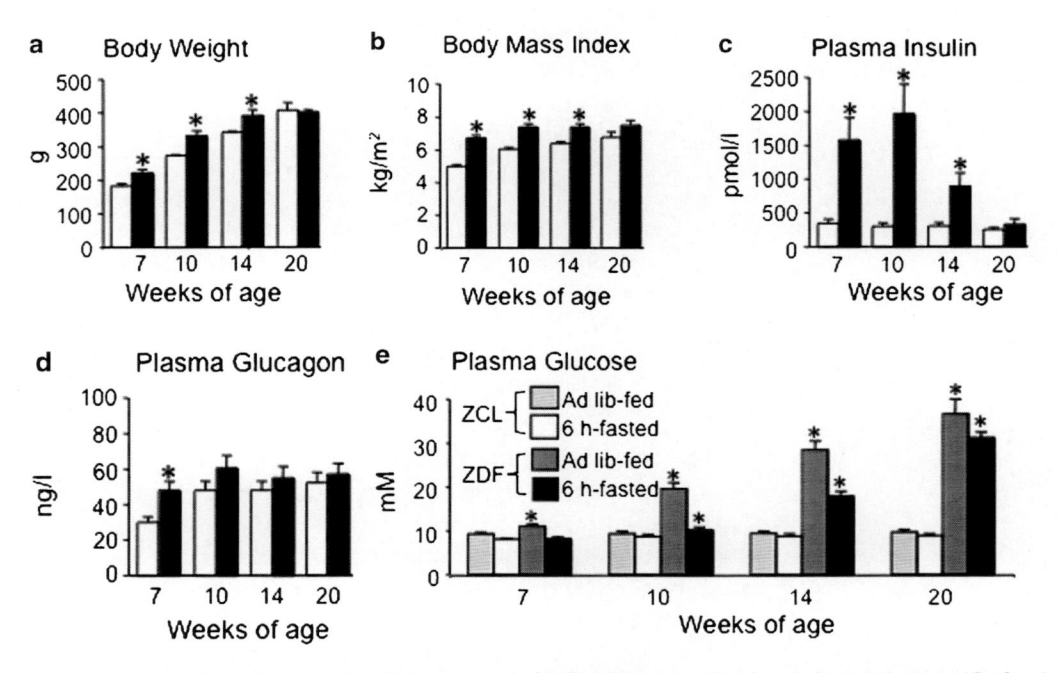

Fig. 1. Changes with aging in body weight (a), body mass index (b), plasma insulin (c) and plasma glucagon (d) after 6 h fasted and plasma glucose levels (e) in ad lib-fed and after 6 h fasted in male Zucker diabetic fatty (ZDF) rats and lean litter mates (ZCL). *Significant difference from the corresponding values of the ZCL group ($P < 0.05$) (adopted from ref. (8)).

2.4. Gluconeogenic Precursors

Blood lactate levels in 6-h-fasted male ZDF rats compared with age-matched ZCL rats are about double (~1 mM) at 10 weeks of age, and like blood glucose levels, progressively rise with aging to 2 mM by 20 weeks (15, 22–24). Blood alanine levels (~0.4 mM) are not significantly different between male ZDF and ZCL rats (15, 22–25). At 5 weeks of age in ZDF rats, plasma concentrations of gluconeogenic amino acids, aspartate, serine, glutamine, glycine, and histidine are lower, whereas taurine, α-aminoadipic acid, methionine, phenylalanine, and tryptophan are higher compared with those of ZCL rats. Even after diabetes develops in ZDF rats, gluconeogenic amino acids remain at lower levels relative to ZCL rats (25). Levels in blood of branched-chain amino acids (leucine, isoleucine, and valine) are higher in male ZDF rats compared with those of ZCL rats (25, 26). These higher branched-chain amino acid levels are associated with higher liver enzyme levels of branched-chain α-keto acid dehydrogenase and branched-chain α-keto acid dehydrogenase kinase (26).

2.5. Hormonal Profiles

Plasma insulin levels in male ZDF rats, compared with ZCL rats, are elevated from approximately 5 weeks of age, progressively rise to approximately 8–12 times higher levels by 8–10 weeks; and then thereafter, progressively decline to levels seen in ZCL rats by 20–25 weeks (Fig. 1c) (3, 15, 17, 19, 21). Plasma glucagon levels in ZDF rats tend to be higher than those of ZCL rats and do not change with aging (Fig. 1d) (15). Plasma corticosterone levels are higher in 10- and 20-week-old ZDF rats compared to aged-matched ZCL rats (27). Levels of plasma thyroid hormones (T3 and T4) in ZDF rats are similar at 10 weeks of age, but 40% lower at 20 weeks compared to aged-matched ZCL rats (27).

2.6. Summary

In the prediabetic stage, patients with obesity exhibit insulin resistance that is compensated by increased insulin secretion to maintain normal glycemia. After which, as diabetes develops in these obese individuals, progressively excessive postprandial hyperglycemia appears while fasting glycemia remains near normal. Fasting hyperglycemia then develops in individuals with long-term obesity, and despite the presence of insulin resistance, plasma insulin levels are reduced to levels lower than lean individuals (28).

In male ZDF rats, progressive obesity, hyperlipidemia, and insulin resistance develop early, before 7 weeks of age. At this early stage, insulin resistance is overcome by greater levels of insulin; as a result, blood glucose levels remain at normal levels. At a later stage, hyperglycemia in male ZDF rats develops between 7 and 9 weeks of age in ad lib-fed male ZDF rats, but fasting glycemia remains normal. Fasting hyperglycemia develops with a progressive decrease in plasma insulin levels after 10 weeks of age. The time period where ZDF rats have a reduced rate of growth appears to coincide with this reduction in plasma insulin and development of fasting hyperglycemia. By 20–25 weeks of age, plasma insulin levels have fallen to levels seen in male ZCL rats and fasting plasma glucose levels reach >30 mM. This progression of diabetic-like features in ZDF rats resembles the development of diabetes as seen in type 2 diabetic patients with obesity.

3. Mechanisms Associated with Glucose Intolerance in Male ZDF Rats

3.1. Gastric Emptying

Male ZDF rats develop dramatically higher rates of gastric emptying of glucose solutions compared to aged-matched ZCL rats after 10 weeks of age (29). This abnormally rapid gastric emptying of glucose solutions is a feature also shared with patients recently diagnosed with type 2 diabetes, which is associated with and thought to contribute to excessive postprandial hyperglycemia (30).

3.2. Skeletal Muscle Glucose Metabolism

Skeletal muscle is the primary site of glucose disposal during an insulin-stimulated state; and thereby, a major tissue that contributes to blood glucose levels (31). Resistance to the action of insulin in skeletal muscle is a major pathogenic factor associated with type 2 diabetes (32). Male ZDF rats at an early (22, 33) and middle stage (24) of diabetes (at ~10 weeks and ~14 weeks of age, respectively), compared to age-matched ZCL rats, have whole-body blood glucose disposal rates that are similar despite six to ten times higher plasma insulin levels, which indicates severe insulin resistance of glucose utilization. Indeed, when glucose disappearance and uptake rates in skeletal muscle are compared between male ZDF and aged-matched ZCL rats at equivalent plasma insulin levels using a hyperinsulinemic-glucose clamp technique, whole-body blood glucose disappearance and skeletal muscle glucose uptake rates are markedly lower (22, 24).

Glucose transport across the plasma membrane is a major regulatory step of glucose utilization in muscle and this process is predominantly regulated by insulin in resting muscle. The glucose transport process resistant to the actions of insulin in skeletal muscle is an early and obligatory defect leading initially to a prediabetic condition and subsequently to overt type 2 diabetes (34–36). In male ZDF rats, insulin (600 pmol/L)-induced glucose transport, as measured using 3-O-methyl-D-glucose in fast-twitch epitrochlearis and slow-twitch soleus muscle strips, is markedly impaired at 7 weeks of age (16). Insulin-induced glucose transport across the plasma membrane is mediated by glucose transporter type 4 (GLUT4). Compared to ZCL rats, GLUT4 protein is reduced by 40, 45, and 19% in red quadriceps, mixed gastrocnemius, and white quadriceps muscles, respectively, in 26-week-old ZDF rats (37). There is also some evidence for a role of glycogen synthase kinase 3 in opposing insulin-induced glucose transport and glycogen synthesis in skeletal muscle of ZDF rats (38–40).

3.3. Kidney Glucose Metabolism

The kidneys contribute to the level of blood glucose via glucose reabsorption and gluconeogenesis. Renal tubular reabsorption of glucose is substantially increased in humans with diabetes mellitus (41). This increased glucose reabsorption has been reported in ZDF rats and contributes towards the maintenance of hyperglycemia. Glucose reabsorption is mediated by two glucose transporters, glucose transporter type 2 (GLUT2) at the basolateral membrane of epithelial cells that line the proximal tubules, and sodium-glucose co-transporters (SGLT) on the luminal surface of epithelial cells that line the S1 and S2 segments of the proximal tubules (41). In the renal proximal tubules of the kidneys in ZDF rats, GLUT2 protein levels are approximately twofold higher than control littermates, while SGLT protein levels remain similar (42).

The post-absorptive synthesis of glucose by the kidneys in humans accounts for 5–25% of total glucose formed by gluconeogenesis in the body (43–45). This metabolic process is stimulated in patients with type 2 diabetes (41, 46, 47). Glucose production from lactate, glutamine, and glycerol is higher by 38%, 51%, and 66%, respectively, in isolated renal proximal tubules from 14 to 17-week-old male ZDF rats compared to age-matched ZCL rats (48). This stimulation of gluconeogenesis is associated with greater activities of key gluconeogenic enzymes, such as phosphoenolpyruvate carboxykinase, fructose-1,6-bisphosphatase, and glucose-6-phosphatase (48).

3.4. Pancreatic β-Cell Function

In patients with type 2 diabetes, β-cell mass is reduced during the early stages of diabetes and declines further with disease progression (49). β-cell mass in patients with obese type 2 diabetes is ~50% of that of obese nondiabetic individuals (50–52). The continuing loss of β-cell function is the underlying cause of deteriorating metabolic control and hyperglycemia in people with type 2 diabetes (53, 54).

In male ZDF rats, β-cell mass at 5–7 weeks of age is approximately twice that of age-matched ZCL animals and islet morphology appears normal (55). In these prediabetic ZDF rats, pancreatic insulin content is twice that of age-matched lean heterozygous and wild-type rats (21). Insulin secretory response to glucose is retained (3) and total pancreatic insulin secreted from isolated perfused pancreas of ZDF rats is greater than that from age-matched ZCL rats (55). However, when adjusted for changes in β-cell mass, insulin secretory responses appear reduced in the prediabetic ZDF rats (55). Thus, even at this early stage in the progression of diabetes in these animals, β-cell dysfunction is present; albeit somewhat concealed by a larger β-cell mass.

Between 8 and 12 weeks of age in male ZDF rats, β-cell mass declines by ~50% and islet morphology appears highly disorganized with significant fibrosis (56). In male ZDF rats between 6 and 10 weeks of age, insulin mRNA levels fall by 70% from their elevated prediabetic levels, and by 12 weeks of age, decrease to that of age-matched lean heterozygous and wild-type rats (21). In response to glucose, potassium chloride, or a rise in intracellular calcium, perfused pancreas or isolated islets from 12-week-old ZDF rats demonstrate a marked reduction or absence of insulin secretion. In contrast, responses to P_{2y} purinoceptor agonists appear to remain normal (57).

At 20 weeks of age, increased islet expression of components of the renin-angiotensin system is observed with increased intra islet fibrosis, apoptosis, and oxidative stress (58). β-cell degradation occurs and β-cell mass falls to below that seen in ZCL rats. The failure to maintain and expand β-cell mass in these older ZDF rats is likely from an increased rate of cell death by apoptosis and not from reduced β-cell proliferation or neogenesis (55).

3.5. Hepatic Glucose Metabolism

After a meal during the post-absorptive period, >90% of glucose produced by the body is derived from liver (59). In humans, 30–60% of total hepatic glucose production is derived from glycogen (60, 61). When blood glucose and insulin levels are raised as occurs postprandially, the liver switches from net glucose production to uptake, which in a healthy human markedly (30–40%) contributes to postprandial glucose disposal (62). A major proportion of glucose taken up by liver is stored as glycogen (63–65). Therefore, liver plays a major role in glucose homeostasis by switching its intermediate metabolism from glucose production to uptake in response to a rise in plasma glucose as well as insulin, and thus changes in blood glucose levels are minimized.

In subjects with type 2 diabetes, net hepatic glucose production correlates with the degree of hyperglycemia after an overnight fast (66–69). Lower hepatic glycogen breakdown and increased gluconeogenesis are found in type 2 diabetic patients compared with normal subjects (70, 71). Increased gluconeogenesis is considered a major contributor to fasting hyperglycemia in patients with type 2 diabetes (72–74). Also postprandially, hepatic glucose production is less suppressed in type 2 diabetic patients compared with normal subjects (69, 73, 75–79). A pronounced transient rise in hepatic glucose production after an oral glucose load is reported in type 2 diabetic patients (80, 81). Additionally, reduced splanchnic glucose uptake (82, 83) and hepatic glycogen synthesis (82) in response to a meal is reported in patients with type 2 diabetes. These patients have blunted levels of hepatic glucose uptake and glycogen synthesis in response to a rise in plasma insulin and/or glucose (78, 84, 85). All together these results characterize hepatic glucose metabolism in patients with type 2 diabetes as having elevated gluconeogenesis as well as blunted effects of insulin and glucose to suppress glucose production and stimulate both glucose uptake and glycogen synthesis.

Male ZDF rats share many of the alterations in hepatic glucose metabolism that are observed in patients with type 2 diabetes. Under a preprandial condition, even in the presence of marked hyperinsulinemia at 10 weeks of age and hyperglycemia combined with hyperinsulinemia at 14 weeks of age (Fig. 1), endogenous glucose production persists in ZDF rats at rates similar to that of age-matched ZCL rats (22, 23, 86). This is in sharp contrast to when plasma glucose and insulin are raised in ZCL rats to levels found in ZDF rats, and endogenous glucose production is completely inhibited. Therefore, the livers of male ZDF rats appear resistant to the effect of elevated insulin as well as glucose to suppress hepatic glucose production. Furthermore, ZDF rats at 20 weeks of age, which are characterized by normal insulin levels but marked hyperglycemia (15), have even higher rates of endogenous glucose production compared with younger male ZDF and age-matched ZCL rats (15).

In normal rats, there is an equal contribution of glycogenolysis and gluconeogenesis to endogenous glucose production (87). As diabetes progresses with age in male ZDF rats, little glycogen synthesis from plasma glucose occurs despite the presence of hyperglycemia and/or hyperinsulinemia during an early stage at ~10 weeks of age (22), a middle stage at ~14 weeks (23, 24), and a late stage at ~20 weeks (15). When plasma glucose and insulin levels in ZCL rats are raised to those of male ZDF rats at 10, 14, and 20 weeks of age, the incorporation of plasma glucose into glycogen via the direct pathway is markedly increased with complete inhibition of net hepatic glucose production (15, 22, 24). In male ZDF rats, the amount of hepatic glycogen is two to three times higher at 10, 14, and 20 weeks of age compared to age-matched ZCL rats. Surprisingly, their hepatic glycogen content does not decrease even after a 20-h fast.

In ZDF rats, measurement of percent contribution of gluconeogenesis, glycogenolysis, and glucose phosphorylation to form glucose-6-phosphate using [2-^{3}H]-glucose, [3-^{3}H]-glucose, and [U-^{14}C]-alanine indicates that ~90% of hepatic glucose production is due to gluconeogenesis, while the contribution of glycogenolysis is <10% (24). van Poelje et al. measured deuterium enrichment at the C2 and C5 position of glucose in 10-week-old ZDF rats after injection of deuterium water and showed results consistent with gluconeogenesis accounting for ~81 and ~88% of endogenous glucose production after an 8-h and 10-h fast, respectively (19).

Based on these sets of results, hepatic glucose metabolism in male ZDF rats is characterized as increased gluconeogenesis, a blunted effect of insulin as well as glucose to suppress glucose production and stimulate both glucose uptake and glycogen synthesis. These characteristics of hepatic carbohydrate metabolism in male ZDF rats resemble those of patients with obese type 2 diabetes.

3.5.1. Mechanisms Associated with Impaired Hepatic Glucose Metabolism in Male ZDF Rats (Glucose Phosphorylation and Glycogen Synthesis)

An acute alteration of net hepatic glucose flux is normally tightly linked to flux between glucose and glycogen (88). The flux from glucose to glycogen has two highly regulated steps, glucose phosphorylation by glucokinase (GK) and the formation of a glycoside bond between C1 of activated glucose uridine-5′-diphosphate (UDPG) and C4 of a terminal glucose residue of glycogen by glycogen synthase. Basu et al. (82, 84) showed that lower net splanchnic glucose uptake measured during a hyperglycemic-hyperinsulinemic clamp in human subjects with type 2 diabetes, when compared with nondiabetic subjects, is associated with a proportionate decrease in both flux through the UDPG pool and percentage of extracellular glucose contributing to glycogen synthesis via the direct pathway. Mevorach et al. (89) reported glucose cycling fails to increase even when the concentration of circulating glucose doubles. These observations suggest that insufficient suppression of net hepatic glucose production and a defect in hepatic glucose uptake in response to increased plasma glucose and insulin as seen with type 2 diabetes results, at least partly, from a failure to enhance glucose phosphorylation mediated by GK.

GK activity in liver is regulated by its 68 kDa regulatory protein (GKRP) (90). GKRP binds to GK and allosterically inhibits the enzyme by decreasing its apparent affinity for glucose (90). The inhibition of GK activity by GKRP is due to competitive inhibition of glucose binding to GK (90). GK is released by fructose-1-phosphate (F-1-P), which binds to GKRP and thereby decreases the affinity of GKRP for GK (91).

The regulation of GK by GKRP is associated with a change in intracellular distribution of GK. In studies using cultured hepatocytes (92, 93), GK and GKRP are predominantly located in the nucleus when hepatocytes are cultured with 5.5 mM glucose. However, catalytic amounts of fructose and sorbitol, precursors of F-1-P, cause GK export from the nucleus (92, 94). These F-1-P precursors also markedly increase the rate of glucose phosphorylation in cultured hepatocytes (91, 95).

Changes in concentrations of plasma glucose and/or insulin are major factors in regulating net hepatic glucose flux through suppression of glucose production and stimulation of glucose uptake (88, 96). Studies using cultured hepatocytes have repeatedly shown that glucose per se is a potent stimulator of GK translocation (92, 96), while the effect of insulin is controversial (92, 95). We reported that increases in plasma glucose and/or insulin levels within the physiological range cause rapid GK translocation from the nucleus to the cytoplasm in conscious normal rats (97).

In ZCL rats, hepatic glycogen synthesis from glucose via the direct pathway (Glucose to glucose-6-phosphate to glucose-1-phosphate to UDP-glucose to Glycogen) and glucose cycling (glucose to glucose-6-phosphate and back to glucose) are increased in response to hyperglycemia and/or hyperinsulinemia. In addition to the suppression of endogenous glucose production, all indicate greater glucose phosphorylation (GK flux). This increased glucose phosphorylation is associated with the translocation of GK from the nucleus to the cytoplasm.

Male ZDF rats at an early stage of diabetes (10 weeks of age), on the other hand, exhibit a markedly lower increment of hepatic glycogen synthesis from glucose via the direct pathway and reduced glucose cycling in response to hyperglycemia and/or hyperinsulinemia, which is associated with an apparent defect in GK translocation (22). In these male ZDF rats, intraportal infusion of a small amount of sorbitol to increase F-1-P content, promotes GK export from the nucleus, and furthermore, promotes hepatic glycogen synthesis from glucose via the direct pathway and increases glucose cycling in response to hyperglycemia and/or hyperinsulinemia (86). Therefore, reduced effectiveness of insulin and/or glucose to suppress hepatic glucose production and stimulate glycogen synthesis from plasma glucose (glucose phosphorylation) may result from a failure of the sugar and/or hormone to activate GK by facilitating its dissociation from GKRP and/or translocation from the nucleus to the cytosol.

At a middle stage of diabetes, 14 weeks of age, male ZDF rats exhibit persistent endogenous glucose production and negligible incorporation of plasma glucose into hepatic glycogen despite marked hyperglycemia and hyperinsulinemia. GK and GKRP are co-localized in the cytoplasm rather than the nucleus of hepatocytes (23). However, an intraportal infusion of a small amount of sorbitol to increase cellular F-1-P content is still able to increase hepatic glycogen synthesis from glucose via the direct pathway and glucose cycling in these animals; albeit in the absence of GK translocation (Shiota et al. unpublished data). These results suggest that at this middle stage of diabetes in male ZDF rats, defects in suppression of endogenous glucose production and failure to increase flux from glucose to glycogen in response to a rise in plasma glucose and insulin result from impaired dissociation of GKRP from GK.

Expression of liver GK in male ZDF rats decreases progressively from the middle stage of diabetes (~14 weeks of age) and reaches about 30% of normal by 20 weeks of age (15). When GK expression at 20 weeks of age in male ZDF rats is normalized by utilizing an adenovirus that encodes for the expression of rat liver GK (AdvCMV-GKL), near normal plasma glucose levels are restored along with endogenous glucose production rates. Normal suppression of endogenous glucose production and increased glucose incorporation into glycogen in response to hyperglycemia were also restored (15). These data suggest that low GK expression in liver is therefore responsible for impaired hepatic glucose flux at this late stage of diabetes in male ZDF rats and thereby contributes to hyperglycemia.

The flux from glucose to glycogen is regulated by glucose phosphorylation catalyzed by GK and glycogen synthase activities. Cline et al. (63) reported that activation of glycogen synthase by treatment with an inhibitor of glycogen synthase kinase-3 improved glucose disposal in an oral glucose tolerance test in ZDF rats, which indicated a defect in net glycogenesis. We observed a defect in glycogen synthesis from plasma glucose with defective activation of glycogen synthase and deactivation of glycogen phosphorylase in response to a rise in plasma glucose and insulin in male ZDF rats at an early, middle, and late stage of diabetes (15, 22, 23, 86). When liver glycogen synthase is activated by inhibition of glycogen phosphorylase, using a glycogen phosphorylase inhibitor in ZDF rats at 14 weeks of age, hyperglycemia is markedly improved along with a net increase in hepatic glycogenesis (24). This study showed that a failure to redirect G-6-P flux from glucose to glycogen due to reduced glycogenic flux is partially responsible for insufficient suppression of net hepatic glucose production, but does not explain the reduction in glucose phosphorylation (24).

The catalytic properties of human GK are similar to that of rat GK (98), as is nuclear localization of GK immunoreactivity, which was shown in parenchymal cells of postmortem human liver samples (99). Human GKRP shares 88% identity with rat GKRP (100). Human GKRP is less dependent upon fructose-6-phosphate (F-6-P) binding for its inhibition of GK, yet has a higher affinity for F-6-P than does rat GKRP (101). F-1-P binding to human GKRP counteracts its inhibition of GK in the presence or absence of F-6-P binding (101). These observations imply that human GK activity compared to that of rat is more tightly regulated by GKRP and the phosphoesters, F-1-P and F-6-P.

The effectiveness of glucose per se to inhibit hepatic glucose production is markedly blunted in subjects with type 2 diabetes (102). In individuals with type 2 diabetes, addition of a catalytic amount of a precursor of F-1-P, fructose or sorbitol, improves the glucose and insulin response profiles in oral glucose tolerance tests (103), and nearly normalizes the ability of hyperglycemia per se to suppress net hepatic glucose production (104). Thus, the impairment of short-term activation of GK by glucose via dissociating this enzyme from GKRP is a possible explanation for decreased effectiveness of elevated plasma glucose to suppress net hepatic glucose production and stimulate hepatic glucose uptake in subjects with type 2 diabetes.

In some obese humans who develop fasting hyperglycemia, in addition to the presence of insulin resistance, plasma insulin levels are reduced to levels below that of lean subjects (28). Additionally, in untreated subjects with type 2 diabetes associated with obesity, lower liver GK activity is associated with a 50% reduction in V_{max} compared with lean controls and subjects with just obesity and no fasting hyperglycemia (105). These findings imply similar impairments of GK regulation by GKRP and lower GK activity contribute to a similar deterioration of hepatic glucose metabolism as seen in both patients with type 2 diabetes and male ZDF rats.

4. Glucotoxicity

In patients with type 2 diabetes, the combination of postprandial and chronic hyperglycemia is sometimes referred to as glucotoxicity, which is proposed as an independent factor in the development of insulin resistance (104, 106–108). Elevated blood glucose per se, glucotoxicity, can reduce insulin action in skeletal muscle, liver, and other tissues. It can also reduce the ability of pancreatic β-cells to respond to an acute glycemic challenge.

4.1. Liver Glucotoxicity

When male ZDF rats are treated with a SGLT inhibitor from 9 weeks of age, a time when fasting hyperglycemia first becomes evident, ZDF rats do not experience marked hyperglycemia nor develop impairment in the ability of insulin to suppress endogenous glucose production (109). Male 14-week-old ZDF rats exhibit persistent endogenous glucose production and negligible incorporation of plasma glucose into hepatic glycogen despite marked hyperglycemia and hyperinsulinemia. The administration of a SGLT inhibitor to these animals normalizes blood glucose levels within a day and maintains blood glucose to near normal levels without altering plasma insulin levels. GK and GKRP are co-localized in the cytoplasm of hepatocytes in the liver of these animals (23).

After 7 days of SGLT inhibitor treatment, GK and GKRP are co-localized in the nuclei of hepatocytes. When plasma glucose is raised to levels seen before SGLT inhibitor treatment in these animals, hepatic glucose production is completely suppressed. GK, but not GKRP, is translocated from the nucleus to the cytoplasm. Glucose cycling, glycogen synthesis from plasma glucose, and fractional contribution of plasma glucose to UDP-glucose flux are markedly increased. These observations suggest that impaired regulation of GK by GKRP in ZDF rats is associated with glucotoxicity (23).

Expression of hepatic GK in male ZDF rats is progressively decreased from ~14 weeks of age and reaches about 30% of ZCL levels by 20 weeks (15). Low GK expression in liver is responsible for impaired hepatic glucose flux and much of the resulting hyperglycemia that occurs at 20 weeks of age in male ZDF rats (15). When male ZDF rats are treated with a SGLT2 inhibitor from 14 weeks of age for 6 weeks, blood glucose levels are maintained at normal levels without significant changes in food intake, body weight, plasma levels of insulin, triglyceride and glucagon, and liver triglyceride content. Additionally, GK expression in liver was not decreased (110, 111). These observations further suggest that chronic hyperglycemia (glucotoxicity), by impairing GK activity, leads to progressive deterioration of hepatic glucose metabolism in male ZDF rats.

4.2. Skeletal Muscle Glucotoxicity

Glucose transport across the plasma membrane is a rate-regulatory step of glucose utilization in muscle and is impaired in ZDF rats. Muscle GLUT4 protein is reduced in 26-week-old ZDF rats (37). This reduction in GLUT4 protein is prevented when blood glucose levels are maintained near normal from 7 weeks of age for 19 weeks by acarbose treatment of ZDF rats (37).

4.3. Pancreatic β-Cells Glucotoxicity

Treatment of ZDF rats with phloridin from 6 weeks of age for 6 weeks normalizes plasma glucose levels and maintains pancreatic insulin content and mRNA to levels found in 6-week-old ZDF rats, but increases plasma free fatty acid and triglyceride levels. Treatment of ZDF rats with Bezafibrate, an anti-lipolytic drug, from 6 weeks of age for 6 weeks decreased plasma free fatty acid and triglyceride levels, but failed to reduce hyperglycemia, lower pancreatic TG content, or maintain pancreatic insulin content and mRNA levels. These data suggest that antecent elevated plasma glucose levels, not plasma lipid levels, are associated with elevated islet TG content and decreased insulin mRNA levels in ZDF rats (21).

5. Complications

Chronic hyperglycemia is a major risk factor for microvascular complications (112), which can cause nephrosis, cataracts, hypertension, neuropathy, and impaired wound-healing. Patients with type 2 diabetes and male ZDF rats share these complications.

5.1. Kidney Complications

Urine output in ZDF rats increases by approximately eightfold as early as 10 weeks of age and eventually plateaus at 16–18-fold greater than ZCL rats (113). The ratio of urinary albumin to creatinine, an indicator of microalbuminurea, is increased significantly in ZDF rats as early as 10 weeks of age and continues to rise between weeks 10 and 36 (113). A marked progression in the severity of hydronephrosis occurs in ZDF rats between 16 and 36 weeks of age (113).

5.2. Eye Complications

ZDF rats have microvascular retinopathy (114). Cataracts develop in 21-week-old male ZDF rats. Apoptosis of lens epithelial cells and alterations related to diabetic cataracts are associated with higher levels of advanced glycation end products, NF-κB signaling and iNOS (115).

5.3. Cardiovascular System Complications

Conflicting results have been reported regarding blood pressure levels in ZDF rats. In ZDF rats compared to age-matched ZCL rats, tail-cuff systolic blood pressures are either similar up to 40 weeks of age (116, 117) or higher in ZDF rats after 13 weeks (118) or 20 weeks of age (58, 119). The intra-arterial blood pressures between ZDF and ZCL rats are similar between 12 and 36 weeks of age while under anesthesia (113, 120), or while conscious between 6 and 24 weeks (121), or lower in ZDF rats at 10 weeks of age (122).

5.4. Neurological Complications

ZDF rats develop neuropathy defined as a slowing of motor nerve conduction velocity (3, 123, 124). Motor nerve conduction velocity is significantly reduced in ZDF rats of 12–14 weeks of age, whereas it is not reduced until 32 weeks of age in ZF rats (125). Motor nerve and sensory nerve conduction velocities, endoneurial blood flow, and vascular relaxation in response to acetylcholine are also impaired in ZDF rats at 28 weeks of age (126).

5.5. Skin Complications

ZDF rats exhibit impairments in wound-size reduction, inflammatory response, tissue organization, and connective tissue turnover (127). ZDF rats may therefore be a new model for the study of impaired wound-healing.

6. Leptin Receptor Defect and Diabetic Phenotypes in Male ZDF Rats

The known inherited deficit in ZDF rats is a leptin receptor mutation. Mutations in leptin or its receptor are associated with profound metabolic abnormalities, which include obesity, dyslipidemia, and perturbations in glucose metabolism together with insulin resistance and hyperinsulinemia (128). In the central nervous system (CNS), a deficit of leptin signaling induces food intake that leads to obesity. These changes in adiposity and/or a reduction in direct peripheral leptin signaling in pancreatic β-cells, liver, and skeletal muscle may affect peripheral insulin sensitivity and result in hyperinsulinemia. In addition to these indirect and direct peripheral effects, leptin can regulate glucose metabolism via signaling in the CNS, independent of its effect on food intake and body weight, by modulating sympathetic and neuroendocrine activity. Nevertheless, it still remains doubtful that the entire diabetic phenotype of male ZDF rats, which includes fasting hyperglycemia and loss of β-cell mass, results from only a deficiency in leptin signaling.

A comparison of male ZF and ZDF rats discriminates between the effects of diabetes in ZDF rats from the effects of insulin resistance and/or obesity in ZF rats. Young male ZF and ZDF rats share in addition to obesity many features of metabolic disorders, such as hyperinsulinemia, insulin resistance, glucose intolerance, and hyperlipidemia (124). Fasting blood glucose levels are near normal at a young age, since compensation for insulin resistance occurs through an increase in pancreatic β-cell insulin production and secretion. However, a conspicuous difference develops with aging between male ZDF and ZF rats in that male ZDF rats, not ZF rats, exhibit progressive development of hyperglycemia. With aging, ZF rats maintain the common metabolic features found in young rats and do not become hyperglycemic. Compared to lean rats, the increased β-cell mass in ZF rats is maintained; and in liver, higher GK and lower glucose-6-phosphatase activities are present (129, 130). In this regard, ZF rats share common characteristics with that of most obese humans.

On the other hand, male ZDF rats develop fasting hyperglycemia, which is associated with progressive loss of pancreatic β-cell mass and function, in addition to a loss of liver GK. It thus appears that ZDF rats also carry a genetic defect in β-cell gene transcription that is inherited independently from the leptin receptor mutation (131). The unique diabetic features in male ZDF rats triggered by additional genetic defect(s) create a vicious cycle of escalating hyperglycemia and glucotoxicity, resulting in an age-related progression of diabetes. Since severe type 2 diabetes develops only in a portion of, not all, patients with obesity, exploring the underlying differences in the metabolic phenotypes of ZF and ZDF rats may assist in the elucidation of the mechanism associated with the evolution of patients from obesity to diabetes.

7. Conclusion

Male ZDF rats possess many common features found in patients with type 2 diabetes, including the progressive development of fasting hyperglycemia in addition to extreme postprandial hyperglycemia, progressive loss of pancreatic β-cell mass in addition to dysfunction, a defect in hepatic glucose uptake likely associated with impaired GK activity, and hyperglycemia-induced and obesity-associated complications. Even though the underlying primary genetic basis for these common diabetic features may differ between humans with obese type 2 diabetes and ZDF rats, their shared secondary complications and defects provide ample justification for the use of ZDF rats as an excellent preclinical animal model for obese type 2 diabetes.

References

1. Phillips MS, Liu Q, Hammond HA et al (1996) Leptin receptor missense mutation in the fatty Zucker rat. Nat Genet 13:18–19
2. Truett GE, Bahary N, Friedman JM et al (1991) Rat obesity gene fatty (fa) maps to chromosome 5: evidence for homology with the mouse gene diabetes (db). Proc Natl Acad Sci U S A 88:7806–7809
3. Peterson RG, Shaw WN, Neel MA et al (1990) Zucker diabetic fatty rat as a model for non-insulin-dependent diabetes mellitus. ILAR News 32:16–19
4. Clark JB, Palmer CJ, Shaw WN (1983) The diabetic Zucker fatty rat. Proc Soc Exp Biol Med 173:68–75
5. Corsetti JP, Sparks JD, Peterson RG et al (2000) Effect of dietary fat on the development of non-insulin dependent diabetes mellitus in obese Zucker diabetic fatty male and female rats. Atherosclerosis 148:231–241
6. Peterson RG (1994) alpha-Glucosidase inhibitors in diabetes: lessons from animal studies. Eur J Clin Invest 24(suppl 3):11–18
7. Kava R, Peterson RG, West DB et al (1990) New rat models of obesity and type II diabetes. ILAR News 32:4–8
8. Aleixandre de Artinano A, Miguel Castro M (2009) Experimental rat models to study the metabolic syndrome. Br J Nutr 102:1246–1253
9. Johnson PR, Greenwood MR, Horwitz BA et al (1991) Animal models of obesity: genetic aspects. Annu Rev Nutr 11:325–353
10. Ikeda H, Shino A, Matsuo T et al (1981) A new genetically obese-hyperglycemic rat (Wistar fatty). Diabetes 30:1045–1050
11. Coleman DL, Hummel KP (1967) Studies with the mutation, diabetes, in the mouse. Diabetologia 3:238–248
12. Naggert JK, Mu JL, Frankel W et al (1995) Genomic analysis of the C57BL/Ks mouse strain. Mamm Genome 6:131–133
13. Leiter EH, Coleman DL, Hummel KP (1981) The influence of genetic background on the expression of mutations at the diabetes locus in the mouse: III. Effect of H-2 haplotype and sex. Diabetes 30:1029–1034
14. Munoz MC, Barbera A, Dominguez J et al (2001) Effects of tungstate, a new potential oral antidiabetic agent, in Zucker diabetic fatty rats. Diabetes 50:131–138
15. Torres TP, Catlin RL, Chan R et al (2009) Restoration of hepatic glucokinase expression corrects hepatic glucose flux and normalizes plasma glucose in Zucker diabetic fatty rats. Diabetes 58:78–86
16. Etgen GJ, Oldham BA (2000) Profiling of Zucker diabetic fatty rats in their progression to the overt diabetic state. Metabolism 49:684–688
17. Johnson JH, Ogawa A, Chen L et al (1990) Underexpression of beta cell high Km glucose transporters in noninsulin-dependent diabetes. Science 250:546–549
18. Tokuyama Y, Sturis J, DePaoli AM et al (1995) Evolution of beta-cell dysfunction in the male Zucker diabetic fatty rat. Diabetes 44:1447–1457
19. van Poelje PD, Potter SC, Chandramouli VC et al (2006) Inhibition of fructose 1,6-bisphosphatase reduces excessive endogenous glucose production and attenuates hyperglycemia in Zucker diabetic fatty rats. Diabetes 55:1747–1754
20. Winter CL, Lange JS, Davis MG et al (2005) A nonspecific phosphotyrosine phosphatase inhibitor, bis(maltolato)oxovanadium(IV), improves glucose tolerance and prevents diabetes in Zucker diabetic fatty rats. Exp Biol Med (Maywood) 230:207–216
21. Harmon JS, Gleason CE, Tanaka Y et al (2001) Antecedent hyperglycemia, not hyperlipidemia, is associated with increased islet triacylglycerol content and decreased insulin gene mRNA level in Zucker diabetic fatty rats. Diabetes 50:2481–2486
22. Fujimoto Y, Donahue EP, Shiota M (2004) Defect in glucokinase translocation in Zucker diabetic fatty rats. Am J Physiol Endocrinol Metab 287:E414–E423
23. Fujimoto Y, Torres TP, Donahue EP et al (2006) Glucose toxicity is responsible for the development of impaired regulation of endogenous glucose production and hepatic glucokinase in Zucker diabetic fatty rats. Diabetes 55:2479–2490
24. Torres TP, Fujimoto Y, Donahue EP et al (2011) Defective glycogenesis contributes toward the inability to suppress hepatic glucose production in response to hyperglycemia and hyperinsulinemia in Zucker diabetic fatty rats. Diabetes 60:2225–2233
25. Wijekoon EP, Skinner C, Brosnan ME et al (2004) Amino acid metabolism in the Zucker diabetic fatty rat: effects of insulin resistance and of type 2 diabetes. Can J Physiol Pharmacol 82:506–514
26. Doisaki M, Katano Y, Nakano I et al (2010) Regulation of hepatic branched-chain

alpha-keto acid dehydrogenase kinase in a rat model for type 2 diabetes mellitus at different stages of the disease. Biochem Biophys Res Commun 393:303–307
27. Sparks JD, Phung TL, Bolognino M et al (1998) Lipoprotein alterations in 10- and 20-week-old Zucker diabetic fatty rats: hyperinsulinemic versus insulinopenic hyperglycemia. Metabolism 47:1315–1324
28. Golay A, Felber JP (1994) Evolution from obesity to diabetes. Diabetes Metab 20:3–14
29. Green GM, Guan D, Schwartz JG et al (1997) Accelerated gastric emptying of glucose in Zucker type 2 diabetic rats: role in postprandial hyperglycaemia. Diabetologia 40:136–142
30. Phillips WT, Schwartz JG, McMahan CA (1992) Rapid gastric emptying of an oral glucose solution in type 2 diabetic patients. J Nucl Med 33:1496–1500
31. DeFronzo RA (1988) Lilly lecture 1987. The triumvirate: beta-cell, muscle, liver. A collusion responsible for NIDDM. Diabetes 37:667–687
32. Petersen KF, Dufour S, Savage DB et al (2007) The role of skeletal muscle insulin resistance in the pathogenesis of the metabolic syndrome. Proc Natl Acad Sci U S A 104:12587–12594
33. Leonard BL, Watson RN, Loomes KM et al (2005) Insulin resistance in the Zucker diabetic fatty rat: a metabolic characterisation of obese and lean phenotypes. Acta Diabetol 42:162–170
34. Henriksen EJ (2002) Invited review: effects of acute exercise and exercise training on insulin resistance. J Appl Physiol 93:788–796
35. Shulman GI (2000) Cellular mechanisms of insulin resistance. J Clin Invest 106:171–176
36. Zierath JR, Krook A, Wallberg-Henriksson H (2000) Insulin action and insulin resistance in human skeletal muscle. Diabetologia 43:821–835
37. Friedman JE, de Vente JE, Peterson RG et al (1991) Altered expression of muscle glucose transporter GLUT-4 in diabetic fatty Zucker rats (ZDF/Drt-fa). Am J Physiol 261:E782–E788
38. Cline GW, Johnson K, Regittnig W et al (2002) Effects of a novel glycogen synthase kinase-3 inhibitor on insulin-stimulated glucose metabolism in Zucker diabetic fatty (fa/fa) rats. Diabetes 51:2903–2910
39. Henriksen EJ, Kinnick TR, Teachey MK et al (2003) Modulation of muscle insulin resistance by selective inhibition of GSK-3 in Zucker diabetic fatty rats. Am J Physiol Endocrinol Metab 284:E892–E900
40. Henriksen EJ, Teachey MK (2007) Short-term in vitro inhibition of glycogen synthase kinase 3 potentiates insulin signaling in type I skeletal muscle of Zucker diabetic fatty rats. Metabolism 56:931–938
41. Gerich JE (2010) Role of the kidney in normal glucose homeostasis and in the hyperglycaemia of diabetes mellitus: therapeutic implications. Diabet Med 27:136–142
42. Kamran M, Peterson RG, Dominguez JH (1997) Overexpression of GLUT2 gene in renal proximal tubules of diabetic Zucker rats. J Am Soc Nephrol 8:943–948
43. Cersosimo E, Garlick P, Ferretti J (2000) Regulation of splanchnic and renal substrate supply by insulin in humans. Metabolism 49:676–683
44. Ekberg K, Landau BR, Wajngot A et al (1999) Contributions by kidney and liver to glucose production in the postabsorptive state and after 60 h of fasting. Diabetes 48:292–298
45. Stumvoll M, Chintalapudi U, Perriello G et al (1995) Uptake and release of glucose by the human kidney. Postabsorptive rates and responses to epinephrine. J Clin Invest 96:2528–2533
46. Meyer C, Stumvoll M, Nadkarni V et al (1998) Abnormal renal and hepatic glucose metabolism in type 2 diabetes mellitus. J Clin Invest 102:619–624
47. Meyer C, Woerle HJ, Dostou JM et al (2004) Abnormal renal, hepatic, and muscle glucose metabolism following glucose ingestion in type 2 diabetes. Am J Physiol Endocrinol Metab 287:E1049–E1056
48. Eid A, Bodin S, Ferrier B et al (2006) Intrinsic gluconeogenesis is enhanced in renal proximal tubules of Zucker diabetic fatty rats. J Am Soc Nephrol 17:398–405
49. Butler AE, Janson J, Bonner-Weir S et al (2003) Beta-cell deficit and increased beta-cell apoptosis in humans with type 2 diabetes. Diabetes 52:102–110
50. Clark A, Wells CA, Buley ID et al (1988) Islet amyloid, increased A-cells, reduced B-cells and exocrine fibrosis: quantitative changes in the pancreas in type 2 diabetes. Diabetes Res 9:151–159
51. Kloppel G, Lohr M, Habich K et al (1985) Islet pathology and the pathogenesis of type 1 and type 2 diabetes mellitus revisited. Surv Synth Pathol Res 4:110–125
52. Stefan Y, Orci L, Malaisse-Lagae F et al (1982) Quantitation of endocrine cell con-

tent in the pancreas of nondiabetic and diabetic humans. Diabetes 31:694–700
53. U.K. Prospective Diabetes Study Group (1995) U.K. prospective diabetes study 16. Overview of 6 years' therapy of type II diabetes: a progressive disease. Diabetes 44: 1249–1258
54. Kahn SE (2000) The importance of the beta-cell in the pathogenesis of type 2 diabetes mellitus. Am J Med 108(suppl 6a):2S–8S
55. Pick A, Clark J, Kubstrup C et al (1998) Role of apoptosis in failure of beta-cell mass compensation for insulin resistance and beta-cell defects in the male Zucker diabetic fatty rat. Diabetes 47:358–364
56. Finegood DT, McArthur MD, Kojwang D et al (2001) Beta-cell mass dynamics in Zucker diabetic fatty rats. Rosiglitazone prevents the rise in net cell death. Diabetes 50: 1021–1029
57. Tang J, Pugh W, Polonsky KS et al (1996) Preservation of insulin secretory responses to P2 purinoceptor agonists in Zucker diabetic fatty rats. Am J Physiol 270:E504–E512
58. Tikellis C, Wookey PJ, Candido R et al (2004) Improved islet morphology after blockade of the renin-angiotensin system in the ZDF rat. Diabetes 53:989–997
59. Cherrington AD, Wasserman DH, McGinness OP (1994) Renal contribution to glucose production after a brief fast: fact or fancy? J Clin Invest 93:2303
60. Petersen KF, Laurent D, Rothman DL et al (1998) Mechanism by which glucose and insulin inhibit net hepatic glycogenolysis in humans. J Clin Invest 101:1203–1209
61. Siler SQ, Neese RA, Christiansen MP et al (1998) The inhibition of gluconeogenesis following alcohol in humans. Am J Physiol 275:E897–E907
62. Radziuk J, Pye S (2001) Hepatic glucose uptake, gluconeogenesis and the regulation of glycogen synthesis. Diabetes Metab Res Rev 17:250–272
63. Cline GW, Rothman DL, Magnusson I et al (1994) ^{13}C-nuclear magnetic resonance spectroscopy studies of hepatic glucose metabolism in normal subjects and subjects with insulin-dependent diabetes mellitus. J Clin Invest 94:2369–2376
64. Petersen KF, Cline GW, Gerard DP et al (2001) Contribution of net hepatic glycogen synthesis to disposal of an oral glucose load in humans. Metabolism 50:598–601
65. Radziuk J (1989) Hepatic glycogen in humans: I. Direct formation after oral and intravenous glucose or after a 24-h fast. Am J Physiol 257:E145–E157

66. Anderwald C, Bernroider E, Krssak M et al (2002) Effects of insulin treatment in type 2 diabetic patients on intracellular lipid content in liver and skeletal muscle. Diabetes 51: 3025–3032
67. Boden G, Chen X, Stein TP (2001) Gluconeogenesis in moderately and severely hyperglycemic patients with type 2 diabetes mellitus. Am J Physiol Endocrinol Metab 280:E23–E30
68. Radziuk J, Pye S (2001) Production and metabolic clearance of glucose under basal conditions in type II (non-insulin-dependent) diabetes mellitus. Diabetologia 44:983–991
69. Singhal P, Caumo A, Carey PE et al (2002) Regulation of endogenous glucose production after a mixed meal in type 2 diabetes. Am J Physiol Endocrinol Metab 283:E275–E283
70. Magnusson I, Rothman DL, Katz LD et al (1992) Increased rate of gluconeogenesis in type II diabetes mellitus. A ^{13}C nuclear magnetic resonance study. J Clin Invest 90: 1323–1327
71. Hundal RS, Krssak M, Dufour S et al (2000) Mechanism by which metformin reduces glucose production in type 2 diabetes. Diabetes 49:2063–2069
72. Consoli A, Nurjhan N, Capani F et al (1989) Predominant role of gluconeogenesis in increased hepatic glucose production in NIDDM. Diabetes 38:550–557
73. Mitrakou A, Kelley D, Veneman T et al (1990) Contribution of abnormal muscle and liver glucose metabolism to postprandial hyperglycemia in NIDDM. Diabetes 39:1381–1390
74. Tayek JA, Katz J (1996) Glucose production, recycling, and gluconeogenesis in normals and diabetics: a mass isotopomer (U-^{13}C)glucose study. Am J Physiol 270:E709–E717
75. Ferrannini E, Simonson DC, Katz LD et al (1988) The disposal of an oral glucose load in patients with non-insulin-dependent diabetes. Metabolism 37:79–85
76. Firth RG, Bell PM, Marsh HM et al (1986) Postprandial hyperglycemia in patients with noninsulin-dependent diabetes mellitus. Role of hepatic and extrahepatic tissues. J Clin Invest 77:1525–1532
77. Kelley D, Mokan M, Veneman T (1994) Impaired postprandial glucose utilization in non-insulin-dependent diabetes mellitus. Metabolism 43:1549–1557
78. Krssak M, Brehm A, Bernroider E et al (2004) Alterations in postprandial hepatic glycogen metabolism in type 2 diabetes. Diabetes 53:3048–3056
79. McMahon M, Marsh HM, Rizza RA (1989) Effects of basal insulin supplementation on

79. disposition of mixed meal in obese patients with NIDDM. Diabetes 38:291–303
80. Proietto J, Nankervis AJ, Traianedes K et al (1992) Identification of early metabolic defects in diabetes-prone Australian aborigines. Diabetes Res Clin Pract 17:217–226
81. Thorburn A, Litchfield A, Fabris S et al (1995) Abnormal transient rise in hepatic glucose production after oral glucose in non-insulin-dependent diabetic subjects. Diabetes Res Clin Pract 28:127–135
82. Basu A, Basu R, Shah P et al (2001) Type 2 diabetes impairs splanchnic uptake of glucose but does not alter intestinal glucose absorption during enteral glucose feeding: additional evidence for a defect in hepatic glucokinase activity. Diabetes 50:1351–1362
83. Felig P, Wahren J, Hendler R (1978) Influence of maturity-onset diabetes on splanchnic glucose balance after oral glucose ingestion. Diabetes 27:121–126
84. Basu A, Basu R, Shah P et al (2000) Effects of type 2 diabetes on the ability of insulin and glucose to regulate splanchnic and muscle glucose metabolism: evidence for a defect in hepatic glucokinase activity. Diabetes 49:272–283
85. Iozzo P, Hallsten K, Oikonen V et al (2003) Insulin-mediated hepatic glucose uptake is impaired in type 2 diabetes: evidence for a relationship with glycemic control. J Clin Endocrinol Metab 88:2055–2060
86. Shin JS, Torres TP, Catlin RL et al (2007) A defect in glucose-induced dissociation of glucokinase from the regulatory protein in Zucker diabetic fatty rats in the early stage of diabetes. Am J Physiol Regul Integr Comp Physiol 292:R1381–R1390
87. Giaccari A, Morviducci L, Pastore L et al (1998) Relative contribution of glycogenolysis and gluconeogenesis to hepatic glucose production in control and diabetic rats. A re-examination in the presence of euglycaemia. Diabetologia 41:307–314
88. Rossetti L, Giaccari A, Barzilai N et al (1993) Mechanism by which hyperglycemia inhibits hepatic glucose production in conscious rats. Implications for the pathophysiology of fasting hyperglycemia in diabetes. J Clin Invest 92:1126–1134
89. Mevorach M, Giacca A, Aharon Y et al (1998) Regulation of endogenous glucose production by glucose per se is impaired in type 2 diabetes mellitus. J Clin Invest 102:744–753
90. Van Schaftingen E, Detheux M, Veiga da Cunha M (1994) Short-term control of glucokinase activity: role of a regulatory protein. FASEB J 8:414–419
91. Davies DR, Detheux M, Van Schaftingen E (1990) Fructose 1-phosphate and the regulation of glucokinase activity in isolated hepatocytes. Eur J Biochem 192:283–289
92. Brown KS, Kalinowski SS, Megill JR et al (1997) Glucokinase regulatory protein may interact with glucokinase in the hepatocyte nucleus. Diabetes 46:179–186
93. Toyoda Y, Miwa I, Kamiya M et al (1994) Evidence for glucokinase translocation by glucose in rat hepatocytes. Biochem Biophys Res Commun 204:252–256
94. Jetton TL, Shiota M, Knobel SM et al (2001) Substrate-induced nuclear export and peripheral compartmentalization of hepatic glucokinase correlates with glycogen deposition. Int J Exp Diabetes Res 2:173–186
95. Agius L, Peak M (1993) Intracellular binding of glucokinase in hepatocytes and translocation by glucose, fructose and insulin. Biochem J 296(pt 3):785–796
96. Pagliassotti MJ, Cherrington AD (1992) Regulation of net hepatic glucose uptake in vivo. Annu Rev Physiol 54:847–860
97. Chu CA, Fujimoto Y, Igawa K et al (2004) Rapid translocation of hepatic glucokinase in response to intraduodenal glucose infusion and changes in plasma glucose and insulin in conscious rats. Am J Physiol Gastrointest Liver Physiol 286:G627–G634
98. Cardenas ML, Rabajille E, Niemeyer H (1984) Suppression of kinetic cooperativity of hexokinase D (glucokinase) by competitive inhibitors. A slow transition model. Eur J Biochem 145:163–171
99. Toyoda Y, Kobayashi S, Ito Y et al (1997) Nuclear location of glucokinase in mammalian livers. Med Sci Res 25:627–629
100. Warner JP, Leek JP, Intody S et al (1995) Human glucokinase regulatory protein (GCKR): cDNA and genomic cloning, complete primary structure, and chromosomal localization. Mamm Genome 6:532–536
101. Brocklehurst KJ, Payne VA, Davies RA et al (2004) Stimulation of hepatocyte glucose metabolism by novel small molecule glucokinase activators. Diabetes 53:535–541
102. Tonelli J, Kishore P, Lee DE et al (2005) The regulation of glucose effectiveness: how glucose modulates its own production. Curr Opin Clin Nutr Metab Care 8:450–456
103. Moore MC, Davis SN, Mann SL et al (2001) Acute fructose administration improves oral glucose tolerance in adults with type 2 diabetes. Diabetes Care 24:1882–1887
104. Hawkins M, Gabriely I, Wozniak R et al (2002) Glycemic control determines hepatic

and peripheral glucose effectiveness in type 2 diabetic subjects. Diabetes 51:2179–2189
105. Caro JF, Triester S, Patel VK et al (1995) Liver glucokinase: decreased activity in patients with type II diabetes. Horm Metab Res 27:19–22
106. Kahn BB, Shulman GI, DeFronzo RA et al (1991) Normalization of blood glucose in diabetic rats with phlorizin treatment reverses insulin-resistant glucose transport in adipose cells without restoring glucose transporter gene expression. J Clin Invest 87:561–570
107. Leahy JL, Bonner-Weir S, Weir GC (1992) Beta-cell dysfunction induced by chronic hyperglycemia. Current ideas on mechanism of impaired glucose-induced insulin secretion. Diabetes Care 15:442–455
108. Rossetti L, Giaccari A, DeFronzo RA (1990) Glucose toxicity. Diabetes Care 13:610–630
109. Nawano M, Oku A, Ueta K et al (2000) Hyperglycemia contributes insulin resistance in hepatic and adipose tissue but not skeletal muscle of ZDF rats. Am J Physiol Endocrinol Metab 278:E535–E543
110. Ueta K, Kuikwon K, Printz RL et al (2011) Glucotoxicity (GTX) contributes to progressive reduction of hepatic glucokinase (GK) in Zucker diabetic fatty rats (ZDF) by affecting a post-transcriptional process. Diabetes 60:A459
111. Ueta K, Torres TP, McCoy GA et al (2010) Normalization of hyperglycemia by inhibiting SGLT2 prevents progressive reduction of hepatic glucokinase (GK) expression and improves hepatic glucose metabolism (HGM) in Zucker diabetic fatty (ZDF) rats. Diabetes 59:A166
112. Abdul-Ghani MA, Norton L, Defronzo RA (2011) Role of sodium-glucose cotransporter 2 (SGLT 2) inhibitors in the treatment of type 2 diabetes. Endocr Rev 32:515–531
113. Baynes J, Murray DB (2009) Cardiac and renal function are progressively impaired with aging in Zucker diabetic fatty type II diabetic rats. Oxid Med Cell Longev 2:328–334
114. Danis RP, Yang Y (1993) Microvascular retinopathy in the Zucker diabetic fatty rat. Invest Ophthalmol Vis Sci 34:2367–2371
115. Kim J, Kim CS, Sohn E et al (2010) Lens epithelial cell apoptosis initiates diabetic cataractogenesis in the Zucker diabetic fatty rat. Graefes Arch Clin Exp Ophthalmol 248: 811–818
116. Fredersdorf S, Thumann C, Ulucan C et al (2004) Myocardial hypertrophy and enhanced left ventricular contractility in Zucker diabetic fatty rats. Cardiovasc Pathol 13:11–19
117. Pamarthi MF, Rudd MA, Bukoski RD (2002) Normal perivascular sensory dilator nerve function in arteries of Zucker diabetic fatty rats. Am J Hypertens 15:310–315
118. Toblli JE, Cao G, Giani JF et al (2011) Long-term treatment with nebivolol attenuates renal damage in Zucker diabetic fatty rats. J Hypertens 29:1613–1623
119. Mizuno M, Sada T, Kato M et al (2002) Renoprotective effects of blockade of angiotensin II AT1 receptors in an animal model of type 2 diabetes. Hypertens Res 25:271–278
120. Hoshi S, Shu Y, Yoshida F et al (2002) Podocyte injury promotes progressive nephropathy in Zucker diabetic fatty rats. Lab Invest 82:25–35
121. Cosson E, Valensi P, Laude D et al (2009) Arterial stiffness and the autonomic nervous system during the development of Zucker diabetic fatty rats. Diabetes Metab 35:364–370
122. Marsh SA, Powell PC, Agarwal A et al (2007) Cardiovascular dysfunction in Zucker obese and Zucker diabetic fatty rats: role of hydronephrosis. Am J Physiol Heart Circ Physiol 293:H292–H298
123. Coppey LJ, Gellett JS, Davidson EP et al (2001) Effect of antioxidant treatment of streptozotocin-induced diabetic rats on endoneurial blood flow, motor nerve conduction velocity, and vascular reactivity of epineurial arterioles of the sciatic nerve. Diabetes 50:1927–1937
124. Shafrir E (1992) Animal models of non-insulin-dependent diabetes. Diabetes Metab Rev 8:179–208
125. Oltman CL, Coppey LJ, Gellett JS et al (2005) Progression of vascular and neural dysfunction in sciatic nerves of Zucker diabetic fatty and Zucker rats. Am J Physiol Endocrinol Metab 289:E113–E122
126. Oltman CL, Davidson EP, Coppey LJ et al (2008) Vascular and neural dysfunction in Zucker diabetic fatty rats: a difficult condition to reverse. Diabetes Obes Metab 10:64–74
127. Slavkovsky R, Kohlerova R, Tkacova V et al (2011) Zucker diabetic fatty rat: a new model of impaired cutaneous wound repair with type II diabetes mellitus and obesity. Wound Repair Regen 19:515–525
128. Morton GJ, Schwartz MW (2011) Leptin and the central nervous system control of glucose metabolism. Physiol Rev 91:389–411

129. Sanchez-Gutierrez JC, Sanchez-Arias JA, Lechuga CG et al (1994) Decreased responsiveness of basal gluconeogenesis to insulin action in hepatocytes isolated from genetically obese (fa/fa) Zucker rats. Endocrinology 134:1868–1873
130. Spydevold SO, Greenbaum AL, Baquer NZ et al (1978) Adaptive responses of enzymes of carbohydrate and lipid metabolism to dietary alteration in genetically obese Zucker rats (fa/fa). Eur J Biochem 89:329–339
131. Griffen SC, Wang J, German MS (2001) A genetic defect in beta-cell gene expression segregates independently from the fa locus in the ZDF rat. Diabetes 50:63–68

Chapter 9

The GK Rat: A Prototype for the Study of Non-overweight Type 2 Diabetes

Bernard Portha, Marie-Hélène Giroix, Cecile Tourrel-Cuzin, Hervé Le-Stunff, and Jamileh Movassat

Abstract

Type 2 diabetes mellitus (T2D) arises when the endocrine pancreas fails to secrete sufficient insulin to cope with the metabolic demand because of β-cell secretory dysfunction and/or decreased β-cell mass. Defining the nature of the pancreatic islet defects present in T2D has been difficult, in part because human islets are inaccessible for direct study. This review is aimed to illustrate to what extent the Goto Kakizaki rat, one of the best characterized animal models of spontaneous T2D, has proved to be a valuable tool offering sufficient commonalities to study this aspect. A comprehensive compendium of the multiple functional GK abnormalities so far identified is proposed in this perspective, together with their time-course and interactions. A special focus is given toward the pathogenesis of defective β-cell number and function in the GK model. It is proposed that the development of T2D in the GK model results from the complex interaction of multiple events: (1) several susceptibility loci containing genes responsible for some diabetic traits; (2) gestational metabolic impairment inducing an epigenetic programming of the offspring pancreas and the major insulin target tissues; and (3) environmentally induced loss of β-cell differentiation due to chronic exposure to hyperglycemia/hyperlipidemia, inflammation, and oxidative stress.

Key words: Type 2 diabetes, GK rat, β-Cell, Insulin action, Glucose tolerance, Hepatic glucose production, Diabetic complications, Glucotoxicity, Lipotoxicity, Hypertension, Quantitative trait locus, Epigenetic

1. Introduction

Syndromes resembling human type 2 diabetes (T2D) can be induced by treating animals with drugs or viruses, excising their pancreases, or manipulating their diet. Alternatively, they can also occur spontaneously in some animal species. Of course, none of the known animal models can be taken to reproduce human diabetes, but they are believed to illustrate various types of etiological and pathogenic mechanisms that could also operate in humans.

Among these models, the Goto Kakizaki (GK) line of the Wistar (W) rat strain can be regarded as one of the best available rodent strains for the study of inherited T2D. During the last three decades, it has been extensively used in experimental diabetes research reported in hundreds of publications (reviews in refs. (1–4)). We and others have found that defects in glucose homeostasis and insulin secretion and action together with long-standing diabetic complications which in many ways resemble those described in human T2D develop in GK rats. Our review aims to describe the method first used by Goto et al. (5, 6) to generate the GK rat, to sum up the informations so far collected in this diabetes model, and to highlight its potential as well as its limitations for future research.

2. The GK (Goto Kakizaki) Model: How to Generate Rats with Spontaneous T2D?

The GK line was established by repeated inbreeding from Wistar (W) rats selected at the upper limit of normal distribution for glucose tolerance (5–7). In the 1970s, Goto and coworkers in Sendai, Japan, initiated the GK substrain. They selected nine animals of each gender from 211 healthy Wistar rats, with the lowest glucose tolerance values, but still within the normal range in response to an oral glucose tolerance test (OGTT) (5, 7). Repeated selection of rats with tendency to lowest glucose tolerance resulted in clear-cut glucose intolerance after five generations (Fig. 1). Until the end of the 1980s, GK rats were bred only in Sendai (GK/Sen) (5). Colonies were then initiated with breeding pairs from Japan, in Paris, France (GK/Par) (8), Dallas, TX, USA (GK/Dal) (9), Stockholm, Sweden (GK/Sto) (1), Cardiff, UK (GK/Card) (10), Coimbra, Portugal (GK/Coi) (11), Tampa, USA (GK/Tamp) (12), at Kuwait city (GK/Kuwait) (13), and at the National Rodent Laboratory Animal Center in Shanghai, China (GK/Shang) (14). Some other colonies existed for shorter periods during the 1990s in London, UK (GK/Lon) (15), Aarhus, Denmark, Seattle, USA (GK/Sea) (16). There are also GK rat colonies derived from Paris in Oxford, UK (GK/Ox) (17) and Brussels, Belgium (GK/Brus) (18). Also, GK rats are available commercially from Japanese breeders Charles River Japan, Yokohama, Oriental Yeast, Tokyo, Clea Japan Inc., Osaka (GK/Clea), Japan SLC, Shizuoka (GK/SLC), Takeda Lab Ltd., Osaka (GK/Taked), and from Taconic, USA (GK/Mol/Tac).

In our colony (GK/Par subline) maintained since 1989, the adult GK/Par body weight is 10–20% lower than that of age- and sex-matched control animals. In male GK/Par rats, non-fasting plasma glucose levels are typically 10–14 mM (6–8 mM in age-matched W inbred controls). Despite the fact that GK rats in the

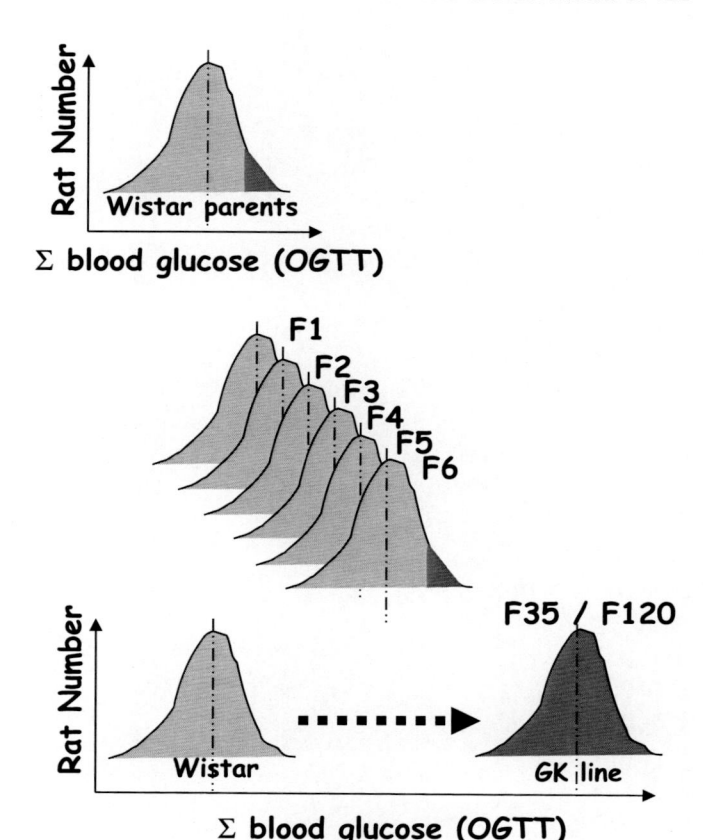

Fig. 1. From the nondiabetic Wistar (W) rat to the spontaneously diabetic GK (Goto-Kakizaki) rat. The inbred GK rat line (Wistar strain) was produced by Goto et al. at Tohoku University, Sendaï, Japan, by selective breeding of normal Wistar rats over many generations using glucose tolerance value (and not basal glucose value only) as a discriminant phenotype (5). Only W rats selected at the upper limit of normal distribution for glucose tolerance were used. The diabetic state (basal hyperglycemia) was reported to become stable after the 30 generations of selective crosses in the original Japanese colony. Here is illustrated the distribution of the sum of blood glucose values (Σ blood glucose) during standardized oral glucose tolerance tests (OGTT) performed in original parent W rats, in rats from generations F1 to F35 in the original Japanese colony and in rats from generations F35 to F120 bred under our conditions in Paris from 1989 to now (subline GK/Par). In the inbred GK/Par rat line, all rats are non-overweight, nonketotic, and display moderate fasting hyperglycemia with strong postprandial glucose intolerance. No attenuation, nor aggravation, of the diabetic phenotype overtime (more than 20 years and 80 generations) was registered in the GK/Par line.

various colonies bred in Japan and outside over 20 years have maintained rather stable degree of glucose intolerance, other characteristics such as β-cell number, insulin content, and islet metabolism and secretion have been reported to differ between some of the different colonies, suggesting that different local breeding environment and/or newly introduced genetic changes account for contrasting phenotypic properties. Presently, it is not clear whether the reported differences are artefactual or true. Careful and extensive identification of GK phenotype within each local subline is therefore necessary when comparing data from different GK sources (review in ref. (19)). As an illustration of this point, we have recently compared insulin and glucagon release by GK/Mol/Tac rats to that of GK/Par rats, using the perfused pancreas technique. Despite no significant difference as far as body weight, basal postabsorptive plasma glucose level, and glucose tolerance to i.v. glucose in vivo are concerned (8 weeks old males), a milder impairment of insulin release in response to glucose (preservation of first phase) or arginine, together with an increased glucagon release in response to arginine, was found in the GK/Mol/Tac as compared to the GK/Par rats.

3. Adult Diabetic GK Rats Have a Perturbed Pancreatic Islet Architecture, Decreased β-Cell Number, and Multiple β-Cell Functional Defects

The adult pancreases of GK/Par, GK/Sto, or GK/Sen exhibit two different populations of islets in situ: large islets with pronounced fibrosis and heterogeneity in the staining of their β-cells, and small islets with heavily stained β-cells and normal architecture (2, 6, 7, 20). The mantle of glucagon and somatostatin cells is disrupted and these cells are found intermingled between β-cells. These changes increase in prevalence with aging (7). No major alteration in pancreatic glucagon content, expressed per pancreatic weight, has been demonstrated in GK/Sto rats (21), although the total α-cell mass was decreased by about 35% in adult GK/Par rats (22). The peripheral localization of glucagon-positive cells in W islets was replaced in GK/Sen, GK/Sto, and GK/Par rats with a more random distribution throughout the core of the islets (23). Pancreatic somatostatin content was slightly but significantly increased in GK/Sto rats (21). Chronic inflammation at the level of the GK/Par islet has recently received demonstration and it is now considered as a pathophysiological contributor in T2D (24–27). Using an Affymetrix microarray approach to evaluate islet gene expression in freshly isolated adult GK/Par islets, we found that 34% of the 71 genes found to be overexpressed belong to inflammatory/immune response gene family and 24% belong to extracellular matrix (ECM)/cell adhesion gene family (24). Numerous macrophages (CD68[+] and MHC class II[+]) and granulocytes were found in/around adult GK/Par islets (24). Upregulation of the MHC class II gene was also reported in a recent study of global expression profiling in GK/Mol/Tac islets (28). Immunolocalization with anti-fibronectin and anti-vWF antibodies indicated that ECM deposition progresses from intra- and peri-islet vessels, as it happens in microangiopathy (24). These data demonstrate that a marked inflammatory reaction accompanies GK/Par islet fibrosis and suggest that islet alterations develop in a way reminiscent of microangiopathy (26). The previous reports by our group and others that increased blood flow and altered vascularization are present in the GK/Par and GK/Sto models (29–31) are consistent with such a view. The increased islet blood flow in GK rats may be accounted for by an altered vagal nerve regulation mediated by nitric oxide, since vagotomy as well as inhibition of NO synthase normalized GK/Sto islet flow (30). In addition, islet capillary pressure was increased in GK/Sto rats (32), a defect reversed after normalization of glycemia by phlorizin treatment. The precise relationship between islet microcirculation and β-cell secretory function remains to be established. Immunohistochemistry on diabetic GK/Par pancreases showed, unlike W islets, the presence of nitrotyrosine and HNE labelings which identify ROS and lipid peroxidation, respectively. Marker-positive cells were predominantly localized at the GK/Par islet periphery or along ducts. Intriguingly, no marker-positive cell was detected within the islets in the same GK/Par pancreases (33). Such was not apparently the case in GK/Taked pancreases, as 8-OHdG and accumulation of HNE-modified proteins accumulation were described within the islets. In this last study, the animals were older as compared to our study and accumulation of markers was correlated to hyperglycemia duration (34). This suggest that the lack of OS-positive cells within islets as found in the young adult diabetic GK/Par is only transient and represents an early stage for a time-dependent evolutive islet adaptation.

In the adult hyperglycemic GK/Par rats (males or females), total pancreatic β-cell mass is decreased (by 60%) (2, 22). This alteration of the β-cell population cannot be ascribed to increased β-cell apoptosis but is related, at least partly, to significantly decreased β-cell replication as measured in vivo, in situ (2). A meaningful set of data from our group (35–38) suggests that the permanently reduced β-cell mass in the GK/Par rat also reflects a permanent limitation of β-cell neogenesis (as discussed below). The islets isolated by standard collagenase procedure from adult GK/Par pancreases show limited decreased β-cell number (by 20% only) and low insulin content compared with control islets (39). The islet DNA content was decreased to a similar extent, consistent with our morphometric data, which indicates that there is no major change in the relative contribution of β-cells to total endocrine cells in the GK islets. In addition, the insulin content, when expressed relative to DNA, remains lower in GK islets than in W islets, which supports some degranulation in the β-cells of diabetic animals (39). Electron microscopy observation of β-cell in GK/SLC pancreas revealed that the number of beta granules is decreased and that of immature granules increased. The Golgi apparatus was developed and the cisternae of the rough endoplasmic reticulum were dilated, indicating cell hyperfunction (40). The distribution of various GK islet cell types appears to differ between some of the GK rat colonies. Thus, in the Stockholm colony, β-cell density and relative volume of insular cells were alike in adult GK/Sto rats and control W rats (1, 21, 22). Similar results were reported in the Dallas colony (GK/Dal) (9). Reduction of adult β-cell mass to an extent similar to that we reported in GK/Par rats was however mentioned in GK/Sen rats (6), in GK/Taked (41), in GK/Clea (42), and in GK/Coi (43). Another element of heterogeneity between the different GK sources is related to the time of appearance of significant β-cell mass reduction when it is observed: it varies from fetal age in GK/Par to neonatal age in GK/Coi (11) or young adult age (8 weeks) in GK/Taked (41) and GK/SLC (40). The reason for such discrepancies in the onset and the severity of the β-cell mass reduction among colonies is not identified, but can be ascribed to differences in islet morphometric methodologies and/or characteristics acquired within each colony and arising from different nutritional and environmental conditions.

As for total pancreatic β-cell mass, there is some controversy regarding the content of pancreatic hormones in GK rats. In the adult hyperglycemic GK/Par rats, total pancreatic insulin stores are decreased by 60–40% (2). In other GK rat colonies (Takeda, Stockholm, Seattle), total insulin store values have been found similarly or more moderately decreased, compared with control rats (16, 21, 44–47). The islets isolated by standard collagenase procedure from adult GK/Par pancreases show lower insulin content compared with control islets (39). In addition, when expressed relative to DNA, the GK/Par islet insulin content remains lower (by 30%) than in W islets, therefore supporting some degranulation in the diabetic β-cells (39). Glucose-stimulated insulin biosynthesis in freshly isolated GK/Par, GK/Jap, or GK/Sto islets has been reported grossly normal (23, 48, 49). The rates of biosynthesis, processing, and secretion of newly synthesized (pro)insulin were comparable (23). This is remarkable in the face of markedly lower prohormone convertase PC2 immunoreactivity and expression in the GK/Sto islets, while the expression patterns of insulin, PC1, and carboxypeptidase E (CPE) remained normal (23). Circulating insulin immunoreactivity in GK/Sto rats was predominantly insulin 1 and 2 in the expected normal ratios with no (pro)insulin evident. The finding that proinsulin biosynthesis and processing of proinsulin appeared normal in adult GK rats suggests that the defective insulin release by β-cells does not arise from a failure to recognize glucose as an activator of prohormone biosynthesis and granule biogenesis. Rather it points to an inability of the β-cell population as a whole to meet the demands on insulin secretion imposed by chronic hyperglycemia in vivo. Although basal circulating GK insulin levels were similar or slightly elevated as compared to W rats, they were always inappropriate for the level of glycemia, indicative of a secretory defect.

Impaired glucose-stimulated insulin secretion (GSIS) has been repeatedly demonstrated in GK rats (whatever the colony), in vivo

(8, 47, 50–52), in the perfused isolated pancreas (1, 8, 21, 45, 53, 54), and in freshly isolated islets (15, 45, 48, 55). A wide panel of alterations or defects has been reported in the stimulus secretion coupling for glucose in GK islets. GLUT2 is underexpressed, but not likely to the extent that it could explain the impairment of insulin release (9). This assumption is supported by the fact that glucokinase/hexokinase activities are normal in GK rat islets (56–58). In addition, glycolysis rates in GK rat islets are unchanged or increased compared with control islets (15, 45, 48, 55, 58–61). Furthermore, oxidation of glucose has been reported decreased (48), unchanged (15, 45, 58, 60, 62, 63), or even enhanced (59). There exists, however, a common message between these data: the ratio of oxidized to glycolysed glucose was always reduced in GK islets compared to W islets. Also, lactate dehydrogenase gene expression (33) and lactate production (59) are increased and pyruvate dehydrogenase activity is decreased (64) in GK rat islets. In GK/Par islets, we showed that mitochondria exhibit a specific decrease in the activities of FAD-dependent glycerophosphate dehydrogenase (48, 58) and branched-chain ketoacid dehydrogenase (39). Similar reduction of the FAD-linked glycerol phosphate dehydrogenase activity was reported in GK/Sto islets (56, 65). These enzymatic abnormalities could work in concert to depress glucose oxidation. An inhibitory influence of islet fatty acid oxidation on glucose oxidation can be eliminated since the islet triglyceride content was found normal and etomoxir, an inhibitor of fatty acid oxidation, failed to restore glucose-induced insulin release in GK/Sto islets (64). We also found that the β-cells of adult GK/Par rats had a significantly smaller mitochondrial volume compared to control β-cells (66). No major deletion or restriction fragment polymorphism could be detected in mtDNA from adult GK/Par islets (66). However, they contained markedly less mtDNA than control islets. The lower islet mtDNA was paralleled by decreased content of some islet mt mRNAs such as cytochrome b (66). In accordance with this, insufficient increase in ATP generation in response to high glucose was shown (58). This supports the hypothesis that the defective insulin response to glucose in GK islet is accounted for by an impaired ATP production, closure of the ATP-regulated K$^+$ channels (57), and impaired elevation of intracellular [Ca^{2+}) (63, 67, 68). Such a view validated in the GK/Par β-cell is however contradictory to the reports in GK/Sto and GK/Sea islets that the ATP production rate is unimpaired (16, 59). Other energy metabolism defects identified in GK/Sto islets include increased glucose cycling due to increased glucose-6-phosphatase activity (45, 59) and decreased pyruvate carboxylase activity (65). It is possible that these alterations may affect ATP concentrations locally. However, the enzyme dysfunctions were restored by normalization of glycemia in GK/Sto rats (65), but with only partial improvement of GSIS. Hence, it is likely that these altered enzyme activities result from a glucotoxic effect rather than being primary causes behind the impaired GSIS. Also, lipotoxic effects leading to defective insulin release have been observed in GK rats on high-fat diet (69, 70), possibly mediated by a mechanism partly involving modulation of UCP-2 expression.

Phosphoinositide (68) and cyclic AMP metabolism (68, 71) are also affected in GK/Par islets. While carbachol was able to promote normal inositol generation in GK/Par islets, high glucose failed to increase inositol phosphate accumulation. The inability of glucose to stimulate IP production is not related to defective phospholipase C activity per se (total activity in islet homogenates is normal) (68). It is rather linked to abnormal targeting of the phosphorylation of phosphoinositides: the activity of phosphatidyl-inositol kinase, which is the first of the two phosphorylating activities responsible for the generation of phosphatidyl-inositol biphosphate, is clearly reduced ((2), Giroix, unpublished data). Moreover, deficient calcium handling and ATP supply in response to glucose probably also contribute to abnormal activation of PI kinases and phospholipase C. A marked decrease in SERCA3 expression has also been described in the GK/Sto islets (72). Concerning cAMP, it is remarkable that its intracellular content is very high in GK/Par β-cells already at low glucose (68, 71). The high basal cAMP level most likely reflects an increased cAMP generation in GK/Par as compared to W islets since: (1) forskolin dose-dependently induced an exaggerated cAMP accumulation; (2) AC2, AC3, and Gαs proteins were overexpressed; (3) IBMX-activated cAMP accumulation was less efficient and PDE3B and PDE1C mRNA were decreased. Moreover, the GK/Par insulin release apparatus appears less sensitive to cAMP, since GK/Par islets released less insulin at submaximal cAMP levels and required five times more cAMP to reach a maximal secretion rate no longer different from W (71). In the GK/Sto rat, it has been shown that increased AC3 is due to functional mutations in the promoter region of the AC3 gene (73). We do not retain this hypothesis in the GK/Par islet since we found that the expressions (mRNA) of AC2 and AC3, and of GαS and Gαolf, are not increased in the prediabetic GK/Par islets (71). Furthermore, cAMP is not further enhanced at increasing glucose concentrations (at variance with the situation in normal β-cells) (68, 71). This suggests that there exists a block in the steps linking glucose metabolism to activation of adenylate cyclase in the GK/Par β-cell. Nevertheless, GLP-1 was able to reactivate GK/Par insulin secretion so that GSIS became indistinguishable from that of W. This GLP-1 effect took place in the absence of any improvement of the $[Ca^{2+}]_i$ response and correlated with an activation of the cAMP-dependent PKA-dependent pathway (71). The increased cAMP production has also offered the possibility to fully restore the β-cell secretory competence to glucose in GK/Sto islets as well (53, 71). This also proves that the glucose incompetence of the GK/Par β-cell is not irreversible and emphasizes the usefulness of GLP-1 as a therapeutic agent in T2D. Also, cholinergic stimulation has been demonstrated to restore GSIS from GK/Sto as well as GK/Par islets (68, 74). We have proposed that such a stimulation is not mediated through activation of the PKC pathway, but via a paradoxical activation of the cAMP/PKA pathway to enhance Ca^{2+}-stimulated insulin release in the GK/Par β-cell (68). In GK/Sto rat islets, other intriguing mechanisms behind defective GSIS have been reported such as: dysfunction of islet lysosomal enzymes (47), excessive NO generation (75, 76), or marked impairment of the glucose–heme oxygenase–carbon monoxide signaling pathway (77). Islet activities of classical lysosomal enzymes, such as acid phosphatase, N-acetyl-beta-D-glucosaminidase, beta-glucuronidase, and cathepsin D, were found reduced by 20–35% in the GK/Sto rat. In contrast, the activities of the lysosomal alpha-glucosidehydrolases (acid glucan-1,4-alpha-glucosidase and acid alpha-glucosidase) were increased by 40–50%. Neutral alpha-glucosidase (endoplasmic reticulum) was unaffected. Since no sign of an acarbose effect on GK alpha-glucosidehydrolase activity (contrarily to W islet) was seen, it was proposed that dysfunction of the islet lysosomal/vacuolar system participates to impairment of GSIS in the GK/Sto rat (47). Electron microscopy analysis from our group has revealed an increased number of autophagosomes in β-cells of diabetic GK/Par rats (unpublished observation) and is suggestive of upregulation of autophagy. Excessive autophagy has also been described in muscles of GK/Shang rats and it was associated with induction of LC3B, Beclin1 and DRP1 (key molecules mediating the autophagy pathway) and it has been proposed that hyperglycemia-associated oxidative stress may induce autophagy through upregulation of the ROS-ERK/JNK-p53 pathway, which may contribute to mitochondrial loss in soleus muscle of diabetic GK rats (78). An abnormally increased NO production in the GK/Sto islets might also be an important factor in the pathogenesis of β-cell dysfunction, since it was associated with abnormal iNOS expression in insulin and glucagon cells, increased ncNOS activity, impaired glucose-stimulated insulin release, glucagon hypersecretion, and impaired glucose-induced glucagon suppression. Moreover, pharmacological blockade of islet NO production by the NOS inhibitor NG-nitro-L-arginine methyl ester greatly improved hormone secretion from GK/Sto islets, and GLP-1 suppressed iNOS and ncNOS expression and activity with almost full restoration of insulin release and partial restoration of glucagon release (75, 76). Also carbon monoxide (CO) derived from β-cell heme oxygenase (HO) might be involved in the secretory dysfunction. A prominent expression of the inducible HO (HO-1) was found in both GK/Sto (77) and GK/Par (33) islets. Decreased HO activity and HO-2 protein expression were reported in GK/Sto islets (77). A diminished pattern of expression and glucose-stimulated activation of several PKC isoenzymes (alpha, theta, and zeta) has been reported in GK/Sto islets, while the novel isoenzyme PKC epsilon not only showed a high expression level but also lacked glucose activation (79, 80). Since broad-range inhibition of the translocation of PKC isoenzymes by BIS increased the exocytotic efficacy of Ca^{2+} to trigger secretion in isolated GK/Sto β-cells (80), perturbed levels and/or activation of some PKC isoforms may be part of the defective signals downstream to glucose metabolism, involved in the GK insulin secretory lesion. Peroxovanadium, an inhibitor of islet protein-tyrosine phosphatase (PTP) activities, was shown to enhance GSIS from GK/Sto islets (81, 82). One possible target for this effect could be PTP sigma that is overexpressed in GK/Sto islets (83). At present, it is not known which exocytosis-regulating proteins are affected by the increased PTPase activity. In addition, defects in islet protein histidine phosphorylation have been proposed to contribute to impaired insulin release in GK/Sea islets (84). Lastly, an increased storage and secretion of amylin relative to insulin was reported in the GK/Sto rat (85) and GLP1 treatment in vivo was recently reported to exert a beneficial effect on the ratio of amylin to insulin mRNA in GK pancreas besides improvement of GSIS (86). This is consistent with hypersecretion of amylin being one of the factors contributing to the impairment of GSIS.

In addition to these upstream abnormalities, important defects reside late in signal transduction, i.e., in the exocytotic machinery. Indeed, GSIS was markedly impaired in GK/Taked, GK/Sto, GK/Sea, and GK/Par islets also when the islets were depolarized by a high concentration of potassium chloride and the ATP-regulated K^+ channels kept open by diazoxide ((16, 34, 87), Szkudelski and Giroix, unpublished data). Similar results were obtained when insulin release was induced by exogenous calcium in electrically permeabilized GK/Jap islets (87). In fact, markedly reduced expressions of the SNARE complex proteins (alpha-SNAP, SNAP-25, syntaxin-1, Munc13-1, Munc18-1, N-ethylmaleimide-sensitive fusion protein, and synaptotagmin 3) have been demonstrated in GK/Sto and GK/Taked islets (49, 88, 89). We also recently found similar results in the GK/Par islets (Tourrel-Cuzin, unpublished data). Thus, a reduced number of docking granules may account for impaired β-cell secretion (90) and this defect should partly be related to glucotoxicity (88). Actin cytoskeleton has also been implicated in regulated exocytosis. The level of total actin protein has been found similar in GK/Par and W islets (91), at variance with reports in other GK rat lines (49, 88). However, confocal analysis of the distribution of phalloidin-stained cortical actin filaments revealed a higher density of the cortical actin web nearby the plasma membrane in GK/Par islets as compared to W. Moreover, preliminary functional results suggest that the higher density of actin cortical web in the GK/Par islets contributes to the defects in GSIS exhibited by GK islets (91).

Among the non-glucidic insulin stimulators, arginine has been shown to induce a normal or even augmented insulin response from perfused pancreases or isolated islets of GK/Clea, GK/Par, GK/Sto, and GK/Lon (8, 16, 53). Insulin responses to leucine and its metabolite, ketoisocaproate (KIC), were found diminished in GK/Par and GK/Sto rats (1, 39, 48). This was attributed to defective mitochondrial oxidative decarboxylation of KIC operated by the branched-chain 2-ketoacid dehydrogenase (BCKDH) complex (39). However, in GK/Lon and GK/Taked islets, KIC induced normal insulin responses (15, 57). Finally, it is of interest that GK islets are duly responsive to non-nutrient stimuli such as the sulfonylureas gliclazide (GK/Par) (48) and mitiglinide (GK/Sto) (92), the combination of Ba^{2+} and theophylline (GK/Par) (48), or high external K^+ concentrations (GK/Lon, GK/Sto, GK/Seat, GK/Par) ((16, 54, 93), Dolz and Portha, unpublished data). However, this does not support the assumption from the molecular biology data that there exists a defect in the late steps of insulin secretion. As a tentative to elucidate this apparent contradiction, exocytosis assessment with high time-resolution membrane capacitance measurement in GK/Sto pancreatic slices showed a decreased efficacy of depolarization-evoked Ca^{2+} influx to trigger rapid vesicle release, contrasting with a facilitation of vesicle release in response to strong sustained Ca^{2+} stimulation (80).

Considerable interest has recently been focused on the putative role of oxidative stress (OS) upon deterioration of β-cell function/survival in diabetes. Recent data from our group indicate that paradoxically GK/Par islets revealed protected against OS since they maintained basal ROS accumulation similar or even lower than nondiabetic islets. Remarkably, GK/Par insulin secretion also exhibited strong resistance to the toxic effect of exogenous H_2O_2 or endogenous ROS exposures. Such adaptation was associated to both high glutathione content and overexpression of a large set of genes encoding antioxidant proteins as well as UCP2 (4, 33). A recent review supplies a compendium of the abnormal intracellular sites so far identified in the β-cells of diabetic GK from the different sources (19).

4. Adult Diabetic GK Rats Have Increased Endogenous Glucose Production and Low Insulin-Stimulated Peripheral Glucose Uptake

Basal (post-absorptive) hepatic glucose production is increased in 2-month-old GK/Par rats (94–97). The clamp studies revealed a decreased insulin-suppressive effect on hepatic glucose production, demonstrating that the liver of adult GK/Par rats was indeed resistant to insulin action (94–96). However, one cannot presently eliminate the possibility that abnormal levels of some blood-borne substances such as corticosterone which is elevated (but not glucagon which is normal) (98) may also contribute to hepatic insulin resistance in the GK/Par rat. In the liver of GK/Tac rats, a time series gene array analysis led to the conclusion that there was a disruption in lipid metabolism together with a chronic activation of natural immunity (99).

In the GK/Par rats, in vivo glucose uptake by the whole body (GUR) in the basal state was increased compared with that in controls (94–97). Such was the tendency in most of the tissues tested individually. Because this was obtained in the presence of high plasma glucose levels, it is difficult to conclude from this sole experiment whether peripheral insulin action is impaired in these diabetic rats. The clear answer was obtained from hyperinsulinemic-euglycemic clamp experiments, which indicated that the whole-body GUR was significantly decreased in 2-month-old GK/Par rats and that in some peripheral tissues (epitrochlearis muscle, periovarian and inguinal white adipose tissues, heart, interscapular brown adipose tissue), but not all, GUR was significantly lower compared with corresponding GUR in control W rats. Therefore, there was no in vivo evidence for a clear-cut decreased skeletal muscle insulin action in adult GK/Par rats (94, 96). Others have also mentioned a minimal impairment of insulin-stimulated muscle glucose uptake in adult hybrid GKSto/Wistar rats (100). However, in vitro studies of soleus muscles from diabetic GK/Sto rats concluded that maximal insulin-stimulated Akt kinase activity and glucose transport were reduced compared with W rats. Importantly, the defects at the level of Akt kinase and glucose transport were completely restored by phlorizin treatment, suggesting that hyperglycemia per se may directly contribute to the development of muscle insulin resistance in this model through alterations in insulin action on Akt kinase and glucose transport (101, 102). Furthermore, insulin resistance occurred in a fiber-type-specific manner in GK/Sto skeletal muscles. Tyrosine phosphorylation of IRS-1 and IRS-1-associated PI 3-kinase activity was severely reduced in oxidative (soleus) muscle, with no impairment in glycolytic (EDL) muscle. In contrast, downstream components of the insulin signal transduction pathway, including Akt and glucose transport, were impaired in oxidative and glycolytic muscle from GK/Sto rats and fully restored to W level with improved glycemic control (103). Insulin resistance and defects in signal transduction have also been noted in skeletal muscle of GK/Sen, GK/Tamp, and GK/Tac rats (104–108). In addition, alterations in muscle fiber type composition in GK/Clea rats have been reported (109). Defects in muscle microvasculature have also been documented in GK/Tac rats, which may be important to both glucose delivery/uptake by muscle as well as its metabolism and function (110–112). Interestingly, array data in GK/Tac suggested increased oxidative capacity in muscles, as well as the presence of chronic inflammation in the musculature (108).

Because in GK/Par rats, the overall decreased insulin-induced GUR could not be supported by a major reduction of the in vivo insulin-induced glucose uptake by the skeletal muscles, we believe that it would not be related to a major defective insulin action, but rather to an impaired proportion of white adipose tissue and/or muscle tissue in the GK/Par rat compared with the W rat. Our assumption is supported by an increased Lee index (body weight/body length^3), a lowered lean body mass and percentage of protein mass, together with an increased percent body fat mass and absolute retroperitoneal fat pad weight, found in 2-month-old GK/Par rats as compared with related W rats (97). No major additional deterioration of both basal hyperglycemia and glucose intolerance could be detected in older GK/Par rats (12- or 18-month-old) compared with 2-month-old GK/Par rats (96).

To elucidate the pathogenesis of hyperglycemia and defective insulin action in the GK model, we studied insulin secretion and insulin action in 4-week-old GK/Par pups at the time of weaning (95). In the postabsorptive state, their basal plasma glucose level was elevated and their tolerance to intravenous glucose was impaired. Their basal glucose production was increased by 40%, and during euglycemic clamp performed at submaximal hyperinsulinemia, suppression of liver glucose production was less effective. However, their whole-body GUR was similar to that of the control W rats. This was correlated with a normal insulin-stimulated GUR by epitrochlearis, soleus, and extensor digitorum longus muscles, diaphragm, and white adipose tissues (95). These data give body to the primacy of the beta-cell defects in the etiology of T2D in the GK/Par rat. They also highlight a possible primary role of the liver defect, while peripheral insulin resistance develops later on at adult age.

We have also studied GK/Par rat glucose homeostasis during aging. None of the following parameters were significantly affected by aging: basal plasma insulin level, insulin secretion in response to glucose in vivo, basal hepatic glucose production, insulin-suppressive effect on hepatic glucose production, and basal whole-body GUR. Only insulin-stimulated GUR and some individual tissue GUR (heart and paraovarian and inguinal white adipose tissues) were significantly decreased during aging. Such a pattern is strikingly different from the situation reported in the aging W nondiabetic rats, in the sense that whereas both insulin secretion (increased) and insulin action (decreased) are profoundly modified by age in the nondiabetic rat (96), they are only marginally affected in the GK/Par rat. Such an adaptation in this T2D model could be related to a limited capacity of these rats to expand their fat mass with age, since it is recognized that the relative contribution of fat mass to whole-body weight gain is largely responsible for the age-related impairment in peripheral insulin action in nondiabetic humans and nondiabetic animal models (113, 114). Supporting this view, the

Lee index significantly increases from 2 to 18 months in W rats, whereas it is not modified during the same period in GK/Par rats (96). The GK/Tac rat also exhibits an age-specific failure to accumulate body fat which was well supported by finding of altered expression of genes involved in adipogenesis and lipogenesis in the white adipose tissue of these animals (115). Furthermore, in this model, chronic inflammation in white adipose tissue was evident from the differential expression of genes involved in inflammatory responses and activation of natural immunity (115).

5. The Prediabetes to Diabetes Transition in Young GK Rats

Follow-up of the animals after delivery revealed that GK/Par pups become overtly hyperglycemic for the first time after 3–4 weeks of age only (i.e., during the weaning period). The occurrence of basal hyperglycemia and diabetes in the GK/Par rat is therefore preceded by a period of prediabetes during which animals are normoglycemic. Despite normoglycemia, total β-cell mass was clearly decreased (by 60%) in the GK/Par pups when compared with age-related W pups (22). This early β-cell growth retardation in the prediabetic GK/Par rat pups can be ascribed neither to decreased β-cell replication nor to increased apoptosis (22). We demonstrated that the recruitment of new β-cells from the precursor pool (β-cell neogenesis) was in fact defective in the young prediabetic GK/Par rat (35, 116). A comparative study of the development of GK/Par and W pancreases indicates that the β-cell deficit (reduced by more than 50%) starts as early as fetal age 16 days (E16) (36). During the time window E16–E20, we detected an unexpected anomaly of proliferation and apoptosis of undifferentiated ductal cells in the GK/Par pancreatic rudiments (36, 38). Therefore, the decreased cell proliferation and survival in the ductal compartment of the pancreas, where the putative endocrine precursor cells localize, suggest that the impaired development of the β-cell in the GK/Par fetus could result from the failure of the proliferative and survival capacities of the endocrine precursor cells. Defective signaling through the IGF2/IGF1-R pathway is involved in this process at this stage (38, 117). Importantly, this represents a primary anomaly since IFG2 and IGF1-R protein expressions are already decreased within the GK/Par pancreatic rudiment at E13, at a time when β-cell mass (first wave of β-cell expansion) is in fact normal (38). Low levels of pancreatic IFG2 associated with β-cell number deficiency are maintained thereafter in the GK/Par fetuses until delivery (117). We have also published data illustrating a poor proliferation and/or survival of the endocrine precursors also during neonatal and adult life (35, 37). Altogether these arguments support the notion that an impaired capacity of β-cell neogenesis (either primary in the fetus or compensatory in the newborn and the adult) results from the permanently decreased pool of endocrine precursors in the GK/Par pancreas (116).

We have also shown that in normoglycemic GK/Par neonates, the basal plasma insulin levels and the insulin-to-glucose ratio are dramatically reduced, and during this prediabetes period, the GSIS in vivo is markedly decreased as measured during glucose tolerance tests (97).

β-cell dysfunction occurred in the absence of glucose intolerance in prediabetic GK/Par rats, whereas after weaning GK/Par rats become clearly glucose intolerant. The basal normoglycemia and the normal glucose tolerance in GK/Par neonates suggest that the impaired insulin secretion was compensated for by an adaptive increased sensitivity to insulin. To assess insulin sensitivity, we performed insulin sensitivity tests in 7-, 14-, and 21-day-old animals, which showed that insulin action was significantly increased in GK/Par rats compared with the age-matched W rats (97). We also assessed in vivo whole-body glucose utilization rate (GUR) in 21-day-old GK/Par rats. When measured in the basal state, GUR obtained through glucose turnover measurement was found greater in prediabetic GK/Par rats than in controls. Because this was obtained in the presence of a low basal plasma insulin level but normal basal plasma glucose, it again suggests that the peripheral tissues are hyperreactive to insulin action in these rats. During hyperinsulinemic and euglycemic conditions, endogenous glucose production in both groups being completely abolished, the whole-body GUR was evaluated by the exogenous glucose infusion rate required to maintain euglycemia. It was found significantly higher in the 21-day-old GK/Par rats compared with W rats (97). This whole set of proofs indicates that before weaning GK/Par rats exhibit a significant insulin hypersensitivity, which is reversed after that time, as adult GK/Par rats develop insulin resistance (94). The underlying mechanism of insulin hypersensitivity in the GK rat before the onset of diabetes is not known. It may reflect an adaptation to the very low circulating insulin levels. However, this adaptive mechanism cannot overcome the lack of appropriate insulin secretion when rats are fed the standard high-carbohydrate diet at and after weaning, resulting in onset of basal hyperglycemia in adult GK/par rats.

In the GK model, the possibility remained, however, for those changes in the metabolic parameters to be caused by qualitative and/or quantitative changes in maternal milk and nursing behavior of diabetic GK/Par dams. To test whether such is the case, we performed cross-fostering experiments from the day of birth and until weaning. Interestingly, our results indicate that GK/Par pups reared with nondiabetic W dams having normal milk composition and normal maternal behavior exhibit similar defects in glucose secretion during an IPGTT and a comparable increase in the whole-body insulin sensitivity to those of GK pups reared with their own diabetic GK/Par mothers (97). This suggests that alteration of metabolic parameters during the prediabetes stage is due prominently to genetic predisposition and that normal postnatal nutrition and nursing behavior cannot significantly affect the occurrence of such abnormalities.

The GK/Par rat is a non-overweight model of T2D. Although T2D in humans is often associated with obesity, all diabetic patients are not obese, and in some populations the prevalence of diabetes increases despite low prevalence of obesity (118). We have explored the postnatal growth, body composition, and adiposity in prediabetic and adult diabetic GK/Par rats. We showed that prediabetic GK/Par rats exhibited a progressive delay in postnatal growth. This decrease in weight gain is attributed to a decreased growth in length. This is reflected by the diminution of both their lean mass and fat mass-to-body mass ratio, at least during the period of 7–14 days (97). At the time of weaning (28 days) and thereafter (56 days), although the lean body mass deficit persisted in the GK/Par rats, their body fat accumulation was unexpectedly turned on. The clear-cut increase in percent body fat mass and retroperitoneal adipose tissue weight in the GK/Par rats (28- and 56-day-old) compared with nondiabetic W rats was a salient finding. As a consequence, the statement that the GK rat is a model for T2D without obesity (1, 5) has to be revisited: despite its low body weight, the GK/Par rat exhibits excessive fat accumulation (in proportion to body weight) especially at the onset of hyperglycemia. The alteration in body composition of GK/Par rats with excessive fat cell number (prediabetic GK/Par rat) and fat cell size (hyperglycemic GK/Par rat) most likely implicate changes in the synthesis and secretion of adipocyte-derived hormones in this model. Indeed, plasma leptin levels are lower in prediabetic GK/Par rats than those in age-matched W rats, whereas in hyperglycemic GK/Par rats circulating leptin is at a higher level than that found in adult W rats (27). To summarize, these data reveal a major, and so far unsuspected, difference in the prediabetic GK/Par fat cell ontogenesis: fat accretion in the GK/Par rat after weaning would be due at first to a more precocious hyperplasia of hypotrophic adipocytes, whereas later on (at and after weaning) increased cellularity is no longer maintained and hypertrophy becomes prominent. The suckling-weaning transition seems to be a very important step for overaccumulation of fat mass in the GK/Par model, and it coincides with the appearance of basal hyperglycemia. The suckling-weaning transition in normal rats is characterized by increased insulin sensitivity and insulin secretion, which underlie the marked increase in size and lipid content that occurs in white adipose tissue at weaning. We suggest that the development of the increased fat mass in the 56-day-old diabetic GK/Par rat could be a consequence of increased

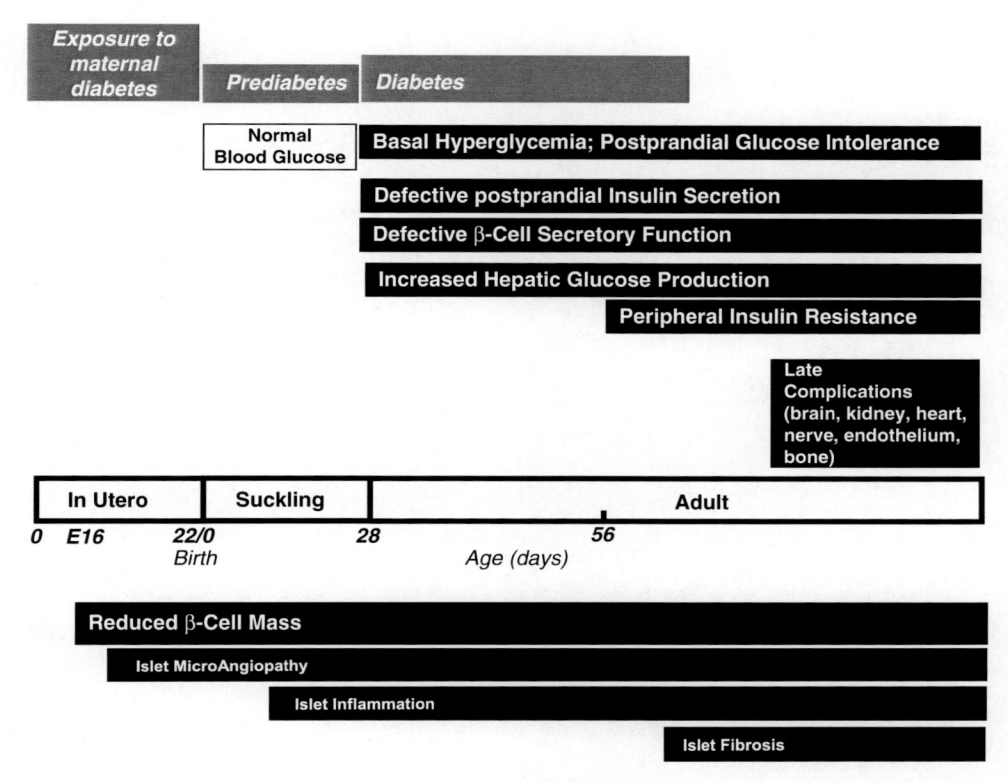

Fig. 2. Time-course of diabetes in the GK/Par rat model. Males and females are similarly affected and their diabetic state is stable over 72 weeks of follow-up (96). In adult GK rats, plasma insulin release in vivo in response to i.v. glucose is abolished. In vitro studies of insulin release with the isolated perfused pancreas or with perfused islets indicate that both the early and late phases of glucose-induced insulin release are markedly affected in the adult GK rat. Concerning insulin action in adult GK rats, increased glucose production and decreased insulin sensitivity have been reported in the liver at early stage (weaning). Moderate insulin resistance in extrahepatic tissues (muscles and adipose tissues) develops later. GK rats exhibit complications of long-standing diabetes. Hyperglycemia is preceded by a period of normoglycemia, ranging from birth to weaning. Therefore, during this period, the young GK/Par rats can be considered to be prediabetic. Hyperglycemic GK fetuses exhibit a similar percentage decrease in islet vascularization and beta-cell mass (BCM). Normoglycaemic GK neonates show systemic inflammation, disturbed angiogenesis, and altered pancreas development. BCM deficiency remains for the whole life of the rats. Islets from adult GK/Par are infiltrated by inflammatory cells and their vascularization is altered. Islet fibrosis becomes prominent with aging.

glucose utilization by adipose tissue in the basal state before weaning. Therefore, it can be inferred that increased body fat mass may indeed result from a primary insulin deficiency and not only from excessive insulin levels, as is more generally recognized.

Figure 2 illustrates our present understanding of how primary and early alteration in the GK/Par beta-cell mass leads to pathogenic progression toward impairment of insulin action in liver and peripheral tissues and sequential appearance of the abnormalities found in T2D. Events are based on comparison of data obtained with nondiabetic W rats.

6. Which Mechanisms Underlie the Programmation of T2D in the GK Model?

Undertaking genetic dissection of the GK diabetes was stimulated not only by the phenotypic traits shown by the GK rat but also by the methodology used successfully for the establishment of the line. Indeed, this methodology implies that genes predisposing to diabetes present in a nondiabetic outbred W strain were concentrated through repeated selective breedings by means of glucose intolerance as a selection index. Search for identification of the morbid genes using a quantitative trait locus (QTL) approach has led to identification of a first set of six independently segregating loci containing genes regulating fasting plasma glucose and insulin levels, glucose tolerance, insulin secretion, and adiposity in GK/Par rats (50). The same conclusion was drawn by Galli et al. (51) using GK/Sto rats. This established the polygenic inheritance of diabetes-related parameters in the GK rats whatever their origin.

In both GK/Sto and GK/Par rats, the strongest evidence of linkage between glucose tolerance and markers spanning a region on rat chromosome 1 is called Niddm1 locus. Recent works using congenic technology have identified a short region on the Niddm1i locus of GK/Sto rats that may contribute to defective insulin secretion (119), while β-cell mass is intact in Niddm1i subcongenics (120). These results are, however, inconsistent with the enhanced insulin release and increased islet size described in a GK/Ox congenic line targeting a similar short region of the GK QTL Niddm1 (121). Recently, QTLs linked to beta-cell mass and plasma concentration of corticosterone, prolactin, and growth hormone were reported in GK/Ox rats (122). The QTL *Bcm1* relevant to pancreas histology does not coincide with previously detected QTLs in the GK/Ox rat. Positional and functional candidate genes for Bcm1 include genes encoding GH, signal transducers and activators of transcription (Stat3, Stat5) which play central roles in mediating the biological effects of prolactin and GH in beta cells, and the suppressor of cytokine signaling Socs-3, which inhibits GH-promoted beta-cell proliferation. In addition, microarray-based gene transcription profiling data showed that Stat3 is significantly overexpressed in GK/Ox (123). No significant linkage to plasma IGF-1 was found, and male-specific genetic effects on the control of plasma GH and prolactin concentrations were detected in chromosomes 6 and 17, respectively. The highly significant QTL *Pcort1* linked to plasma corticosterone was detected in a region of rat chromosome 1 which maps more than 30 cM away from QTLs linked to glucose tolerance, adiposity, insulin secretion (50), and cholesterol metabolism (124). This QTL is distinct to the locus *Scort1* for serum corticosterone identified in an hypertensive rat strain, which maps to the telomeric end of chromosome 1 (125).

A fine mapping of the major diabetes susceptibility locus in the GK/Sto rat 52-Mb locus Niddm1 (126) has recently been reported. A 16-Mb portion of Niddm1, Niddm1i, confers defective insulin secretion without insulin resistance (119) and is homologous to a region on human chromosome 10 that is associated with T2D (127) and includes Tcf7l2, the strongest candidate gene for T2D to date (128). However, Tcf7l2 RNA levels were not different in the GK/Sto Niddm1i congenics displaying reduced insulin secretion compared with controls (120). In congenic strains harboring different parts of GK-derived Niddm1i on the genetic background of normoglycemic F344 rats, two distinct regions within Niddm1i have been identified that confer impaired glucose metabolism and aberrant β-cell exocytosis, respectively (129). The 4.5-Mb locus conferring aberrant exocytosis is fully contained in the congenic strain N1I12 and was further dissected by generation of the congenic strains N1I5 and N1I11 that have reduced extent of GK/Sto genotype in the locus. GSIS measured in batch-incubated islets was normal in N1I11 islets. By contrast, N1I5 islets had a reduced GSIS compared with N1I11 and control islets. These observations suggest major differences in the secretory machineries of the two strains. These are not secondary to hyperglycemia, as the animals investigated had no overt diabetes. Instead, the impaired β-cell exocytosis in N1I5 was caused by the additional 1.4-Mb GK/Sto-derived genetic segment. The segment contains five known protein-coding genes: *Pdcd4, Lysmd3, Shoc2, Adra2a, and ENSR NOG00000036577*. Expression analysis revealed an upregulation of Adra2a mRNA in pancreatic islets from N1I5 compared with N1I11 but no differences for the other genes. This was paralleled by a 90% increase in alpha2A-adrenergic receptor [alpha(2A)AR] protein in both islets and brain in N1I5 relative to N1I11 (129). Pharmacological receptor antagonism, silencing of receptor expression, or blockade of downstream effectors rescued insulin secretion in N1I5 congenic islets. On the basis of these findings, SNP analysis of the human ADRA2A gene was undertaken and demonstrated a linkage between the minor allele of rs553668, located in the 3′URD region of ADRA2A, and impaired insulin secretion in humans. In addition, studies with a large cohort of nondiabetic and diabetic individuals indicated that ADRA2A rs553668 was associated with increased risk of T2D (129). Moreover, two functional point mutations in the promoter region of the adenyl cyclase type III (AC-III) gene (located on rat chromosome 6) have also been reported in GK/Sto islets and they are associated to GK/Sto β-cell AC-III overexpression and increased cAMP generation (73).

Of course, contribution of other susceptibility loci is required for the development of the full GK diabetic phenotype. This important notion is illustrated by the discovery of mutations in the genes for IDE (an insulin degrading activity) and SHIP2 (a phospholipid phosphatase), two genes localized in the GK/Sto QTL Niddm1 and whose mutations slightly impair insulin action (130, 131).

While most disease-association studies of genetic variation focus on individual nucleotide sequences, large-scale changes like copy number variations generally defined as the copy number differences of DNA stretches larger than 1 kb have also been linked to complex human diseases. Utilizing array comparative genome hybridization technology, 137 nonredundant copy number variation regions have been recently identified in GK/Shang rat genome, using normal W rats as control. These CNV regions (CNVRs) covered approximately 36 Mb nucleotides, accounting for about 1% of the whole genome. By integrating information from gene annotations and disease knowledge, comprehensive analysis of the CNVRs resulted in the identification of several novel diabetes susceptibility loci involving 16 putative protein-coding genes and two microRNA genes (14).

Given the critical roles miRNAs are suggested to play in several aspects of glucose homeostasis, it has been hypothesized that miRNA expression profiles of insulin target tissues is altered in the GK model. Indeed, a comprehensive assessment of miRNA expression in three insulin target tissues of GK/Ox rats identified significantly altered miRNA expression patterns in GK/Ox muscle, liver, and adipose tissue as compared to corresponding tissues from nondiabetic rats (132). Moreover, a global profiling of miRNAs in the GK/Sto islets revealed a perturbed miRNA network and the authors have suggested that the reduced insulin secretion may be partly due to upregulated miRNA expression leading to decreased production of key proteins of the insulin exocytotic machinery (133).

Besides the role of GK susceptibility loci, the possibility exists that the GK maternal diabetic environment per se causes early changes in the structure and function of several organs in the offspring, including the endocrine pancreas, and has profound influence on glucose handling in the fetus, which persists into adult life and the subsequent generation offsprings. It is now acknowledged that hyperglycemia experienced during the fetal and/or early postnatal life may contribute to programming of the endocrine pancreas and that gestational diabetes may pass from one generation to the next one (134, 135). Such a scenario potentially applies to the GK/Par rat, as GK/Par mothers are slightly hyperglycemic through their gestation and during the suckling period (136) (Fig. 3). It offers a rationale to elucidate several clues: (1) the initiation of pancreas programming in the F1 offspring of the first founders (F0), since the GK line is issued from intercrosses between W females and males with borderline IGT but otherwise normal basal blood glucose level (5); (2) the progression of the IGT phenotype until a stable mild diabetic phenotype was reached among the generations $n = 30$ (5); (3) the lack of attenuation of the

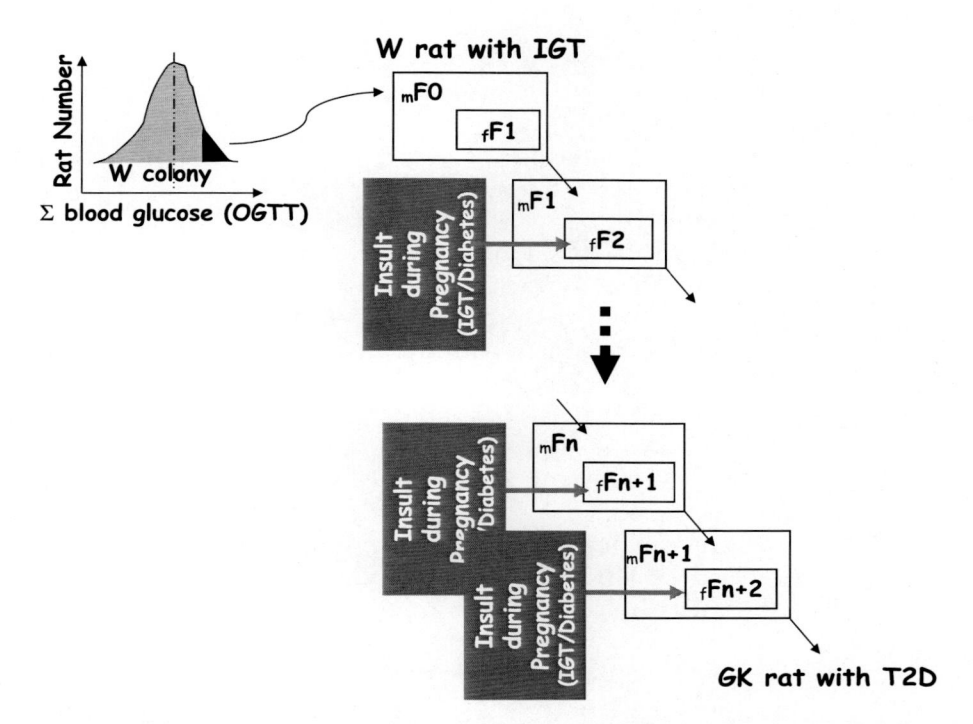

Fig. 3. Mechanisms for the installation and intergenerational transmission of programmed beta-cell mass disruption and T2D in the GK/Par rat model of type 2 diabetes. Maternal IGT/diabetes during gestation induces BCM programming in the first (F1) and the subsequent rat generations. Metabolic modifications in the pups, during the in utero and suckling periods, are followed by the onset of pathological conditions in adulthood (glucose intolerance and type 2 diabetes) and the transmission of programmed endocrine/metabolic capacities to the next generation. *W* Wistar strain.

diabetic GK phenotype overtime (along more than 20 years and 100 generations for the GK/Par subline), since offspring of GK female/W male crosses were more hyperglycemic than those of W female/GK male crosses (52). We have preliminary data using an embryo transfer strategy first described by Gill-Randall et al. (137), suggesting that GK/Par embryos transferred in the uterus of euglycemic W mother still develop deficiency of β-cell mass when adults, to the same extent as the GK/Par rats from our stock colony (138). While this preliminary conclusion rather favors a major role for inheritance of morbid genes, additional studies are needed to really eliminate the option that the gestational diabetic pattern of the GK/Par mothers does not contribute to establish and/or maintain the transmission of endocrine pancreas programming from one GK/Par generation to the next one. Moreover, studies on the offspring in crosses between GK/Par and W rats demonstrated that F1 hybrid fetuses, regardless of whether the mother was a GK or a W rat, exhibit decreased beta-cell mass and GSIS closely resembling those in GK/GK fetuses (136). This finding indicates that conjunction of GK genes from both parents is not required for defective β-cell mass to be fully expressed. We have also shown that to have one GK parent is a risk factor for a low β-cell mass phenotype in young adults, even when the other parent is a normal W rat (139).

The subsequent question to be answered now is whether or not epigenetic perturbation of gene expression occurs in the developing fetal GK/Par pancreas and programs a durable alteration of the β-cell mass as seen in the adult. igf2 and igf1r genes are good candidates for such a perspective.

Finally, since the loss of GK/Taked β-cells was mitigated by in vivo treatment with the alpha-glucosidase inhibitors voglibose (62) or miglitol (42), or enhanced when the animals are fed sucrose (41, 140), pathological progression (β-cell loss, fibrosis) of the GK β-cell mass is also dependent on the metabolic (glycemic) control.

Concerning the GK β-cell secretory failure, there are several arguments indicating that there are at least partially, related to the abnormal metabolic environment (glucotoxicity and lipotoxicity). When studied under in vitro static incubation conditions, islets isolated from normoglycemic (prediabetic) GK/Par pups amplified their secretory response to high glucose, leucine, or leucine plus glutamine to the same extent as age-related W islets (2). This suggests that there does not exist a major intrinsic secretory defect in the prediabetic GK/Par β-cells which can be considered as normally glucose competent at this stage, at least when tested in vitro. In the GK/Par rat, basal hyperglycemia and mild hypertriglyceridemia with hyperlipoproteinemia are observed only after weaning (2). The onset of a profound alteration in GSIS by the GK/Par β-cell (after weaning) is time correlated with the exposure to the diabetic milieu. These changes in islet function could be ascribed, at least in part, to a loss of differentiation of β-cells chronically exposed to even mild chronic hyperglycemia and elevated plasma nonesterified fatty acids. This view is supported by the reports that chronic treatments of adult GK rats (from various sublines) with phlorizin (4, 49, 60, 88), T-1095 (141), glinides (92, 142), glibenclamide (142), gliclazide (143), JTT-608 (144, 145), voglibose (146), or insulin (142) partially improved glucose-induced insulin release, while hyperlipidemia induced by high-fat feeding markedly impaired their insulin secretion (69, 70).

In conclusion, taking into account the diverse informations so far available from the GK model through its different phenotype variants, the early pathogenic items are proposed: multiple morbid genes causing impaired β-cell mass, early epigenetic programming of the β-cell mass by gestational diabetes which is transmitted from one generation to the other and acquired loss of β-cell differentiation due to chronic exposure to hyperglycemia/hyperlipidemia. The abnormalities so far detected in the diabetic GK β-cell population and those found in the T2D human β-cell population put into the front stage a number of striking commonalities (19).

7. GK Rats Exhibit Complications of Long-Standing T2D

GK/Sen rats were first used for studies of late diabetic complications. Signs of neuropathy were noted as reduced motor nerve conduction velocity (MNCV) in the tail nerve as early as in 2-month-old GK/Sen relative to W rats (4, 7, 147). In addition, morphological alterations such as axonal degeneration and segmental demyelination as well as increased sorbitol and decreased myoinositol levels were observed in sciatic nerves in 6-month-old GK/Sen rats. Some of these defects were prevented by treatment with aldose reductase inhibitor (147). Moreover, administration of nateglinide to GK/Clea rats normalized the delayed MNCV while glibenclamide had only a partial effect (148). Reduced motor conduction velocity in the femoral nerve was also reported in 8-month-old GK/Sto rats (1) and more detailed studies of peripheral nerve morphology and function were performed in 2- and 18-month-old GK/Sto rats (149).

Morphological changes indicating retinopathy seem to develop rather late in GK rats: an altered retinal endothelial cell/pericyte ratio was demonstrated in animals more than 1 year old, but not in 8-month-old GK/Sto rats (150, 151). Biochemical and functional alterations in the GK/Sto rat retina have been described as earlier phenomena, such as reduced glutathion levels (151), increased tissue levels of vascular endothelial growth factor (VEGF) (152), and impaired retinal blood flow (153). An increased production of nitric oxide in GK/Coi rat retinas has been suggested to account for increased blood–retinal barrier permeability and breakdown (154).

Metabolic and vascular consequences of GK/Par diabetes induce CNS complications. We have recently shown that neurogenesis is impaired in the GK/Par dentate gyrus (DG) of the hippocampus, a neurogenic area associated with memory and learning processes. GK/Par DG is characterized by increased proliferation of progenitor cells and differentiation into immature neurons, but deficient survival ability (98). However, it is not associated with changes in the number or shape of astrocytes. These data confirm those obtained in 18-week-old diabetic GK/Tac rats (155). These authors also showed that neurogenesis is not modified in younger normoglycemic GK/Tac rats, indicating the deleterious effect of chronic hyperglycemia itself. In addition, they demonstrated that diabetic GK/Tac progenitors fail to respond in vitro to growth factors. These alterations might be responsible for longer-lasting cognitive impairments, which have been observed following ischemia in diabetic GK/Sto rats (156, 157). We also found a net reduction in blood vessel area and branching in DG from diabetic GK/Par rats, together with decreased glucocorticoid receptor immunolabeling in CA1 hippocampal area, associated with higher corticosteronemia. We have proposed that the aberrant DG neurogenesis in diabetic GK/Par rats could be secondary to mild neurodegeneration, acting as a brain compensatory strategy. Despite a small initial upregulation of cell proliferation, complex interactions of metabolic and endothelial dysfunctions render the neurogenic GK/Par microenvironment unable to preserve the survival of newborn cells (98). The GK rat can also be considered a suitable model to study the impact of diabetic hyperglycemia on the development of secondary brain injuries following focal ischemia: severe cognitive impairments and recovery of motor and cognitive functions of GK/Sto rats were examined following extradural compression of the sensorimotor cortex. Scores for tests of vestibulomotor function (beam-walking) and combined tests of motor function and learning (locomotor activity) were found consistently impaired after extradural compression of the sensorimotor cortex which mimics focal ischemia resulting from decreased blood flow supply to the cortex owing to stroke (157). Irreversible post-compression neuronal degeneration in the ipsilateral cortex, hippocampus, and thalamus was detected and the amount of degeneration in these structures was considerably higher in GK/Sto rats (157). Under basal conditions, adult diabetic GK/Sto rats showed significantly higher mRNA expression of antioxidant and proinflammatory genes, suggesting that oxidative stress and neuroinflammation already developed (158). Results obtained in the GK/Coi brain are consistent with the view that there exists a diabetes-related mitochondrial dysfunction in the brain and it is exacerbated by aging and the presence of neurotoxic agents, such as β-amyloid (159). This study supports the idea that the GK rat could be a suitable model to study the correlation between age-related neurodegeneration/Alzheimer's disease and diabetes.

Several studies have revealed GK rats are not hypertensive (160). In GK/Par rats, Valensi et al. (161) reported slightly but not significantly elevated systolic blood pressure levels in 3–18-month-old GK/Par rats as assessed by telemetric measures. In contrast, Witte et al. have described the development of mild hypertension in GK/Mol/Tac rats that was associated with a reduction in vascular nitric-oxide-sensitive guanylyl cyclase (162). More recently, GK/Mol/Tac rats were reported already moderately hypertensive on a low-sodium diet and showed marked impairment of endothelium-mediated vascular relaxation and perivascular inflammation (163). A high-sodium diet for 8 weeks increased blood pressure further (163). It also induced the development of cardiac hypertrophy, marked kidney damages, and aggravated endothelial dysfunction and the inflammatory response associated with increased oxidative stress. Under these conditions, the beneficial cardiovascular and renal effects of valsartan indicated the involvement of increased renin-angiotensin system activity in the pathogenesis of diabetic nephropathy and vascular complications in the GK/Mol/Tac rats (163).

The GK model allows one to study the effect of diabetes on the heart without other complications such as obesity. It was previously demonstrated that the heart of 10-month-old male GK/Ox rats is insulin-resistant with a decreased insulin-stimulated glucose uptake and an impaired insulin signaling pathway (164). A diabetic cardiomyopathy phenotype was present in the GK/Par rat, as far as left ventricular wall thickness was increased, left ventricular ejection fraction was reduced, and isovolumic relaxation time was increased compared with W rats (165). Systolic blood pressure was normal (165). The hypertrophy phenotype was accompanied by an increase in myocardial Na^+/H^+ exchanger (NHE1) activity in left ventricular GK/Par myocytes and it can be prevented by chronic treatment with the NHE1 inhibitor cariporide. Activation of the Akt pathway likely underlies the hypertrophic effect of increased NHE1 activity (165). GK/Card rats have also been shown to display mild cardiomyopathy, evident as exaggerated diastolic dysfunction during hypoxia (166). No difference in cardiac function was found before ischemia in GK/Mol/Tac rat hearts compared with their controls, as reported either in younger (167, 168) or in older rats (169, 170). Recently, we reported an increased susceptibility of diabetic GK/Par rat heart to ischemic injury that is not associated with impaired energy metabolism (171). Modifications in the NO pathway may play a major role in ischemia-reperfusion injury in the diabetic GK/Par rat heart, since decreased coronary flow, upregulation of eNOS expression, and increased total NOx levels confirmed NO pathway modifications (171) which are presumably related to increased oxidative stress. There are, however, some discrepancies in the literature concerning the modifications of the NO pathway in the GK model: Bitar et al. (13) have shown increased eNOS expression in the aortas of young GK/Kuwait rats compared with W rats. Kazuyama et al. (172) showed an increase in eNOS and a decrease in nNOS mRNA expression in 12-week-old GK/SLC rat aortas compared with age-matched controls. Some other studies have rather shown decreased NOx content in GK/Sto hearts (173) or in the aortas of GK/Kuwait rats (13) together with upregulation of eNOS. In contrast to upregulation of eNOS, a significant decrease of eNOS, iNOS, and nNOS mRNA expressions was observed in the 70-week-old GK/SLC rat aortas compared with those in the younger GK/SLC rats (172), while El-Omar et al. (174) have shown that eNOS expression was similar in control and diabetic GK/Card hearts, whereas only diabetic hearts expressed iNOS protein. Lack of antioxidant coenzyme Q9 has been suggested to be responsible for an increased susceptibility of GK/Coi heart mitochondria to oxidative damage and subsequent impaired myocardial function (175).

GK rats have been used in several studies of diabetic nephropathy (160, 176, 177). Phillips et al. did not detect any significant proteinuria or renal function impairment up to 52 weeks of age (176).

Others have described a 1.5-fold increase in albuminuria as compared to W rats (163). A gradual increase in glomerular basal membrane with aging has been shown in GK/Sen rats from 3 months of age (148). GK/Tamp rats have also been found to develop impaired renal function (by 50–75%), reflected as increased serum creatinine and urea nitrogen levels as compared with W rats (178). Age-dependent morphological changes consist of thickening of the glomerular (176, 179) and tubular basement membranes as well as the development of marked glomerular hypertrophy at 35 weeks of age (176). Glomerular hypertrophy was the consequence of an increase in both the total mesangial volume and glomerular capillary luminal volume, while fractional capillary and mesangial volumes remained unchanged. Signs of podocyte injury as assessed by their de novo expression of desmin were observed in GK/Card rats from 20 weeks on, while there was no evidence of mesangial activation as assessed by their de novo expression of a smooth muscle actin. Moreover, increased interstitial monocyte/macrophage infiltration at 12 weeks, as well as elevated glomerular monocyte/macrophage infiltration at 35 weeks could be demonstrated (176). Monocyte/macrophage infiltration in the renal perivascular space as well as increased expression of ICAM1 in the interstitium, intima, and adventitia of the small renal vessels were also reported in GK/Mol/Tac rats on low-sodium diet and were prevented by valsartan treatment (163). Long-standing GK/Card diabetes was not associated with the appearance of glomerulosclerosis or interstitial fibrosis (176). Only at 2 years, close to the maximal rat life span, segmental glomerulosclerosis and interstitial fibrosis associated with an increased urinary protein excretion were reported (180). Induction of moderate hypertension in GKMol/Tac rats by administration of 6% NaCl over 8 weeks resulted in a 3.5-fold increase in albuminuria and increased perivascular monocyte/macrophage infiltration (163). Some mesangial thickening and a slight thickening of the afferent arterioles were observed. There was no sign of glomerulosclerosis or interstitial fibrosis in these GK/Mol/Tac rats on high-salt diet (163). Valsartan treatment had no effect on blood pressure or endothelial dysfunction but protected against albuminuria, inflammation, and oxidative stress in GK/Mol/Tac rats on high-salt diet (163). Ventromedial hypothalamic (VMH) lesions in GK/Clea rats induced accentuated hyperglycemia and hypertriglyceridemia with visceral fat accumulation and reduced pancreatic insulin content (181). In addition, the VMH lesion enhanced proteinuria and glomerular basal membrane thickening as well as induced morphological changes in the aortic intima characteristic of an early stage of atherosclerosis (182). Thus, the VMH-lesioned GK/Clea rat has been suggested to be a model of microangiopathy and macroangiopathy. An atherogenic diet in GK/Coi rats was also reported to increase blood glucose, total cholesterol, triglycerides, and induced renal injuries that may be prevented by insulin or metformin administration (183). Therefore, a wide set of observations support the notion that long-standing GK diabetes alone may not be sufficient to induce progressive nephropathy unless secondary injurious mechanisms are present.

Signs of diabetic osteopathy (184–186) and impaired bone morphogenesis around dental implants (187) were also noted in GK/Sto rats.

8. Conclusion

The study of the GK model and its different inbred sublines has provided new insights into the pathogenesis of T2D as the rats develop spontaneous defects in insulin secretion and action and long-standing diabetic complications that, in many ways, resemble those described in human T2D. The advantages of these easily produced rodent models are several fold.

They provide interesting models for the study of onset of chronic hyperglycemia and its pathogenesis. Since the rats can be easily kept for more than 2 years under standard breeding conditions, they allow study in the adult of the long-term consequences of a primary reduction of the beta-cell mass.

The wealth of phenotypic information that can be collected in the GK rats makes them a powerful tool for genetic studies of quantitative traits underlying complex T2D phenotypes.

They are suitable to evaluate the effect of the major modulators of diabetes, such as composition of the diet, aging, gestation, and obesity. They have proved to be useful for studies related to the pathogenesis of nephropathy, vascular complications, hypertension, or osteopenia under conditions of chronic hyperglycemia.

They are valuable for testing hypoglycemic drugs and identifying their mechanisms of action.

They are particularly suitable to assess the effectiveness of therapeutics aimed to enhance beta-cell growth and/or survival and to understand the mechanisms for compensation growth of the beta-cell mass.

Of course, the GK model is not a blueprint for the diseased T2D human. There are, however, sufficient similarities with high value, to justify more efforts to understand the etiopathogenesis of T2D in this rat model now widely used and, more specifically, the pivotal role played by the GK islet cells in the onset of T2D.

Acknowledgments

The GK/Par studies done at Lab B2PE, BFA Unit, have been funded by the CNRS, the University Paris-Diderot, the French ANR (programme Physio 2006—Prograbeta), the EFSD/MSD European

Foundation, SERVIER, MERCK-SERONO, NOVO-Nordisk, PFIZER, MetaBrain Research, NESTLE-France, the SFD/French Diabetes Association, the FRM/Medical Research Foundation and NEB Research Foundation.

References

1. Östenson CG (2001) The Goto-Kakizaki rat. In: Sima AAF, Shafrir E (eds) Animal models of diabetes: a primer. Harwood Academic, Amsterdam, pp 197–211
2. Portha B, Giroix MH, Serradas P et al (2001) Beta-cell function and viability in the spontaneously diabetic GK rat. Information from the GK/Par colony. Diabetes 50(suppl 1): A89–A93
3. Portha B (2005) Programmed disorders of beta-cell development and function as one cause for type 2 diabetes? The GK rat paradigm. Diabetes Metab Res Rev 21:495–504
4. Portha B, Lacraz G, Dolz M et al (2007) Issues surrounding beta-cells and their roles in type 2 diabetes. What tell us the GK rat model. Expert Rev Endocrinol Metab 2:785–795
5. Goto Y, Kakizaki M, Masaki N (1975) Spontaneous diabetes produced by selective breeding of normal Wistar rats. Proc Jpn Acad 51:80–85
6. Goto Y, Suzuki KI, Sasaki M et al (1988) GK rat as a model of nonobese, noninsulindependent diabetes. Selective breeding over 35 generations. In: Shafrir E, Renold AE (eds) Lessons from animal diabetes. Libbey, London, pp 301–303
7. Suzuki KI, Goto Y, Toyota T (1992) Spontaneously diabetic GK (Goto-Kakizaki) rats. In: Shafrir E (ed) Lessons from animal diabetes. Smith-Gordon, London, pp 107–116
8. Portha B, Serradas P, Bailbé D et al (1991) β-Cell insensitivity to glucose in the GK rat, a spontaneous nonobese model for type II diabetes. Dissociation between reductions in glucose transport and glucose-stimulated insulin secretion. Diabetes 40:486–491
9. Ohneda M, Johnson JH, Inman LR et al (1993) GLUT2 expression and function in β-cells of GK rats with NIDDM. Diabetes 42:1065–1072
10. Lewis BM, Ismail IS, Issa B et al (1996) Desensitisation of somatostatin, TRH and GHRH responses to glucose in the diabetic Goto-Kakizaki rat hypothalamus. J Endocrinol 151:13–17
11. Duarte AI, Santos MS, Seiça R et al (2004) Oxidative stress affects synaptosomal γ- aminobutyric acid and glutamate transport in diabetic rats. The role of insulin. Diabetes 53:2110–2116
12. Villar-Palasi C, Farese RV (1994) Impaired skeletal muscle glycogen synthase activation by insulin in the Goto-Kakizaki (GK) rat. Diabetologia 37:885–891
13. Bitar MS, Wahid S, Mustafa S et al (2005) Nitric oxide dynamics and endothelial dysfunction in type II model of genetic diabetes. Eur J Pharmacol 511:53–64
14. Ye ZQ, Niu S, Yu Y et al (2010) Analyses of copy number variation of GK rat reveal new putative type 2 diabetes susceptibility loci. PLoS One 5:e14077
15. Hughes SJ, Suzuki K, Goto Y (1994) The role of islet secretory function in the development of diabetes in the GK Wistar rat. Diabetologia 37:863–870
16. Metz SA, Meredith M, Vadakekalam J et al (1999) A defect late in stimulus secretion coupling impairs insulin secretion in Goto–Kakizaki diabetic rats. Diabetes 48:1754–1762
17. Wallis RH, Wallace KJ, Collins SC et al (2004) Enhanced insulin secretion and cholesterol metabolism in congenic strains of the spontaneously diabetic (type 2) Goto-Kakizaki rat are controlled by independent genetic loci in rat chromosome 8. Diabetologia 47: 1096–1106
18. Sener A, Ladrière L, Malaisse WJ et al (2001) Assessment by D-[(3)H]mannoheptulose uptake of B-cell density in isolated pancreatic islets from Goto-Kakizaki rats. Int J Mol Med 8:177–180
19. Portha B, Lacraz G, Kergoat M et al (2009) The GK rat beta-cell: a prototype for the diseased human beta-cell in type 2 diabetes? Mol Cell Endocrinol 297:73–85
20. Guenifi A, Abdel-Halim SM, Höög A et al (1995) Preserved beta-cell density in the endocrine pancreas of young, spontaneously diabetic Goto-Kakizaki (GK) rats. Pancreas 10:148–153
21. Abdel-Halim SM, Guenifi A, Efendic S et al (1993) Both somatostatin and insulin responses to glucose are impaired in the perfused pancreas of the spontaneously non-insulin dependent diabetic GK (Goto-Kakizaki) rat. Acta Physiol Scand 1482:19–26

22. Movassat J, Saulnier C, Serradas P et al (1997) Impaired development of pancreatic beta-cell mass is a primary event during the progression to diabetes in the GK rat. Diabetologia 40:916–925
23. Guest PC, Abdel-Halim SM, Gross DJ et al (2002) Proinsulin processing in the diabetic Goto–Kakizaki rat. J Endocrinol 175:637–647
24. Homo-Delarche F, Calderari S, Irminger JC et al (2006) Islet Inflammation and fibrosis in a spontaneous model of type 2 diabetes, the GK rat. Diabetes 55:1625–1633
25. Ehses JA, Perren A, Eppler E et al (2007) Increased number of islet-associated macrophages in type 2 diabetes. Diabetes 562:356–370
26. Ehses JA, Calderari S, Irminger JC et al (2007) Islet Inflammation in type 2 diabetes (T2D): from endothelial to beta-cell dysfunction. Curr Immunol Rev 3:216–232
27. Giroix MH, Irminger JC, Lacraz G et al (2011) Hypercholesterolaemia, signs of islet microangiopathy and altered angiogenesis precede onset of type 2 diabetes in the Goto–Kakizaki (GK) rat. Diabetologia 54:2451–2462
28. Ghanaat-Pour H, Huang Z, Lehtihet M et al (2007) Global expression profiling of glucose-regulated genes in pancreatic islets of spontaneously diabetic Goto-Kakizaki rats. J Mol Endocrinol 39:135–150
29. Atef N, Portha B, Penicaud L (1994) Changes in islet blood flow in rats with NIDDM. Diabetologia 37:677–680
30. Svensson AM, Östenson CG, Sandler S et al (1994) Inhibition of nitric oxide synthase by NG-nitro-L-arginine causes a preferential decrease in pancreatic islet blood flow in normal rats and spontaneously diabetic GK rats. Endocrinology 135:849–853
31. Svensson AM, Östenson CG, Jansson L (2000) Age-induced changes in pancreatic islet blood flow: evidence for an impaired regulation in diabetic GK rats. Am J Physiol Endocrinol Metab 279:E1139–E1144
32. Carlsson PO, Jansson L, Östenson CG et al (1997) Islet capillary blood pressure increase mediated by hyperglycemia in NIDDM GK rats. Diabetes 46:947–952
33. Lacraz G, Figeac F, Movassat J et al (2009) Diabetic rat beta-cells can achieve self-protection against oxidative stress through an adaptive up-regulation of their antioxidant defenses. PLoS One 4(8):e6500
34. Ihara Y, Toyokuni S, Uchida K et al (1999) Hyperglycemia causes oxidative stress in pancreatic beta-cells of GK rats, a model of type 2 diabetes. Diabetes 48:927–932
35. Movassat J, Portha B (1999) Beta-cell growth in the neonatal Goto-Kakizaki rat and regeneration after treatment with streptozotocin at birth. Diabetologia 42:1098–1106
36. Miralles F, Portha B (2001) Early development of beta-cells is impaired in the GK rat model of type 2 diabetes. Diabetes 50(suppl 1):84–88
37. Plachot C, Movassat J, Portha B (2001) Impaired beta-cell regeneration after partial pancreatectomy in the adult Goto-Kakizaki rat, a spontaneous model of type 2 diabetes. Histochem Cell Biol 116:131–139
38. Calderari S, Gangnerau MN, Thibault M et al (2007) Defective IGF-2 and IGFR1 protein production in embryonic pancreas precedes beta cell mass anomaly in Goto-Kakizaki rat model of type 2 diabetes. Diabetologia 50:1463–1471
39. Giroix MH, Saulnier C, Portha B (1999) Decreased pancreatic islet response to L-leucine in the spontaneously diabetic GK rat: enzymatic, metabolic and secretory data. Diabetologia 42:965–977
40. Momose K, Nunomiya S, Nakata M et al (2006) Immunohistochemical and electron-microscopic observation of beta-cells in pancreatic islets of spontaneously diabetic Goto-Kakizaki rats. Med Mol Morphol 39:146–153
41. Koyama M, Wada R, Sakuraba H et al (1998) Accelerated loss of islet beta-cells in sucrose-fed Goto-Kakizaki rats, a genetic model of non-insulin-dependent diabetes mellitus. Am J Pathol 153:537–545
42. Goda T, Suruga K, Komori A et al (2007) Effects of miglitol, an alpha-glucosidase inhibitor, on glycaemic status and histopathological changes in islets in non-obese, non-insulin-dependent diabetic Goto-Kakizaki rats. Br J Nutr 98:702–710
43. Seiça R, Martins MJ, Pessa PB et al (2003) Morphological changes of islet of Langerhans in an animal model of type 2 diabetes. Acta Med Port 16:381–388
44. Keno Y, Tokunaga K, Fujioka S et al (1994) Marked reduction of pancreatic insulin content in male ventromedial hypothalamic-lesioned spontaneously non-insulin-dependent diabetic (Goto-Kakizaki) rats. Metabolism 43:32–37
45. Östenson CG, Khan A, Abdel-Halim SM et al (1993) Abnormal insulin secretion and glucose metabolism in pancreatic islets from the spontaneously diabetic GK rat. Diabetologia 36:3–8
46. Suzuki N, Aizawa T, Asanuma N et al (1997) An early insulin intervention accelerates pancreatic β-cell dysfunction in young Goto-Kakizaki

rats, a model of naturally occurring noninsulin-dependent diabetes. Endocrinology 138: 1106–1110
47. Salehi A, Henningsson R, Mosén H et al (1999) Dysfunction of the islet lysosomal system conveys impairment of glucose-induced insulin release in the diabetic GK rat. Endocrinology 140:3045–3053
48. Giroix MH, Vesco L, Portha B (1993) Functional and metabolic perturbations in isolated pancreatic islets from the GK rat, a genetic model of non-insulin dependent diabetes. Endocrinology 132:815–822
49. Nagamatsu S, Nakamichi Y, Yamamura C et al (1999) Decreased expression of t-SNARE, syntaxin 1, and SNAP-25 in pancreatic beta-cells is involved in impaired insulin secretion from diabetic GK rat islets: restoration of decreased t-SNARE proteins improves impaired insulin secretion. Diabetes 48:2367–2373
50. Gauguier D, Froguel P, Parent V et al (1996) Chromosomal mapping of genetic loci associated with non-insulin dependent diabetes in the GK rat. Nat Genet 12:38–43
51. Galli J, Li LS, Glaser A et al (1996) Genetic analysis of non-insulin dependent diabetes mellitus in the GK rat. Nat Genet 12:31–37
52. Gauguier D, Nelson I, Bernard C et al (1994) Higher maternal than paternal inheritance of diabetes in GK rats. Diabetes 43:220–224
53. Kimura K, Toyota T, Kakizaki M et al (1982) Impaired insulin secretion in the spontaneous diabetes rats. Tohoku J Exp Med 137: 453–459
54. Abdel-Halim SM, Guenifi A, Khan A et al (1996) Impaired coupling of glucose signal to the exocytotic machinery in diabetic GK rats; a defect ameliorated by cAMP. Diabetes 45:934–940
55. Giroix MH, Sener A, Portha B et al (1993) Preferential alteration of oxidative relative to total glycolysis in pancreatic islets of two rats models of inherited or acquired type 2 (non-insulin dependent) diabetes mellitus. Diabetologia 36:305–309
56. Östenson CG, Abdel-Halim SM, Rasschaert J et al (1993) Deficient activity of FAD-linked glycerophosphate dehydrogenase in islets of GK rats. Diabetologia 36:722–728
57. Tsuura Y, Ishida H, Okamoto Y et al (1993) Glucose sensitivity of ATP-sensitive K+ channels is impaired in beta-cells of the GK rat A new genetic model of NIDDM. Diabetes 42:1446–1453
58. Giroix MH, Sener A, Bailbé D et al (1993) Metabolic, ionic and secretory response to D-glucose in islets from rats with acquired or inherited non-insulin dependent diabetes. Biochem Med Metab Biol 50:301–321
59. Ling ZC, Efendic S, Wibom R et al (1998) Glucose metabolism in Goto–Kakizaki rat islets. Endocrinology 139:2670–2675
60. Ling ZC, Hong-Lie C, Östenson CG et al (2001) Hyperglycemia contributes to impaired insulin response in GK rat islets. Diabetes 50(suppl 1):108–112
61. Fradet M, Giroix MH, Bailbé D et al (2008) Glucokinase activators modulate glucose metabolism and glucose-stimulated insulin secretion in islets from diabetic GK/Par rats (Abstract). Diabetologia 51(suppl 1):A198–A199
62. Koyama M, Wada R, Mizukami H et al (2000) Inhibition of progressive reduction of islet beta-cell mass in spontaneously diabetic Goto-Kakizaki rats by alpha-glucosidase inhibitor. Metabolism 49:347–352
63. Hughes SJ, Faehling M, Thorneley CW et al (1998) Electrophysiological and metabolic characterization of single beta-cells and islets from diabetic GK rats. Diabetes 47:73–81
64. Zhou YP, Östenson CG, Ling ZC et al (1995) Deficiency of pyruvate dehydrogenase activity in pancreatic islets of diabetic GK rats. Endocrinology 136:3546–3551
65. MacDonald MJ, Efendic S, Östenson CG (1996) Normalization by insulin treatment of low mitochondrial glycerol phosphate dehydrogenase and pyruvate carboxylase in pancreatic islets of the GK rat. Diabetes 45:886–890
66. Serradas P, Giroix MH, Saulnier C et al (1995) Mitochondrial deoxyribonucleic acid content is specifically decreased in adult, but not fetal, pancreatic islets of the Goto-Kakizaki rat, a genetic model of non-insulin-dependent diabetes. Endocrinology 136:5623–5631
67. Marie JC, Bailbé D, Gylfe E et al (2001) Defective glucose-dependent cytosolic Ca2+ handling in islets of GK and nSTZ rat models of type2 diabetes. J Endocrinol 169:169–176
68. Dolz M, Bailbé D, Giroix MH et al (2005) Restitution of defective glucose-stimulated insulin secretion in diabetic GK rat by acetylcholine uncovers paradoxical stimulatory effect of beta cell muscarinic receptor activation on cAMP production. Diabetes 54:3229–3237
69. Shang W, Yasuda K, Takahashi A et al (2002) Effect of high dietary fat on insulin secretion in genetically diabetic Goto-Kakizaki rats. Pancreas 25:393–399
70. Briaud I, Kelpe CL, Johnson LM et al (2002) Differential effects of hyperlipidemia on insulin secretion in islets of Langerhans from hyperglycemic versus normoglycemic rats. Diabetes 51:662–668

71. Dolz M, Movassat J, Bailbé D et al (2011) cAMP-secretion coupling is impaired in diabetic GK/Par rat β-cells. A defect counteracted by GLP-1. Am J Physiol Endocrinol Metab 301:E797–E806
72. Váradi A, Molnár E, Östenson CG et al (1996) Isoforms of endoplasmic reticulum Ca2+-ATPase are differentially expressed in normal and diabetic islets of Langerhans. Biochem J 319:521–527
73. Abdel-Halim SM, Guenifi A, He B et al (1998) Mutations in the promoter of adenylyl cyclase (AC)-III gene, overexpression of AC-III mRNA, and enhanced cAMP generation in islets from the spontaneously diabetic GK rat model of type 2 diabetes. Diabetes 47:498–504
74. Guenifi A, Simonsson E, Karlsson S et al (2001) Carbachol restores insulin release in diabetic GK rat islets by mechanisms largely involving hydrolysis of diacylglycerol and direct interaction with the exocytotic machinery. Pancreas 22:164–171
75. Mosén H, Östenson CG, Lundquist I et al (2008) Impaired glucose-stimulated insulin secretion in the rat is associated with abnormalities in islet nitric oxide production. Regul Pept 151:139–146
76. Salehi A, Meidute AS, Jimenez-Feltstrom J et al (2008) Excessive islet NO generation in type 2 diabetic GK rats coincides with abnormal hormone secretion and is counteracted by GLP1. PLoS One 3(5):e2165
77. Mosén H, Salehi A, Alm P et al (2005) Defective glucose-stimulated insulin release in the diabetic Goto-Kakizaki (GK) rat coincides with reduced activity of the islet carbon monoxide signaling pathway. Endocrinology 146:1553–1558
78. Yan J, Feng Z, Liu J et al (2012) Enhanced autophagy plays a cardinal role in mitochondrial dysfunction in type 2 diabetic Goto-Kakizaki (GK) rats: ameliorating effects of (−)-epigallocatechin-3-gallate. J Nutr Biochem. 23(7):716–724
79. Warwar N, Efendic S, Östenson CG et al (2006) Dynamics of glucose-induced localization of PKC isoenzymes in pancreatic beta-cells. Diabetes-related changes in the GK rat. Diabetes 55:590–599
80. Rose T, Efendic S, Rupnik M (2007) Ca2+-secretion coupling is impaired in diabetic Goto Kakizaki rats. J Gen Physiol 129:493–508
81. Abella A, Marti L, Camps M et al (2003) Semicarbazide-sensitive amine oxidase/vascular adhesion protein-1 activity exerts an antidiabetic action in Goto–Kakizaki rats. Diabetes 52:1004–1013
82. Chen J, Östenson CG (2005) Inhibition of protein-tyrosine phosphatases stimulates insulin secretion in pancreatic islets of diabetic Goto–Kakizaki rats. Pancreas 30:314–317
83. Östenson CG, Sandberg-Nordqvist AC, Chen J et al (2002) Overexpression of protein tyrosine phosphatase PTP sigma is linked to impaired glucose-induced insulin secretion in hereditary diabetic Goto–Kakizaki rats. Biochem Biophys Res Commun 291:945–950
84. Kowluru A (2003) Defective protein histidine phosphorylation in islets from the Goto–Kakizaki diabetic rat. Am J Physiol 285:E498–E503
85. Leckström A, Östenson CG, Efendic S et al (1996) Increased storage and secretion of islet amyloid polypeptide relative to insulin in the spontaneously diabetic GK rat. Pancreas 13:259–267
86. Weng HB, Gu Q, Liu M et al (2008) Increased secretion and expression of amylin in spontaneously diabetic Goto-Kakizaki rats treated with rhGLP1(7–36). Acta Pharmacol Sin 29:573–579
87. Okamoto Y, Ishida H, Tsuura Y et al (1995) Hyperresponse in calcium-induced insulin release from electrically permeabilized pancreatic islets of diabetic GK rats and its defective augmentation by glucose. Diabetologia 38:772–778
88. Gaisano HY, Östenson CG, Sheu L et al (2002) Abnormal expression of pancreatic islet exocytotic soluble N-ethylmaleimide-sensitive factor attachment protein receptors in Goto-Kakizaki rats is partially restored by phlorizin treatment and accentuated by high glucose treatment. Endocrinology 143:4218–4226
89. Zhang W, Khan A, Östenson CG et al (2002) Down-regulated expression of exocytotic proteins in pancreatic islets of diabetic GK rats. Biochem Biophys Res Commun 291:1038–1044
90. Ohara-Imaizumi M, Nishiwaki C, Kikuta T et al (2004) TIRF imaging of docking and fusion of single insulin granule motion in primary rat pancreatic beta cells: different behaviour of granule motion between normal and Goto–Kakizaki diabetic rat beta-cells. Biochem J 381:13–18
91. Movassat J, Deybach C, Bailbé D et al (2005) Involvement of cortical actin cytoskeleton in the defective insulin secretion in Goto-Kakizaki rats (Abstract). Diabetes 54:A1
92. Kaiser N, Nesher R, Oprescu A et al (2005) Characterization of the action of S21403 (mitiglinide) on insulin secretion and biosynthesis in normal and diabetic beta-cells. Br J Pharmacol 146:872–881

93. Katayama N, Hughes SJ, Persaud SJ et al (1995) Insulin secretion from islets of GK rats is not impaired after energy generating steps. Mol Cell Endocrinol 111:125–128
94. Bisbis S, Bailbe D, Tormo MA et al (1993) Insulin resistance in the GK rat: decreased receptor number but normal kinase activity in liver. Am J Physiol 265(5):E807–E813
95. Picarel-Blanchot F, Berthelier C, Bailbé D et al (1996) Impaired insulin secretion and excessive hepatic glucose production are both early events in the diabetic GK rat. Am J Physiol 271(4):E755–E762
96. Berthelier C, Kergoat M, Portha B (1997) Lack of deterioration of insulin action with aging in the GK rat: a contrasted adaptation as compared with nondiabetic rats. Metabolism 46:890–896
97. Movassat J, Bailbé D, Lubrano-Berthelier C et al (2008) Follow-up of GK rats during prediabetes highlights increased insulin action and fat deposition despite low insulin secretion. Am J Physiol Endocrinol Metab 294(1):E168–E175
98. Beauquis J, Homo-Delarche F, Giroix MH et al (2010) Hippocampal neurovascular and hypothalamic pituitary adrenal axis alterations in spontaneously type 2 diabetic GK rats. Exp Neurol 222:125–134
99. Almon RR, DuBois DC, Lai W et al (2009) Gene expression analysis of hepatic roles in cause and development of diabetes in Goto-Kakizaki rats. J Endocrinol 200(3):331–346
100. Nolte LA, Abdel-Halim SM, Martin IK et al (1995) Development of decreased insulin-induced glucose transport in skeletal muscle of glucose-intolerant hybrids of diabetic GK rats. Clin Sci (Lond) 88(3):301–306
101. Krook A, Kawano Y, Song XM et al (1997) Improved glucose tolerance restores insulin-stimulated Akt kinase activity and glucose transport in skeletal muscle from diabetic Goto-Kakizaki rats. Diabetes 46(12):2110–2114
102. Steiler TL, Galuska D, Leng Y et al (2003) Effect of hyperglycemia on signal transduction in skeletal muscle from diabetic Goto-Kakizaki rats. Endocrinology 144(12):5259–5267
103. Song XM, Kawano Y, Krook A et al (1999) Muscle fiber type-specific defects in insulin signal transduction to glucose transport in diabetic GK rats. Diabetes 48(3):664–670
104. Farese RV, Standaert ML, Yamada K et al (1994) Insulin-induced activation of glycerol-3-phosphate acyltransferase by a chiro-inositol-containing insulin mediator is defective in adipocytes of insulin-resistant, type II diabetic, Goto-Kakizaki rats. Proc Natl Acad Sci U S A 91(23):11040–11044
105. Begum N, Ragolia L (1998) Altered regulation of insulin signaling components in adipocytes of insulin-resistant type II diabetic Goto-Kakizaki rats. Metabolism 47:54–62
106. Dadke SS, Li HC, Kusari AB et al (2000) Elevated expression and activity of protein-tyrosine phosphatase 1B in skeletal muscle of insulin-resistant type II diabetic Goto-Kakizaki rats. Biochem Biophys Res Commun 274(3):583–589
107. Kanoh Y, Bandyopadhyay G, Sajan MP et al (2001) Rosiglitazone, insulin treatment, and fasting correct defective activation of protein kinase C-zeta/lambda by insulin in vastus lateralis muscles and adipocytes of diabetic rats. Endocrinology 142(4):1595–1605
108. Nie J, Xue B, Sukumaran S et al (2011) Differential muscle gene expression as a function of disease progression in Goto-Kakizaki diabetic rats. Mol Cell Endocrinol 338(1–2):10–17
109. Yasuda K, Nishikawa W, Iwanaka N et al (2002) Abnormality in fibre type distribution of soleus and plantaris muscles in non-obese diabetic Goto-Kakizaki rats. Clin Exp Pharmacol Physiol 29(11):1001–1008
110. Copp SW, Hageman KS, Behnke BJ et al (2010) Effects of type II diabetes on exercising skeletal muscle blood flow in the rat. J Appl Physiol 109(5):1347–1353
111. Padilla DJ, McDonough P, Behnke BJ et al (2006) Effects of type II diabetes on capillary hemodynamics in skeletal muscle. Am J Physiol Heart Circ Physiol 291(5):H2439–H2444
112. Padilla DJ, McDonough P, Behnke BJ et al (2007) Effects of type II diabetes on muscle microvascular oxygen pressures. Respir Physiol Neurobiol 156(2):187–195
113. Barzilai N, Rossetti L (1995) Relationship between changes in body composition and insulin responsiveness in models of the aging rat. Am J Physiol 1269:E591–E597
114. De Fronzo RA (1979) Glucose intolerance and aging. Diabetes 28:1095–1101
115. Xue B, Sukumaran S, Nie J et al (2011) Adipose tissue deficiency and chronic inflammation in diabetic Goto-Kakizaki rats. PLoS One 6(2):e17386
116. Movassat J, Calderari S, Fernández E et al (2007) Type 2 diabetes—a matter of failing beta-cell neogenesis? Clues from the GK rat model. Diabetes Obes Metab 9(suppl 2):187–195
117. Serradas P, Goya L, Lacorne M et al (2002) Fetal insulin-like growth factor-2 production is impaired in the GK rat model of type 2 diabetes. Diabetes 51:392–397

118. Katakura M, Komatsu M, Sato Y et al (2004) Primacy of beta-cell dysfunction in the development of hyperglycemia: a study in the Japanese general population. Metabolism 53:949–953
119. Lin JM, Ortsäter H, Fakhraid-Ra H et al (2001) Phenotyping of individual pancreatic islets locates genetic defects in stimulus secretion coupling to Niddm1i within the major diabetes locus in GK rats. Diabetes 50:2737–2743
120. Granhall C, Rosengren AH, Renström E et al (2006) Separately inherited defects in insulin exocytosis and beta-cell glucose metabolism contribute to type 2 diabetes. Diabetes 55:3494–3500
121. Wallis RH, Collins SC, Kaisaki PJ et al (2008) Pathophysiological, genetic and gene expression features of a novel rodent model of the cardio-metabolic syndrome. PLoS One 3(8):e2962
122. Finlay C, Argoud K, Wilder SP et al (2010) Chromosomal mapping of pancreatic islet morphological features and regulatory hormones in the spontaneously diabetic (type 2) Goto-Kakizaki rat. Mamm Genome 21:499–508
123. Hu Y, Kaisaki P, Argoud K et al (2009) Functional annotations of diabetes nephropathy susceptibility loci through analysis of genome-wide renal gene expression in rat models of diabetes mellitus. BMC Med Genomics 2:41
124. Argoud K, Wilder SP, McAteer MA et al (2006) Genetic control of plasma lipid levels in a cross derived from normoglycaemic Brown Norway and spontaneously diabetic Goto-Kakizaki rats. Diabetologia 49:2679–2688
125. Bilusic M, Bataillard A, Tschannen MR et al (2004) Mapping the genetic determinants of hypertension, metabolic diseases, and related phenotypes in the lyon hypertensive rat. Hypertension 44:695–701
126. Galli J, Fakhrai-Rad H, Kamel A et al (1999) Pathophysiological and genetic characterization of the major diabetes locus in GK rats. Diabetes 48(12):2463–2470
127. Duggirala R, Blangero J, Almasy L et al (1999) Linkage of type 2 diabetes mellitus and of age at onset to a genetic location on chromosome 10q in Mexican Americans. Am J Hum Genet 64:1127–1140
128. Grant SF, Thorleifsson G, Reynisdottir I et al (2006) Variant of transcription factor 7-like 2 (TCF7L2) gene confers risk of type 2 diabetes. Nat Genet 38:320–323
129. Rosengren AH, Jokubka R, Tojjar D et al (2010) Overexpression of alpha2A-adrenergic receptors contributes to type 2 diabetes. Science 327:217–220
130. Fakhrai-Rad H, Nikoshkov A, Kamel A et al (2000) Insulin-degrading enzyme identified as a candidate diabetes susceptibility gene in GK rats. Hum Mol Genet 9(14):2149–2158
131. Marion E, Kaisaki PJ, Pouillon V et al (2002) The gene INPPL1, encoding the lipid phosphatase SHIP2, is a candidate for type 2 diabetes in rat and man. Diabetes 51(7):2012–2017
132. Herrera BM, Lockstone HE, Taylor JM et al (2010) Global microRNA expression profiles in insulin target tissues in a spontaneous rat model of type 2 diabetes. Diabetologia 53(6):1099–1109
133. Esguerra JL, Bolmeson C, Cilio CM et al (2011) Differential glucose-regulation of microRNAs in pancreatic islets of non-obese type 2 diabetes model Goto-Kakizaki rat. PLoS One 6(4):e18613
134. Simmons R (2006) Developmental origins of adult metabolic disease. Endocrinol Metab Clin North Am 35:193–204
135. Portha B, Chavey A, Movassat J (2011) Early-life origins of type 2 diabetes: fetal programming of the beta-cell mass. Exp Diabetes Res 2011:105076
136. Serradas P, Gangnerau MN, Giroix MH et al (1998) Impaired pancreatic beta cell function in the fetal GK rat. Impact of diabetic inheritance. J Clin Invest 101:899–904
137. Gill-Randall R, Adams D, Ollerton RL et al (2004) Type 2 diabetes mellitus—genes or intrauterine environment? An embryo transfer paradigm in rats. Diabetologia 47:1354–1369
138. Chavey A, Gangnerau MN, Maulny L et al (2008) Intrauterine programming of beta-cell development and function by maternal diabetes. What tell us embryo-transfer experiments in GK/Par rats? (Abstract). Diabetologia 51(suppl 1):A151
139. Calderari S, Gangnerau MN, Meile MJ et al (2006) Is defective pancreatic beta-cell mass environmentally programmed in Goto Kakizaki rat model of type 2 diabetes: insights from cross breeding studies during suckling period. Pancreas 33:412–417
140. Mizukami H, Wada R, Koyama M et al (2008) Augmented beta-cell loss and mitochondrial abnormalities in sucrose-fed GK rats. Virchows Arch 452:383–392
141. Yasuda K, Okamoto Y, Nunoi K et al (2002) Normalization of cytoplasmic calcium response in pancreatic beta-cells of spontaneously diabetic GK rat by the treatment with T-1095, a specific inhibitor of renal Na+-glucose co-transporters. Horm Metab Res 34:217–221
142. Kawai J, Ohara-Imaizumi M, Nakamichi Y et al (2008) Insulin exocytosis in Goto-Kakizaki

rat beta-cells subjected to long-term glinide or sulfonylurea treatment. Biochem J 412: 93–101

143. Dachicourt N, Bailbé D, Gangnerau MN et al (1998) Effect of gliclazide treatment on insulin secretion and beta-cell mass in non-insulin dependent diabetic Goto-Kakizaki rats. Eur J Pharmacol 361:243–251

144. Ohta T, Furukawa N, Komuro G et al (1999) JTT-608 restores impaired early insulin secretion in diabetic Goto-Kakizaki rats. Br J Pharmacol 126:1674–1680

145. Ohta T, Miyajima K, Komuro G et al (2003) Antidiabetic effect of chronic administration of JTT-608, a new hypoglycaemic agent, in diabetic Goto-Kakizaki rats. Eur J Pharmacol 476:159–166

146. Ishida H, Kato S, Nishimura M et al (1998) Beneficial effect of long-term combined treatment with voglibose and pioglitazone on pancreatic islet function of genetically diabetic GK rats. Horm Metab Res 30:673–678

147. Goto Y, Kakizaki M, Yagihashi S (1982) Neurological findings in spontaneously diabetic rats. Excerpta Med Int Congr Ser 581: 26–38

148. Kitahara Y, Miura K, Takesue K et al (2002) Decreased blood glucose excursion by nateglinide ameliorated neuropathic changes in Goto Kakizaki rats, an animal model of non-obese type 2 diabetes. Metabolism 5: 1452–1457

149. Murakawa Y, Zhang W, Pierson CR et al (2002) Impaired glucose tolerance and insulinopenia in the GK-rat causes peripheral neuropathy. Diabetes Metab Res Rev 18(6):473–483

150. Agardh CD, Agardh E, Zhang H, Östenson CG (1997) Altered endothelial/pericyte ratio in Goto–Kakizaki rat retina. J Diabetes Complications 11:158–162

151. Agardh CD, Agardh E, Hultberg B et al (1998) The glutathione levels are reduced in Goto-Kakizaki rat retina, but are not influenced by aminoguanidine treatment. Curr Eye Res 17(3):251–256

152. Sone H, Kawakami Y, Okuda Y et al (1997) Ocular vascular endothelial growth factor levels in diabetic rats are elevated before observable retinal proliferative changes. Diabetologia 40(6):726–730

153. Miyamoto K, Ogura Y, Nishiwaki H et al (1996) Evaluation of retinal microcirculatory alterations in the Goto-Kakizaki rat. A spontaneous model of non-insulin-dependent diabetes. Invest Ophthalmol Vis Sci 37:898–905

154. Carmo A, Cunha-Vaz JG, Carvalho AP et al (2000) Nitric oxide synthase activity in retinas from non-insulin-dependent diabetic Goto–Kakizaki rats: correlation with blood-retinal barrier permeability. Nitric Oxide 4:590–596

155. Lang BT, Yan Y, Dempsey RJ et al (2009) Impaired neurogenesis in adult type-2 diabetic rats. Brain Res 1258:25–33

156. Moreira T, Malec E, Ostenson CG et al (2007) Diabetic type II Goto-Kakizaki rats show progressively decreasing exploratory activity and learning impairments in fixed and progressive ratios of a lever-press task. Behav Brain Res 180:28–41

157. Moreira T, Cebers G, Pickering C et al (2007) Diabetic Goto-Kakizaki rats display pronounced hyperglycemia and longer-lasting cognitive impairments following ischemia induced by cortical compression. Neuroscience 144(4):1169–1185

158. Moreira TJ, Cebere A, Cebers G et al (2007) Reduced HO-1 protein expression is associated with more severe neurodegeneration after transient ischemia induced by cortical compression in diabetic Goto-Kakizaki rats. J Cereb Blood Flow Metab 27(10):1710–1723

159. Moreira PI, Santos MS, Moreno AM et al (2003) Increased vulnerability of brain mitochondria in diabetic (Goto-Kakizaki) rats with aging and amyloid-beta exposure. Diabetes 52:1449–1456

160. Janssen U, Vassiliadou A, Riley SG et al (2004) The quest for a model of type II diabetes with nephropathy: the Goto Kakizaki rat. J Nephrol 17(6):769–773

161. Valensi P, Mesangeau D, Paries J et al (1996) Erythrocyte rheology and heart hypertrophy in diabetes mellitus. J Mal Vasc 21:185–187

162. Witte K, Jacke K, Stahrenberg R et al (2002) Dysfunction of soluble guanylyl cyclase in aorta and kidney of Goto-Kakizaki rats: influence of age and diabetic state. Nitric Oxide 6:85–95

163. Cheng ZJ, Vaskonen T, Tikkanen I et al (2001) Endothelial dysfunction and salt-sensitive hypertension in spontaneously diabetic Goto-Kakizaki rats. Hypertension 37:433–439

164. Desrois M, Sidell RJ, Gauguier D et al (2004) Initial steps of insulin signaling and glucose transport are defective in the type 2 diabetic rat heart. Cardiovasc Res 61:288–296

165. Darmellah A, Baetz D, Prunier F et al (2007) Enhanced activity of the myocardial Na^+/H^+ exchanger contributes to left ventricular hypertrophy in the Goto-Kakizaki rat model of type 2 diabetes: critical role of Akt. Diabetologia 50:1335–1344

166. El-Omar MM, Yang ZK, Phillips AO et al (2004) Cardiac dysfunction in the Goto–Kakizaki rat. A model of type II diabetes mellitus. Basic Res Cardiol 99:133–141

167. Chandler MP, Morgan EE, McElfresh TA et al (2007) Heart failure progression is accelerated following myocardial infarction in type 2 diabetic rats. Am J Physiol Heart Circ Physiol 293:H1609–H1616
168. Kristiansen SB, Lofgren B, Stottrup NB et al (2004) Ischaemic preconditioning does not protect the heart in obese and lean animal models of type 2 diabetes. Diabetologia 47:1716–1721
169. Howarth FC, Shafiullah M, Qureshi MA (2007) Chronic effects of type 2 diabetes mellitus on cardiac muscle contraction in the Goto-Kakizaki rat. Exp Physiol 92:1029–1036
170. Howarth FC, Jacobson M, Shafiullah M et al (2008) Long-term effects of type 2 diabetes mellitus on heart rhythm in the Goto-Kakizaki rat. Exp Physiol 93:362–369
171. Desrois M, Clarke K, Lan C et al (2010) Upregulation of eNOS and unchanged energy metabolism in increased susceptibility of the aging type 2 diabetic GK rat heart to ischemic injury. Am J Physiol Heart Circ Physiol 299:H1679–H1686
172. Kazuyama E, Saito M et al (2009) Endothelial dysfunction in the early- and late-stage type-2 diabetic Goto-Kakizaki rat aorta. Mol Cell Biochem 332:95–102
173. Bulhak AA, Jung C, Ostenson CG et al (2009) PPAR-alpha activation protects the type 2 diabetic myocardium against ischemia-reperfusion injury: involvement of the PI3-Kinase/Akt and NO pathway. Am J Physiol Heart Circ Physiol 296:H719–H727
174. El-Omar MM, Lord R, Draper NJ et al (2003) Role of nitric oxide in posthypoxic contractile dysfunction of diabetic cardiomyopathy. Eur J Heart Fail 5:229–239
175. Santos DL, Palmeira CM, Seiça R et al (2003) Diabetes and mitochondrial oxidative stress: a study using heart mitochondria from the diabetic Goto-Kakizaki rat. Mol Cell Biochem 246(1–2):63–70
176. Phillips AO, Baboolal K, Riley S et al (2001) Association of prolonged hyperglycemia with glomerular hypertrophy and renal basement membrane thickening in the Goto Kakizaki model of non-insulin-dependent diabetes mellitus. Am J Kidney Dis 37(2):400–410
177. Schrijvers BF, De Vriese AS, Van de Voorde J et al (2004) Long-term renal changes in the Goto-Kakizaki rat, a model of lean type 2 diabetes. Nephrol Dial Transplant 19:1092–1097
178. Vesely DL, Gower WR Jr, Dietz JR, Overton RM, Clark LC, Antwi EK, Farese RV (1999) Elevated atrial natriuretic peptides and early renal failure in type 2 diabetic Goto-Kakizaki rats. Metabolism 48(6):771–778
179. Yagihashi S, Goto Y, Kakizaki M et al (1978) Thickening of glomerular basement membrane in spontaneously diabetic rats. Diabetologia 15:309–312
180. Sato N, Komatsu K, Kurumatani H (2003) Late onset of diabetic nephropathy in spontaneously diabetic GK rats. Am J Nephrol 23:334–342
181. Yoshida S, Yamashita S, Tokunaga K et al (1996) Visceral fat accumulation and vascular complications associated with VMH lesioning of spontaneously non-insulin-dependent diabetic GK rat. Int J Obes Relat Metab Disord 20(10):909–916
182. Nishida M, Miyagawa JI, Tokunaga K et al (1997) Early morphologic changes of atherosclerosis induced by ventromedial hypothalamic lesion in the spontaneously diabetic Goto-Kakizaki rat. J Lab Clin Med 129(2):200–207
183. Louro TM, Matafome PN, Nunes EC et al (2011) Insulin and metformin may prevent renal injury in young type 2 diabetic Goto-Kakizaki rats. Eur J Pharmacol 25(653):89–94
184. Östenson CG, Fière V, Ahmed M et al (1997) Decreased cortical bone thickness in spontaneously non-insulin-dependent diabetic GK rats. J Diabetes Complications 11(6):319–322
185. Ahmad T, Ohlsson C, Sääf M et al (2003) Skeletal changes in type-2 diabetic Goto-Kakizaki rats. J Endocrinol 178(1):111–116
186. Ahmad T, Ugarph-Morawski A, Li J et al (2004) Bone and joint neuropathy in rats with type-2 diabetes. Regul Pept 119(1–2):61–67
187. Wang F, Song YL, Li DH et al (2010) Type 2 diabetes mellitus impairs bone healing of dental implants in GK rats. Diabetes Res Clin Pract 88:e7–e9

Chapter 10

Experimentally Induced Rodent Models of Type 2 Diabetes

Md. Shahidul Islam and Rachel Dorothy Wilson

Abstract

Diabetes is one of the major global public health problems and is gradually getting worse particularly in developing nations where 95% of patients are suffering from type 2 diabetes (T2D). Animal models in diabetes research are very common where rodents are the best choice of use due to being smaller in size, easy to handle, omnivorous in nature, and non-wild tranquil behavior. Normally rodent models are classified into two major classes namely: (1) genetic or spontaneously induced models and (2) non-genetic or experimentally induced models. Non-genetic models are more popular compared to genetic models due to lower cost, wider availability, easier to induce diabetes, and of course easier to maintain compared to genetic models. A number of non-genetic models have been developed in last three decades for diabetes research including adult alloxan/streptozotocin (STZ) models, partial pancreatectomy model, high-fat (HF) diet-fed models, fructose-fed models, HF diet-fed STZ models, nicotinamide–STZ models, monosodium-glutamate (MSG) induced models, and intrauterine growth retardation (IUGR) models. A T2D model should have the all major pathogenesis of the disease usually found in humans; however, none of the above-mentioned models are without limitations. This chapter comparatively evaluates most of the experimentally induced rodent models of T2D with their limitations, advantages, disadvantages, and criticality of development in order to help diabetes research groups to more appropriately select the animal models to work on their specific research question.

Key words: Streptozotocin, Alloxan, Nicotinamide, High-fat diet, Fructose, Intrauterine growth retardation, Monosodium glutamate

1. Introduction

By 2030, the World Health Organization (WHO) predicts that over 330 million people worldwide will have diabetes, and the percentages of national health care budget to diabetes alone, are estimated at 5–10% (1). Between two major types of diabetes, type 2 is the most prevalent in adults with different range of age and gradually increasing in young children and adolescents. In a recent comprehensive review (2), it has been clearly summarized that type 2 diabetes (T2D) is increasing among the children in all over the world, and appears that have increased significantly in last 20 years. It was also reported that T2D accounts for up to 45% in new cases among adolescents. In Japan, 80% of new cases of pediatric diabetes (3) and 70% of new cases among Native Americans are identified as T2D (3, 4). T2D is a heterogeneous disorder characterized by a progressive decline in insulin action (insulin resistance), followed by the inability of β-cells to compensate for insulin resistance (β-cell dysfunction) (5). The prevalence of T2D is more than type 1 and it is about 95% of total existing diabetic cases in the world. With the prevalence of T2D on the rise, drug development research and intensive studies into disease mechanistic has sharply increased; with the majority of work being performed on animal models (6).

To date, an extensive range of animal models has been developed which includes non-human primates, large mammals such as pigs, dogs, and cats and smaller animals such as rabbits, rats, and mice. Larger animals are naturally difficult to maintain, require higher maintenance costs and hence are not as commonly used as the smaller animals. Among the smaller animal models, rodents are the first choice of use due to their smaller body size, omnivorous nature, and non-wild tranquil behavior, which allows for an ease of handling for researchers as well as significantly reduced dietary and housing costs. Rodent models are subdivided into two major categories: genetic or spontaneously induced models and non-genetic or non-spontaneously or experimentally induced models (7). This chapter has been designed to discuss only the non-genetic or experimentally induced rodent models of T2D.

2. Experimentally Induced Rodent Models of Diabetes

Experimentally or non-spontaneously induced or non-genetic models are so-named as they make use of non-genetic animal strains those that are not diabetic under normal conditions (7). These animals are much cheaper in price and far more widely available to researchers worldwide compared to genetically or spontaneously induced diabetic models. Experimentally induced models can be induced either by chemical means or by dietary manipulation or by their combination. Besides the cost factor, these models have become highly popular in recent years due to the resemblance of the pathogenesis of diabetes in humans. No single model presents the full pathophysiology of T2D. However, rodent models are available that present one or both of the two major pathogenic features of T2D—these being insulin resistance and, subsequently, the development of pancreatic beta cell dysfunction. A number of approaches have been used to induce these two major pathogenesis of T2D in rodents including partial pancreatectomy, neonatal streptozotocin (STZ) or alloxan injection, single dose of STZ/alloxan injection, long-term high-fat (HF) diet or fructose feeding, combination of nicotinamide and STZ injections, combination of HF diet feeding and STZ injection, combination of fructose feeding and STZ injection, injection of monosodium glutamate (MSG), and intrauterine growth reduction (IUGR). Although many of these approaches could not successfully induce the full pathogenesis of T2D, some recent models were almost successful in this regard. Although a number of approaches have been used to develop the animal models of T2D, this chapter will discuss the most widely used approaches for the development of experimentally induced rodent models of T2D including their advantages, disadvantages, limitations, and difficulties faced during the development of each model in order to help researchers to choose an appropriate model for a specific study.

2.1. Adult Streptozotocin/Alloxan Models

Alloxan was used for the first time in 1943 to induce T2D in animals by Goldner and Gomori (8). It is a uric acid derivative that selectively destroys pancreatic beta cells by oxidative stress mechanisms (9). However, the use of alloxan nowadays is significantly lower compared to STZ due to its lesser efficacy and some proven side effects in animals e.g., liver and kidney damage. The STZ, on the other hand, is a natural antibiotic produced by the bacterial species *Streptomyces achromogenes* (10). It is a structural analogue of N-acetyl glucosamine that acts as a potent alkylating agent which results in disrupted glucose transport, glucokinase activity as well as the breakdown of multiple DNA strands (11). Over the decades, various combinations have been used to develop animal models by using STZ or alloxan; including single high dose STZ injection (>65 mg/kg BW), multiple low dose STZ injections (<35 mg/kg BW) or its combination with HF diets. It is, however, known that single high dose STZ injection (>60 mg/kg BW) results in massive pancreatic beta cell destruction, more characteristic of T1D, whereas intermediate dosages of STZ injections (between 40 and 55 mg/kg BW) cause only partial impairment to insulin secretory mechanisms seen in T2D (5). A single dose lower than 35 mg/kg BW in rats fed a normal commercial diet usually fails to elicit any hyperglycemic effect (5). The STZ is usually injected intraperitoneally at varying dosages to rats (35–65 mg/kg BW) and mice (100–200 mg/kg BW) and in the case of alloxan, 40–200 mg/kg BW to rats and 50–200 mg/kg BW to mice (7). These models are usually characterized by fasting or non-fasting hyperglycemia, lowered serum insulin levels with hyperlipidemia; however, insulin resistance is often absent in these models. Due to this limitation, although these models cannot be considered as appropriate models for T2D but they can be used for the screening of antihyperglycemic or insulinotropic drugs and natural medicines.

2.2. Neonatal Streptozotocin/Alloxan Models

Neonatal STZ and alloxan diabetic models have been employed since mid 1970s (12, 13). Thereafter, several attempts at refining this model have been made, most successfully using dosages of STZ between 25 and 50 mg/kg BW in male spontaneously hypertensive rats (SHR) (14). In these models, STZ is most commonly delivered intraperitoneally to neonatal rats 2 days after birth. Initially until the 4th week, NFBG levels appear normal to moderately hyperglycemic. As adulthood approaches, hyperglycemia progressively develops, leading to adult-onset T2D mellitus (15). It is important to note the discrepancies of these models when using different rodent strains. Two days old male Wister rats have been shown to develop diabetes only when injected with a significantly higher dose of STZ (90 mg/kg BW i.p.) (16); however, Fischer 344 rats develop a stable and optimal diabetic state when injected with a STZ dose of 80 mg/kg BW (i.p.). Apart from STZ, alloxan was also used to develop this model with a dose of 200 mg/kg BW (i.p.) in male SD rats of 2, 4 and 6 days of age (17) and has been found as a better model in terms of sustaining diabetic condition compared to a STZ-induced model. In these models, diabetes was characterized by mild to moderate hyperglycemia, increased blood glycated hemoglobin, urinary glucose excretion, and increased food intake. In a long-term study, it has been noted that the diabetic condition induced by this method can be maintained for a significantly longer period of time (52 weeks) (18). Hence, this model can be used to study the detailed pathogenesis of various diabetic complications.

However, this model takes quite a long time (at least 12 weeks) to induce diabetes so it may not be suitable for quick and routine pharmacological screening of anti-type 2 diabetic drugs or natural medicines. Additionally, many of these models have not been validated by anti-diabetic drugs and thus limit their suitability as an appropriate model for T2D (7).

2.3. Partial Pancreatectomized Models

As a means to avoid liver and kidney damage induced by alloxan, Pauls and Bancroft (19) developed a new method to induce T2D in mice through partial pancreatectomy. In 1983, Bonner-Weir et al. (20) aimed to study the consequences of reduced pancreatic beta cell masses in rats through removal of 85–90% of the pancreas. These animals displayed mild to moderate hyperglycemia from day 4 post-surgery and was maintained for a further 6 week period. During this 6 week period, no significant differences were noted in serum insulin or BW compared to the control group; however, after 7 weeks they had a normal FBG and insulin concentrations, and only became hyperglycaemic post-prandially or after an intraperitoneal glucose load. A major limitation of this model is the regeneration of the remnant pancreas for some researchers, so studies into the adaptive mechanisms of pancreatic beta cells may be required, for which this model may be particularly useful (21).

Srinivasan and Ramarao (22) noted the advantages of this model being the resemblance of T2D through reduced pancreatic beta cell mass and that this model avoids any cytotoxic effect of chemical-inducers of T2D in other organs. Kurup and Bhonde (23) developed a more stable form of diabetes by the combination of partial pancreatectomy and the injection of chemical inducers such as STZ. This model was accomplished by 50% pancreatectomy in combination of a 350 mg/kg BW nicotinamide injection prior to and after intraperitoneal injection of 200 mg/kg BW STZ in BALB/c mice. This model demonstrated stable and significantly elevated FBG with reduced serum insulin; however, a drastic loss in BW was observed which is similar to that seen in case of type 1 diabetes.

The overall disadvantage is the advanced technical and surgical skill required to develop this model. Another disadvantage may be the occurrence of digestive problems due to the excision of exocrine portions of the pancreas leading to a deficiency in amylase enzymes (22). For this reason, this model has not become that popular to researchers in recent years.

2.4. High-Fat Diet-Fed Models

The approach of feeding HF diet for the induction of T2D was first described during late 1980s (24). Subsequently, a number of researchers used this approach to develop rodent models of T2D by using different strains of mice or rats and different amounts of dietary calories from fat. Obesity is one of the major factors for the development of T2D, and obesity usually develops when rodents are fed a diet containing high amounts of fat (40–60% of the total calories). Several researchers have developed this model by using C57BL/6 J mice (24–26). However, it should be noted that this model presents insulin resistance but no beta cell failure, and that insulin resistance in the C57BL/6 J strain is compensated by a marked beta cell proliferation.

The high-fat diet models are usually characterized by overweight, obesity, impaired glucose tolerance, and insulin resistance. An important consideration when high-fat diet is used in rodents to induce insulin resistance, is the initiation of feeding the high-fat diets at a younger age (6–8 weeks), as this has been shown as the most effective age to develop obesity (27). The C57BL/6 J mice are typically fed a diet containing 40–60% of calories from fat, approximately eight times higher fat content than that of control mice for 8–16 weeks. Although some of the diabetic features were noted just after 4 weeks; however, the longer duration of fat-feeding enhances the features of insulin resistance, impaired glucose tolerance revealing elevated serum insulin and glucose, abnormal lipid profile, and mild to moderate hyperglycemia. The degree of hyperglycemia largely depends on the type and amount of fat and the duration of feeding (25, 27) and it takes a considerably longer period of time (16 weeks) to develop fasting hyperglycemia. Because of the marked beta cell proliferation, diabetes with plasma glucose levels >16.6 mM and glucosuria does not develop in the C57BL/6 J strain.

The approach of HF diet feeding to induce T2D has also been implicated to out bred Sprague–Dawley (SD) rats as it has remarkable sensitivity to HF diets to induce insulin resistance and diabetes as opposed to some other strains of rats (27, 28). At a longer stage of feeding this model can also develop hyperlipidemia and hyperinsulinemia leading to T2D; however, the major disadvantage of this model is also the duration of time (>10 weeks) required to induce the all major pathogenesis of T2D particularly hyperglycemia and insulin resistance (22), which is not suitable for many researchers, as this increases the cost of the experiment.

2.5. Fructose-Fed Models

Zavaroni et al. (29) and Tobey et al. (30) first demonstrated that *fructose* feeding in rats induced symptoms of hypertriglyceridemia, hyperinsulinemia, and insulin resistance including some recent investigators (31). To develop these pathogeneses, calorie intake in diets contained between 35 and 72% fructose in diet, or 10–15% *fructose* solutions in drinking water (31) ad libitum for 2–12 weeks. Dai et al. (31) demonstrated that rats fed a 5–10% *fructose* solution showed dose-dependent increases in fluid intake, as commonly seen in type 2 diabetics as polydipsia. Furthermore, over the 14-week period, these rats experienced progressive weight gain. Their experiment also revealed that feeding a 10% fructose solution (the equivalent of approximately 52.5% calories in a diet) in drinking water for 1 week or more was the most suitable time for developing a common secondary complication of T2D known as hypertension with increases in systolic blood pressure of 20–25 mmHg.

Benado et al. (32) fed a varying concentration of fructose (0–45%) in diet for a period of 28 days in order to study their effects on lipid levels in normal SD rats. Their diet consisted of both fat and carbohydrate levels reflecting those typically seen in an average American diet. The fructose levels varied between 0, 10, 20 and 45% fructose. Their results indicated no significant difference in total cholesterol, non-HDL cholesterol, and triglycerides in 10%-fructose-fed rats; however, significant differences in the 20% and 45% groups were seen when compared to the control (0% fructose). A significant mean BW gain was only, however, noted in the 45%-fructose-fed group. The fructose consumption at "normal" levels i.e. 10% of energy intake did not produce any adverse effect on lipid levels, which might be due to the shorter period of experiment.

The prevalence of overweight, obesity followed by insulin resistance, and diabetes in Americans are largely associated with the consumption of higher amounts of fructose particularly from simple carbohydrates, soft drinks, and high-fructose corn syrup (32). It has been also reported that long-term feeding of high fructose containing diet causes hyperlipidemia which is directly linked to the development of insulin resistance, the first major pathogenesis of T2D (33, 34). Research indicates that fructose is more hyperlipidemic than both glucose and starch due to its unique metabolism and high-fructose diets have been shown to significantly increase total cholesterol levels through increases in very-low-density lipoprotein (VLDL) and low-density lipoprotein (LDL) concentrations in rats (32).

So fructose can be used as an inducer for T2D but the major limitation of this model is that it takes quite longer period of time to induce the all major pathogenesis of T2D which may not be suitable for many researchers for routine and rapid pharmacological screening of anti-type 2 diabetic drugs or natural products.

2.6. Fat-Fed Streptozotocin Models

Diet induced diabetes was first described in 1947 (35). In fat-fed STZ-injected models, animals are usually fed with HF diet to induce insulin resistance followed by injection with STZ to induce partial pancreatic beta cell dysfunction. This model has a major advantage over genetic models because it replicates the natural pathogenesis with producing several characteristics that are in parallel to the human pathogenesis of T2D (36).

In 2000, Reed et al. (37) developed a fat-fed-STZ-injected rat model by feeding 40% of total calories from animal originated fat for 2 weeks followed by a single injection (i.p.) of STZ (50 mg/kg BW) in Sprague–Dawley rats. The animals developed both insulin resistance and reduced plasma insulin concentrations leading to hyperglycemia. Later, a similar approach was used by Zhang et al. (38) by feeding 30% HF (mostly from animal origin) containing diet with a lower dose of STZ injection (15 mg/kg BW) via caudal vein and reported that impaired glucose tolerance was observed after 2 months and significant hyperglycemia, hyperinsulinemia, hyperlipidemia were noticed after another 2 months period. The major disadvantage of this particular model is the longer induction time which might be due to the relatively lower dietary fat and lower dose of STZ injection (i.p.) to the animals.

Recently, a similar, but modified approach was used by Srinivasan et al. (5). They fed a HF diet containing 58% calories from lard to SD rats for 2 weeks prior to STZ injection (i.p.) with a varying dosage of 25, 35, 45, 55 mg/kg BW and continued ad libitum feeding of HF diet throughout the experimental period. The animals injected with 35 mg/kg STZ dose showed frank hyperglycemia, significantly elevated total serum cholesterol, and serum triglycerides. Serum insulin concentration was significantly lower in this group compared to the rats fed only a HF diet. Advantageously, this model was also sensitive to two anti-diabetic drugs confirming its suitability as a model for T2D. So this model appears to be a good choice for use as a rodent model for T2D either for rapid and routine pharmacological screening of anti-diabetic drugs and natural products.

Further modification on this model has been reported by Zhang et al. (38). They used a combination of HF diet with multiple low-dose STZ injections. Their HF diet consisted of 22% fat, 48% carbohydrates, and 20% protein. After 4 weeks feeding of HF diet, the rats were injected (i.p.) twice with STZ at a dose of 30 mg/kg BW, with a 1 week interval. Diabetes was characterized by fasting hyperglycemia, insulin resistance and blood lipid disorders and 85% of the animal became diabetic after the 8 weeks experimental period. Although it has not been mentioned what kind of fat has been used in this study and it takes quite long time (8 weeks) to develop diabetes, HF diet-fed with a couple of low-dose STZ-injected rats can be an alternative to develop the rat model of T2D.

In spite of different approaches used for the development of T2D models by using HF diet with a lower to intermediate dose of STZ; however, the overall success rate of this approach is better compared to many other approaches. Although some approaches take relatively longer periods of time to induce all major pathogenesis of the disease; many of them can induce diabetes in a shorter period of time. Hence, HF diet feeding followed by STZ injection can be an excellent approach for the development of T2D in rats.

2.7. Nicotinamide–Streptozotocin Models

The STZ–nicotinamide model was originally developed by Masiello et al. (39) and later, Nakamura et al. (40) adapted this to resemble a non-obese non-genetic model of T2D in mice. The basis for this model relies on the theory that STZ-induced DNA damage stimulates DNA repair mechanisms that consume large quantities of nicotinamide adenine dinucleotide (NAD). The supplementation of nicotinamide serves as a partial protection against excessive pancreatic beta cell damage caused by STZ. Masiello et al. (39) developed this model by injecting (i.p.) a dose of 230 mg/kg BW nicotinamide 15 min prior to a STZ injection (i.p.) at a dose of 65 mg/kg BW in 3 month old male Wistar rats. This model showed features of non-fasting hyperglycemia, abnormal glucose tolerance and insulin responses as well as a 40% preservation of pancreatic insulin stores.

By using a similar approach, another model was developed by Nakamura et al. (40) in male C57BL/6 J mice at 5–6 weeks of age. The STZ was injected (i.p.) twice with a dose of 100 mg/kg BW at day 0 and 2 of experiment 15 min after the injection (i.p.) of nicotinamide (240 mg/kg BW) in each case. To this combination they also investigated the effects of a HF diet (34% calories mostly from lard) on this model. After 6 weeks, this model revealed significantly elevated BW, glucose intolerance, insulin resistance, total cholesterol, triglycerides, and HDL-cholesterol compared to normal pellet diet-fed mice. This model is advantageous as it resembles closely the diabetic pattern particularly seen in East Asian diabetic patients, a large percentage of which are non-obese. Both models by Masiello et al. (39) and Nakamura et al. (40) were validated by anti-diabetic drugs and thus are suitable for drug screening and pharmacological studies particularly for non-obese T2D.

2.8. Monosodium Glutamate (MSG) Induced Models

MSG is the sodium salt of glutamic acid and is frequently used as a flavor enhancer (41). Studies of the effects of subcutaneous injections of MSG on neonatal rats began in 1970s where the preliminary results showed detrimental effects on rat growth, brain, and reproductive function as well as impaired glucose tolerance (42). In the late 1990s numerous studies revealed that feeding MSG develops central obesity and hyperinsulinemia in experimental animals (43–47).

Iwase et al. (44) reported that neonatal treatment of MSG glutamate with a dose of 4 mg/kg BW for 5 consecutive days increased serum triglycerides in female SHR; however, total cholesterol results remained statistically insignificant even after a 14-month period. However, they have been reported to have significantly elevated glycated hemoglobin (HbA1c), mesenteric fat and BW, serum blood glucose and insulin as well as elevated systolic blood pressure at this period of treatment.

Nagata et al. (48) developed a novel ICR (Institute of Cancer Research) mouse model for T2D induced by MSG. Subcutaneous MSG injections (2 mg/kg BW) were delivered on the day of birth until the 4th day of age in both male and female mice, whilst normal saline was injected accordingly to the control mice. Their results revealed a significantly higher BW in both sexes compared to the respective controls after 7 weeks of age; however, no significant differences were noted between food and fluid intake compared to the control group, indicating the absence of polyphagia and polydipsia and concluding that obesity was not caused through polyphagia. These two characteristic features, however, are common symptoms of the diabetes. Male-MSG-treated mice developed glucosuria after 8 weeks, whilst females only developed this symptom after 19 weeks. After 12 weeks of age, the male mice demonstrated significantly impaired glucose tolerance and insulin resistance indicating a diabetic state. Furthermore the male mice demonstrated an abnormal liver enzyme profile, which is indicative of hepatic insulin resistance. Disadvantageously, this model developed small liver tumors, which could interfere in the interpretation of results when being used as a model for T2D. It was also shown that male mice serve as a better model as the females appear to be less susceptible for the induction of diabetes with MSG.

Morrison et al. (47) injected MSG at a dose of 4 g/kg BW (i.p) from the first day of birth until the 7th day. Their results revealed central obesity in the MSG-treated rats as well as all rats over the age of 65 weeks having developed cataracts, a common complication of T2D. At 32 weeks of age, no significant differences were noted in glucose tolerance tests compared to control rats; however, differences were noted after 65 weeks between these two groups. Whilst this comparatively new model for T2D offers both the major and minor pathogeneses, the major limitation is that it takes a significantly longer period of time to develop diabetes and most of these models have not been validated by anti-diabetic drugs (7).

2.9. Intrauterine Growth Retardation Models

Intrauterine growth retardation (IUGR) is the low-birth weight of infants due to the limited availability of nutrients to the fetus during gestation and is a relatively common complication of pregnancies (49, 50). Barker et al. (51) were the first to speculate that IUGR was linked to the development of disease later in life, specifically the development of obesity, hypertension, and T2D. Nutrient deficits to the fetus result in modifications to the gene expression and functionality of cells within the pancreas, liver, and muscle (52). This is confirmed by earlier work by Hales et al. (53) who demonstrated that poor fetal and neonatal growth is directly linked to T2D in adulthood. IUGR causes significant reductions in pancreatic beta cell mass in neonates, which cannot be recovered in adulthood, resulting in impaired glucose tolerance and can lead to the development of T2D. Advantageously, these animals follow the natural pattern of disease by developing insulin resistance as an early feature in life and later developing hyperglycemia and subsequent pancreatic beta cell dysfunction (49).

In 2001, Simmons et al. (49) developed an IUGR rat model through bilateral uterine artery ligation such that blood flow to the fetus is not fully diminished but rather reflecting the human complication seen in some pregnancies. After 19 days of gestation, bilateral uterine artery ligation was done after an injection (i.p.) of xylazine (8 mg/kg BW) and ketamine (40 mg/kg BW) anesthesia. Neonatally these rats displayed decreases in insulin compared to controls and significantly decreased BW. However, by week 26, IUGR rats were obese, having a significantly higher fat pad mass around the body compared to the control rats. One week after birth, no significant difference was observed in FBG or insulin among the offspring; however, after week 7, both FBG and insulin were significantly higher compared to the control. Significantly increased insulin levels were sustained only until week 15, after which they remained non-significantly different from the control, having demonstrated a decline in insulin secretion. On the other hand, increases in FBG seen in the IUGR group continued to rise, even after 26 weeks up to >200 mg/dl, indicating a state of T2D. In another study, Vuguin et al. (50) demonstrated that IUGR permanently alters hepatic glucose metabolism through oxidative stress mechanisms in the fetal development, thus occurring prior to the onset of obesity and hyperglycemia, which represents an early defect, similar to insulin resistance seen in humans.

The major advantages of this model are the successful induction of insulin resistance, hyperglycemia, hyperinsulinemia, obesity, and reduced beta cell mass. However, many additional diabetic parameters including lipid profiling, liver and kidney functioning, and responses to anti-diabetic agents have not yet been reported and hence remain unknown, thus compromising its suitability as a model for T2D as a whole. Moreover, the surgical ligation of uterine arteries requires advanced technical skills and the development of T2D is only seen after 3 months of age (49, 50) thus requiring a long induction period which may not be suitable for some researchers. Further investigations are required to confirm the suitability of this model; however, the literature reported thus far, indicates that it may be an appropriate model for T2D if one can ignore the longer induction time.

3. Concluding Remarks

Over the decades, a multitude of experimental animal models have been developed through chemical, dietary, and combination treatments. Each model provides unique advantages specific for an area of T2D study or its complications. No one model contains all clinical pathogeneses of T2D, to which the extent of this disadvantage is dependent on the purpose of the study intended. An ideal model should typically, however, mimic the natural disease pattern as closely as possible with the two major pathogeneses, insulin resistance, and partial pancreatic beta cell dysfunction. Symptoms of hyperglycemia, hyperlipidemia, and impaired insulin responses are also critical to the success of the model. A number of models have been discussed in this chapter of which many of them are routinely used by researchers, where some of their uses are very seldom due to numerous reasons or limitations. Although a moderate to higher (50–65 mg/kg BW) single injection (i.p.) of alloxan or STZ to rats can induce hyperglycemia, it cannot induce insulin resistance, one of the two major pathogenesis of T2D. On the other hand, although HF or high-fructose diet can induce insulin resistance as well as hyperglycemia followed by T2D it takes significantly longer time to develop the complete pathogenesis of T2D which is not suitable for most of the researchers. For this reason, the combination of HF or high-fructose diet with a diabetic inducer particularly STZ is considered as a better option for the development of rodent models of T2D. However, the type and amount of fat or fructose and the dose of diabetic inducer are fully involved in determining the success of model development. Apart from these, nicotinamide–STZ model is only suitable as a model for non-obese type 2 diabetic patients. Neonatal alloxan/STZ models require a significantly longer period of time for the induction of diabetes and

MSG causes hepatic tumors during the induction of diabetes. Although partial pancreatectomy and IUGR have been considered as some better approaches for the development of T2D; however, pancreatic regeneration, longer induction time, and sophisticated surgical procedures reduced the popularity of these models.

Acknowledgments

This work was supported by a Competitive Research Grant from the Research Office, University of KwaZulu-Natal, Durban; an Incentive Grant for rated researchers and a Grant for Female and Young researchers from National Research Foundation (NRF), Pretoria, South Africa. Some information of this chapter has been taken from one of the publications of the first author with permission from publisher of Methods and Findings in Experimental and Clinical Pharmacology 2009; 31(4): 249–261. Copyright © 2011 Prous Science, S.A.U. or its licensors. All rights reserved.

References

1. World Health Organization (2010) Facts and figures about diabetes. http://www.who.int/diabetes/facts/en/ Accessed 5 Dec 2011
2. Pinhas-Hamiel O, Zeitler O (2005) The global spread of type 2 diabetes mellitus in children and adolescents. J Pediatr 146:693–700
3. Moore KR et al (2003) Three-year prevalence and incidence of diabetes among American Indian youth in Montana and Wyoming 1999 to 2001. J Pediatr 143:368–371
4. Krosnick A (2000) The diabetes and obesity epidemic among the Pima Indians. N J Med 97:31–37
5. Srinivasan K et al (2005) Combination of high-fat diet-fed and low-dose streptozotocin-treated rat: a model for type 2 diabetes and pharmacological screening. Pharmacol Res 52:313–320
6. Wall RJ, Shani M (2008) Are animal models as good as we think? Theriogenology 69:2–9
7. Islam MS, Loots DT (2009) Experimental rodent models of type 2 diabetes: a review. Methods Find Exp Clin Pharmacol 31:249–261
8. Goldner MG, Gomori G (1943) Alloxan diabetes in the dog. Endocrinology 33:297–308
9. Rerup CC (1970) Drugs producing diabetes through damage of the insulin secreting cells. Pharmacol Rev 22:485–518
10. Rees DA, Alcolado JC (2005) Animal models of diabetes mellitus. Diabet Med 22:359–370
11. Bolzan AD, Bianchi MS (2002) Genotoxicity of streptozotocin. Mutat Res 512:121–134
12. Portha B et al (1974) Diabetogenic effect of streptozotocin in the rat during the perinatal period. Diabetes 23:889–895
13. Portha B, Picon L, Rosselin G (1979) Chemical diabetes in the adult rat as the spontaneous evolution of neonatal diabetes. Diabetologia 17:371–377
14. Iwase M et al (1986) A new model of type 2 (non-insulin-dependent) diabetes mellitus in spontaneously hypertensive rats: diabetes induced by neonatal streptozotocin injection. Diabetologia 29:808–811
15. Giddings SJ et al (1985) Impaired insulin biosynthetic capacity in a rat model for non-insulin-dependent diabetes. Studies with dexamethasone. Diabetes 34:235–240
16. Shinde UA, Goyal RK (2003) Effect of chromium picolinate on histopathological alterations in STZ and neonatal STZ diabetic rats. J Cell Mol Med 7:322–329
17. Kodama T et al (1993) A new diabetes model induced by neonatal alloxan treatment in rats. Diabetes Res Clin Pract 20:183–189
18. Iwase M (1991) A new animal model of non-insulin dependent diabetes mellitus with

hypertension: neonatal streptozotocin treatment in spontaneously hypertensive rats. Fukuoka Igaku Zasshi 82:415–427
19. Pauls F, Bancroft RW (1949) Production of diabetes in the mouse by partial pancreatectomy. Am J Physiol 160:103–106
20. Bonner-Weir S, Trent DF, Weir GC (1983) Partial pancreatectomy in the rat and subsequent defect in glucose-induced insulin release. J Clin Invest 71:1544–1553
21. Masiello P (2006) Animal models of type 2 diabetes with reduced pancreatic β-cell mass. Int J Biochem Cell Biol 38:873–893
22. Srinivasan K, Ramarao P (2007) Animal models in type 2 diabetes research: an overview. Indian J Med Res 125:451–472
23. Kurup S, Bhonde RR (2000) Combined effect of nicotinamide and streptozotocin on diabetic status in partially pancreatectomized adult BALB/c mice. Horm Metab Res 32:330–334
24. Surwit RS et al (1988) Diet-induced type II diabetes in C57BL/6J mice. Diabetes 37:1163–1167
25. Winzel MS, Ahrén B (2004) The high-fat diet-fed mouse: a model for studying mechanisms and treatment of impaired glucose tolerance and type 2 diabetes. Diabetes 53:S215–S219
26. Kobayashi M et al (2004) Characterization of diabetes-related traits in MSM and JF1 mice on high-fat diet. J Nutr Biochem 15:614–621
27. Reuter TY (2007) Diet-induced models for obesity and type 2 diabetes. Drug Discov Today Dis Models 4:3–8
28. Chang S et al (1990) Metabolic differences between obesity-prone and obesity-resistant rats. Am J Physiol 259:R1103–R1110
29. Zavaroni I et al (1980) Effect of fructose feeding on insulin secretion and insulin action in the rat. Metabolism 29:970–973
30. Tobey TA et al (1982) Mechanism of insulin resistance in fructose-fed rats. Metabolism 31:608–612
31. Dai S et al (1994) Fructose-loading induces cardiovascular and metabolic changes in non-diabetic and diabetic rats. Can J Physiol Pharmacol 72:771–781
32. Benado M et al (2004) Effects of various levels of dietary fructose on blood lipids in rats. Nutr Res 24:565–571
33. Trujillo ME, Scherer PE (2006) Adipose tissue-derived factors: impact on health and disease. Endocr Rev 27:762–778
34. Barnes KM, Miner JL (2009) Role of resistin in insulin sensitivity in rodents and humans. Curr Protein Pept Sci 10:96–107
35. Houssay BA, Martinez C (1947) Experimental diabetes and diet. Science 105:548–549
36. Chen D, Wang M-W (2005) Development and application of rodent models for type 2 diabetes. Diabetes Obes Metab 7:307–317
37. Reed MJ et al (2000) A new rat model of type 2 diabetes: the fat-fed, streptozotocin-treated rat. Metabolism 49:1390–1394
38. Zhang M et al (2008) The characterization of high-fat and multiple low-dose streptozotocin induced type 2 diabetes rat model. Exp Diabetes Res 2008:7074045. doi:10.1155/2008/704045
39. Masiello P et al (1998) Experimental NIDDM: development of a new model in adult rats administered streptozotocin and nicotinamide. Diabetes 47:224–229
40. Nakamura T et al (2006) Establishment and pathophysiological characterization of type 2 diabetic mouse model produced by streptozotocin and nicotinamide. Biol Pharm Bull 29:1167–1174
41. Jinap S, Hajeb P (2010) Glutamate: its applications in food and contribution to health. Appetite 55:1–10
42. Lengvari I (1977) Effect of perinatal monosodium glutamate treatment on endocrine functions of rats in maturity. Acta Biol Acad Sci Hung 28:133–141
43. Hirata AE et al (1997) Monosodium glutamate (MSG)-obese rats develop glucose intolerance and insulin resistance to peripheral glucose uptake. Braz J Med Biol Res 30:671–674
44. Iwase M et al (1998) Obesity induced by neonatal monosodium glutamate treatment in spontaneously hypertensive rats: an animal model of multiple risk factors. Hypertens Res 21:1–6
45. Ito M et al (1999) New model of progressive non-insulin-dependent diabetes mellitus in mice induced by streptozotocin. Biol Pharm Bull 22:988–989
46. Ribeiro EB et al (1997) Hormonal and metabolic adaptations to fasting in monosodium glutamate-obese rats. J Comp Physiol B 167:430–437
47. Morrison JFB et al (2007) Sensory and autonomic nerve changes in the monosodium glutamate-treated rat: a model of type II diabetes. Exp Physiol 93:213–222
48. Nagata M et al (2006) Type 2 diabetes mellitus in obese model induced by monosodium glutamate. Exp Anim 55:109–115

49. Simmons RA, Templeton LJ, Gertz SJ (2001) Intrauterine growth retardation leads to the development of type 2 diabetes in the rat. Diabetes 50:2279–2286
50. Vuguin P et al (2004) Hepatic insulin resistance precedes the development of diabetes in a model of intrauterine growth retardation. Diabetes 53:2617–2622
51. Barker DJP et al (1993) Type 2 (non-insulin-dependent) diabetes mellitus, hypertension and hyperlipidemia (syndrome X): relation to reduced fetal growth. Diabetologia 36:62–67
52. Peterside IE, Selak MA, Simmons RA (2003) Impaired oxidative phosphorylation in hepatic mitochondria in growth-retarded rats. Am J Physiol Endocrinol Metab 285: E1258–E1266
53. Hales CN et al (1991) Fetal and infant growth and impaired glucose tolerance at age 64. Br Med J 303:1019–1022

Part III

Other Species

Chapter 11

Investigation and Treatment of Type 2 Diabetes in Nonhuman Primates

Barbara C. Hansen

Abstract

Nonhuman primates provide the ideal animal model for discovering and examining further the mechanisms underlying human type 2 diabetes mellitus. In all aspects studied to date the nonhuman primate has been shown to develop the same disease with the same features that develop in overweight middle-aged humans. This includes the progressive development of the known complications of diabetes, all of which are extraordinarily like those identified in humans. In addition, for the development and evaluation of new therapeutic agents, the translation of findings from nonhuman primates to application in humans has been highly predictable. Both therapeutic efficacy and identification of potential adverse responses can be effectively examined in nonhuman primates due to their great similarity to humans at the molecular, biochemical, and physiological levels. This chapter provides guidance for the development and management of a colony of monkeys with naturally occurring type 2 diabetes mellitus.

Key words: Prediabetes, Metabolic syndrome, Type 2 diabetes, Nonhuman primates, Monkeys, Rhesus (*Macaca mulatta*), Cynomolgus (*Macaca fascicularis*), Insulin therapy, Complications of diabetes

1. Introduction

Naturally occurring spontaneous type 2 diabetes very frequently develops in middle-aged monkeys and has been extensively studied in rhesus (*Macaca mulatta*) (1–9) and more recently in cynomolgus (*Macaca fascicularis*) (10, 11) monkeys. In addition, type 2 diabetes has been identified in baboons (*Papio hamadryas*) (12–14), chimpanzees (*Pan troglodytes*) (15), and many other primate species (cases described mostly in the zoological literature). In recent years, the most common uses of diabetic monkeys in biomedical research have been for the examination of therapeutic efficacy of new and emerging therapies (16–22), the improvement of islet transplant protocols (23–26), and the study of the long-term complications of overt type 2 diabetes (9, 27–29). Here we discuss the diagnosis of prediabetes and of overt diabetes as it develops naturally in primates and then provide guidelines for the therapeutic management and treatment of diabetic monkeys.

2. Materials

1. Middle-aged, overweight, nonhuman primates (maintained in a protective environment).
2. Environmental enrichment (toys, videos, mirrors, treats, human interactions).
3. Diabetes management supplies including glucose testing materials: glucose meters, glucose testing strips for those meters, urine testing strips, HbA1c (hemoglobin A1c) kits, insulin, insulin syringes, metformin, or other oral antidiabetic agents.
4. Anesthetic agents such as ketamine hydrochloride.
5. Other clinical therapy and surgical supplies.

3. Methods

3.1. Maintenance of Laboratory Housed Nonhuman Primates

1. Single housing for optimal care and management of diabetic primates. Although prediabetes and diabetes can develop in free ranging primates, such as those maintained on a protected and chow-provisioned island by the Caribbean Primate Research Center in Puerto Rico, it is difficult to provide an early diagnosis or preventive therapy in such colony management arrangements. Therefore, in order to study both the early stages of prediabetes and to effectively evaluate, treat, and study overt diabetes, it is recommended that the animals be singly housed in cages meeting the *Guide for the care and use of laboratory animals* (30) or in accord with expert recommendations and performance indices concerning the housing of obese primates (OLAW, 2012) (see Note 1).
2. The characteristics of the ideal environment for care and study of diabetic monkeys include (a) the ability to provide 24 h/day continuous food availability (usually a primate specific diet formulated as a chow although other nutritionally complete diets may be selected). (b) The ability to measure the actual food intake (within ± 10%) for each individual animal (essential to preventing insulin overdosing—see below). (c) The ability to monitor blood and urine glucose as often as two times/day.

3. Environmental enrichment, particularly of a nonnutritive sort that will enhance the health and welfare of these precious animals.

4. A caring and attentive laboratory animal technical support team including the care-givers and the veterinary staff.

3.2. Diagnosis of "Prediabetes" and Overt Type 2 Diabetes Mellitus in Nonhuman Primates

1. "Prediabetes" refers to the period of mildly elevated glucose, usually only appreciated if multiple longitudinal (carefully overnight fasted) blood glucose levels are obtained over a 2–3-month period (see Note 2).

2. We use a 16 h ± 1–2 h overnight fast to assure the animal's glucose is not the result of recent food intake.

3. The glucose levels ranging from 80 to about 100 mg/dL suggest prediabetes if obtained on at least two and usually multiple overnight fasted morning samples.

4. For humans overnight fasted normal glucose levels are usually around 85–90 mg/dL. In monkeys (both rhesus and cynomolgus) fasting blood glucose levels are much lower, usually averaging between 60 and 65 mg/dL but often with levels as low as 45–50. We consider the upper 70s to be a time to watch the monkey carefully for conversion to prediabetes.

3.3. Evaluation of the Progression from Normal to Overt Diabetes

1. Diagnosis of overt diabetes in monkeys is made at a level lower than for humans due to the lower basal fasting glucose in monkeys. For humans the agreed upon diagnostic level for diabetes is currently ≥126 mg/dL, (and prediabetes is often considered to be the range of 100–125 mg/dL (5.6–6.9 mmol/L) fasting glucose level) (Blood glucose must be repeated at least once on another day to assure the diagnosis is not spurious due to stress.) Since monkeys have about a 25 mg/dL lower fasting glucose level, it is reasonable to diagnose type 2 diabetes in monkeys at a glucose level of about 100 mg/dL (see Note 3). Overt type 2 diabetes is characterized by a failure of glucose-stimulated insulin secretion as revealed by the intravenous glucose tolerance test (Fig. 1).

2. Age contributes heavily to the risk of developing diabetes in both monkeys and humans, with greatly increased risk at middle age. In humans the peak age of diagnosis is in the 50s and 60s to mid 70s, although even teenagers who are obese or people in their 80s can develop type 2 diabetes. The comparable ages in rhesus monkeys for whom the greatest number of diabetes "onsets" have been documented, the average age of diabetes onset (while under study) is about 18 years (the great majority of overt diabetes conversions taking place between ages 15 and 23 years). The earliest documented onset (studied before and after onset longitudinally) in the rhesus was 10 years

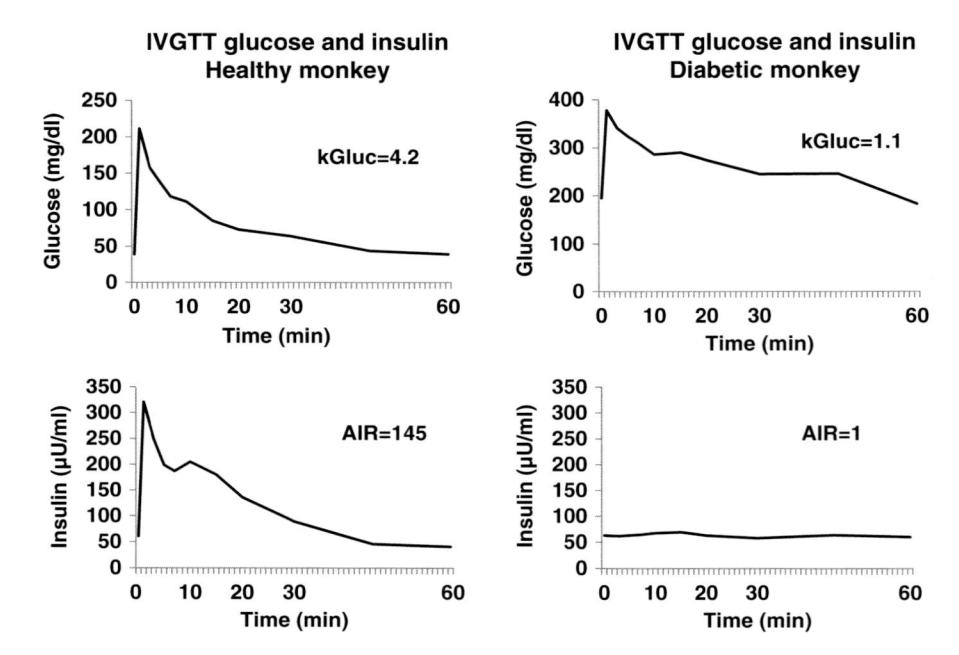

Fig. 1. Intravenous glucose tolerance test showing the change in glucose induced by the IV glucose and the associated beta cell response to secrete insulin into the circulation. This later response has two phases, the acute phase usually considered to be the rise above basal from 0 to 10 min, and the late phase including those points from 10 min onward.

while the oldest longitudinal conversion to overt diabetes yet documented was age 29 years. For cynomolgus monkeys these ages appear to be slightly younger by 2–4 years.

3.4. Management of Early Diabetes or Its Prevention

1. Symptoms of impending or undiagnosed diabetes include increased water drinking usually noticed as increased wet bedding and urination. The overweight or obese monkey may start to lose weight even while ingesting normal amounts of chow (see Note 4). Triglyceride levels are likely to be rising, and if measured, HDL cholesterol levels are likely to be declining (see Note 5).

2. Halting or slowing of the progression to overt diabetes can be achieved by restricting the amount of food available to a monkey. Generally a reduction of about 20% of calories will result in a return to normal glucose levels. While this modest reduction may or may not produce weight loss, eventually the monkey will gradually develop increased glucose levels (see Note 6).

3.5. Therapeutic Treatment of Overt Type 2 Diabetes in Nonhuman Primates

1. When diabetes is first diagnosed, the monkey is likely to gradually and slowly lose weight, a loss sometimes attributed to glucosuria (loss of glucose in the urine—the cause of the increased drinking and increased urination). No treatment is necessary in this early stage unless the goal is to halt the development of the disease (see above 3.4-2 and Note 6).

2. Oral agents, just as used in humans, can be used in monkeys to reduce the weight loss and control the symptoms for a period of a year or more. Most commonly, metformin may be used, but other oral antidiabetic agents are also effective in delaying the overt disease (see Note 7). Eventually, as in humans, insulin therapy will be required to prevent excessive weight loss and stabilize the monkey.

3. Insulin dosing is usually required within 1–2 years of the onset of overt diabetes, although some monkeys progress to this stage more slowly. The initiation and adjustment of insulin doses are carried out in the same way and using the same insulin types as for humans (see Note 8).

4. Hypoglycemia, where glucose levels decline below ~35 mg/dL, is usually the result of the administration of insulin with little or no subsequent food intake. Generally this is prevented by assuring that the monkey has ingested food and is taking food well before the administration of the daily insulin. The counter to hypoglycemia is the administration of glucose by whatever means is available. If the monkey is alert, fruit or another source of sugar is offered. If the animal is unresponsive glucose is given by vein or by gavage. The blood glucose levels are monitored closely until full recovery (glucose >120 mg/dL). All procedures are exactly as used for humans with hypoglycemia, including administration of glucagon if needed.

3.6. Evaluation and Management of the Complications of Diabetes in Primates

The complications of diabetes can be observed in most organs, but some carry more significant and discernible morbidity. Rhesus monkeys have been shown to develop evidence of diabetic kidney disease even present at the time of diagnosis, and increasing in severity with duration of diabetes. Diabetic nephropathy is assessed by collecting spot or timed or 24 h urine samples for the determination of urine glucose and albumin excretion. Albumin excretion rate (AER) is a good indicator of progressive nephropathy (9, 29). Peripheral neuropathy and microvascular disease are also common complications of diabetes in both humans and monkeys (28, 31, 32) (see Note 9). Retinopathy and choroidopathy are prominent features of diabetic eye disease and also are early and progressive disorders resulting from diabetes.

4. Notes

1. Although monkeys and other primates can be trained to present a limb or other skin location for the testing of blood glucose, (such as is done in corral maintained diabetic chimpanzees), it is difficult to provide the daily monitoring of energy intake, and the adjustment of insulin dosing regimen in an

optimal manner without a full knowledge of the food intake of the animal. It is also essential to following the progress of the disease to be able to provide an overnight fast to assess basal glucose and insulin levels, a process facilitated by individual housing. There are many other reasons that support the importance of single housing, including amplification of the quality of care and monitoring. We have maintained successfully one of the world's oldest rhesus monkeys under these optimal conditions during more than 10 years of insulin therapy, with the animal becoming frail at age 40, leading to elective euthanasia due to disability.

2. It is very easy to obtain an invalid elevated blood glucose level if the squeezing of a monkey to the front of the cage is handled roughly or by an inexperienced and insensitive person. Stress immediately induces a rise in epinephrine that leads to the output of glucose from the liver, resulting in an apparent, but erroneous, increased glucose. In the initial training of a monkey to present a limb or body surface for the lancet touch, it is important to reward the monkey with a small treat such as a raisin, grape, peanut, or other tiny snack. Show the monkey the treat and give it to him immediately after the glucose strip has been swiped into the blood droplet. Sometimes it is necessary to massage the puncture area with two fingers to bring up a droplet. The meter must be very close and already prepared with the strip inserted. If the monkey moves, this often wipes off the blood droplet and requires a bit more massaging. We use a carefully planned 16 h fast preceding the blood test. Blood can also be tested without fasting but results in much higher variability, and less accurate assessment of diabetes progression. It is however useful in assessing the effectiveness of the insulin therapy or the need to implement this treatment (see Note 3).

3. Spurious blood glucose levels may be obtained for several reasons. The monkey may not have learned to come to the front of the cage for his treat *after* the obtaining of the droplet sample, and therefore be stressed by the procedure. The monkey may have obtained a biscuit or snack, possibly from a well-meaning animal technician or from a neighboring monkey! Only repeated measures (on different days) help to validate the level. We like to see 3 or 4 determinations before we are confident of the diabetes diagnosis.

4. To date under our longitudinal studies, all monkeys showing initial progression from normal to prediabetes have excessive adiposity (are obese or overweight). For rhesus, females are generally over 8.5 kg and males are nearly always over 13.5 kg at the time of onset of diabetes. Note however that if the early progression has not been monitored closely, the monkey may lose a considerable amount of weight before the diagnosis of

diabetes has been applied. Thus it might appear that a lean monkey has developed diabetes, but in all cases to date, where diagnosis occurred in a lean animal, it was an animal that had previously be considerably heavier with excess adipose tissue—especially abdominal in location. Such overweight monkeys also carry increased adiposity on their backs and shoulders, but the most obvious area is the abdominal "pouching." This is true for both males and females.

5. Dyslipidemia is very common in middle-aged monkeys that are progressing toward diabetes (7, 33). The vast majority show elevated triglyceride levels (>100 mg/dL) and often these elevations can be severe (>300 mg/dL). HDL cholesterol generally moves downward but not with the magnitude of change seen with triglyceride levels. LDL cholesterol may or may not be elevated and elevated levels generally occur in middle-age in normal as well as in monkeys developing diabetes. Diabetes does not appear to be a significant contributor to this increase in LDL cholesterol.

6. Our long-term (average 23 year) study of calorie restriction, beginning with monkeys 10–12 years old, has shown that if one prevents the development of obesity by titrating the calories allowed to assure stable healthy weight (what we call the bathroom scale model) one can entirely prevent the development of overt diabetes in rhesus (34).

7. Concerning doses used in monkeys, we most often start with the same dose as in humans and evaluate its effects for a given monkey. In the case of metformin this is a dose of 500–1,000 mg/day in divided doses (supplied under many drug names). These doses can be doubled if glucose remains elevated. Monkeys are also treated orally with drugs in the PPAR agonist category, currently limited to pioglitazone (Actos). GLP-1 agonists and DPPIV inhibitors, both supporting increased insulin output, may also be used. All of these drugs have been studied in rhesus monkeys (16, 21, 22, 35, 36).

8. Insulin dosing is usually initiated with a long-acting insulin (e.g., glargine or insulin detemir). These can be initiated with one or two units of insulin but usually much more is required. Depending upon the attainment of glucose control, or lack thereof, insulin dosing is adjusted. NPH (intermediate acting) insulin is used if mid-day glucose levels are excessively elevated (>160 mg/dL), as an add-on to the long-acting insulin, sometimes referred to as basal insulin. A morning dose of 70/30 type insulin may also be used, thus targeting lowering of glucose during the prandial period (10 to 12 hours of lights on).

9. Every complication of diabetes can be followed longitudinally using minimally invasive or noninvasive means described in our prior studies. The nonhuman primate is the only animal that

serves as a valid reflection of the same pathophysiology in humans that result from diabetes, and thus serve as the best model to test reversibility or halting of these major causes of diabetic morbidity.

Acknowledgments

This work was supported by NIH grants and contracts including NIA HHSN253200800C and NIA N01AG31012 and by past support from various foundations and industry. The extraordinary quality of care was based on the work of Drs. Noni Bodkin, Heidi Ortmeyer, and Cathy Kai-Lin Jen. The work on the complications of diabetes has had many critical collaborators and coworkers, particularly the dedicated efforts of Dr. Xenia Tigno.

References

1. Hansen BC, Bodkin NL (1986) Heterogeneity of insulin responses: phases leading to type 2 (non-insulin-dependent) diabetes mellitus in the rhesus monkey. Diabetologia 29:713–719
2. Hansen BC, Bodkin NL (1990) Beta-cell hyperresponsiveness: earliest event in development of diabetes in monkeys. Am J Physiol 259:R612–R617
3. Ortmeyer HK, Bodkin NL, Hansen BC (1993) Insulin-mediated glycogen synthase activity in muscle of spontaneously insulin-resistant and diabetic rhesus monkeys. Am J Physiol 265:R552–R558
4. Hotta K, Funahashi T, Bodkin NL et al (2001) Circulating concentrations of the adipocyte protein adiponectin are decreased in parallel with reduced insulin sensitivity during the progression to type 2 diabetes in rhesus monkeys. Diabetes 50:1126–1133
5. Bodkin NL, Alexander TM, Ortmeyer HK et al (2003) Mortality and morbidity in laboratory-maintained Rhesus monkeys and effects of long-term dietary restriction. J Gerontol A Biol Sci Med Sci 58:212–219
6. Tigno XT, Gerzanich G, Hansen BC et al (2004) Age-related changes in metabolic parameters of nonhuman primates. J Gerontol A Biol Sci Med Sci 59:1081–1088
7. Ding SY, Tigno XT, Hansen BC et al (2007) Nuclear magnetic resonance-determined lipoprotein abnormalities in nonhuman primates with the metabolic syndrome and type 2 diabetes mellitus. Metabolism 56:838–846
8. Cnop M, Hughes SJ, Igoillo-Esteve M et al (2010) The long lifespan and low turnover of human islet beta cells estimated by mathematical modelling of lipofuscin accumulation. Diabetologia 53:321–330
9. Cusumano AM, Bodkin NL, Hansen BC et al (2002) Glomerular hypertrophy is associated with hyperinsulinemia and precedes overt diabetes in aging rhesus monkeys. Am J Kidney Dis 40:1075–1085
10. Bauer SA, Leslie KE, Pearl DL et al (2010) Survey of prevalence of overweight body condition in laboratory-housed cynomolgus macaques (Macaca fascicularis). J Am Assoc Lab Anim Sci 49:407–414
11. Bauer SA, Leslie KE, Pearl DL et al (2010) Retrospective case–control study of hyperglycemia in group-housed, mature female cynomolgus macaques (Macaca fascicularis). J Med Primatol 39:408–416
12. Chavez AO, Lopez-Alvarenga JC, Tejero ME et al (2008) Physiological and molecular determinants of insulin action in the baboon. Diabetes 57:899–908
13. Guardado-Mendoza R, Dick EJ Jr, Jimenez-Ceja LM et al (2009) Spontaneous pathology of the baboon endocrine system. J Med Primatol 38:383–389
14. Perez VL, Caicedo A, Berman DM et al (2011) The anterior chamber of the eye as a clinical transplantation site for the treatment of diabetes: a study in a baboon model of diabetes. Diabetologia 54:1121–1126

15. McTighe MS, Hansen BC, Ely JJ et al (2011) Determination of hemoglobin A1c and fasting blood glucose reference intervals in captive chimpanzees (Pan troglodytes). J Am Assoc Lab Anim Sci 50(2):165–170
16. Winegar DA, Brown PJ, Wilkison WO et al (2001) Effects of fenofibrate on lipid parameters in obese rhesus monkeys. J Lipid Res 42(10):1543–1551
17. Schafer SA, Hansen BC, Völkl A et al (2004) Biochemical and morphological effects of K-111, a peroxisome proliferator-activated receptor (PPAR) alpha activator, in non-human primates. Biochem Pharmacol 68:239–251
18. Ding SY, Tigno XT, Braileanu GT et al (2007) A novel peroxisome proliferator–activated receptor alpha/gamma dual agonist ameliorates dyslipidemia and insulin resistance in prediabetic rhesus monkeys. Metabolism 56:1334–1339
19. Kharitonenkov A, Wroblewski VJ, Koester A et al (2007) The metabolic state of diabetic monkeys is regulated by fibroblast growth factor-21. Endocrinology 148:774–781
20. Kavanagh K, Brown KK, Berquist ML et al (2010) Fluid compartmental shifts with efficacious pioglitazone therapy in overweight monkeys: implications for peroxisome proliferator-activated receptor-gamma agonist use in prediabetes. Metabolism 59:914–920
21. Wagner JD, Shadoan MK, Zhang L et al (2010) A selective peroxisome proliferator-activated receptor alpha agonist, CP-900691, improves plasma lipids, lipoproteins, and glycemic control in diabetic monkeys. J Pharmacol Exp Ther 333:844–853
22. Hansen BC, Tigno XT, Bénardeau A et al (2011) Effects of aleglitazar, a balanced dual peroxisome proliferator-activated receptor alpha/gamma agonist on glycemic and lipid parameters in a primate model of the metabolic syndrome. Cardiovasc Diabetol 10:7
23. Casu A, Bottino R, Balamurugan AN et al (2008) Metabolic aspects of pig-to-monkey (Macaca fascicularis) islet transplantation: implications for translation into clinical practice. Diabetologia 51:120–129
24. Bottino R, Criscimanna A, Casu A et al (2009) Recovery of endogenous beta-cell function in nonhuman primates after chemical diabetes induction and islet transplantation. Diabetes 58(2):442–447
25. Rogers SA, Mohanakumar T, Liapis H et al (2010) Engraftment of cells from porcine islets of Langerhans and normalization of glucose tolerance following transplantation of pig pancreatic primordia in nonimmune-suppressed diabetic rats. Am J Pathol 177:854–864
26. Hammerman MR (2011) Engraftment of insulin-producing cells from porcine islets in non-immune-suppressed rats or nonhuman primates transplanted previously with embryonic pig pancreas. J Transplant 2011:261352
27. Kim SY, Johnson MA, McLeod DS et al (2005) Neutrophils are associated with capillary closure in spontaneously diabetic monkey retinas. Diabetes 54:1534–1542
28. Pare M, Albrecht PJ, Noto CJ et al (2007) Differential hypertrophy and atrophy among all types of cutaneous innervation in the glabrous skin of the monkey hand during aging and naturally occurring type 2 diabetes. J Comp Neurol 501:543–567
29. Najafian B, Masood A, Malloy PC et al (2011) Glomerulopathy in spontaneously obese rhesus monkeys with type 2 diabetes: a stereological study. Diabetes Metab Res Rev 27:341–347
30. National Research Council (2011) Guide for the care and use of laboratory animals, 8th edn. The National Academies Press, Washington, DC
31. Tigno XT, Ding SY, Hansen BC (2006) Paradoxical increase in dermal microvascular flow in pre-diabetes associated with elevated levels of CRP. Clin Hemorheol Microcirc 34:273–282
32. Tigno XT, Hansen BC, Nawang S et al (2011) Vasomotion becomes less random as diabetes progresses in monkeys. Microcirculation 18:429–439
33. Shamekh R, Linden EH, Newcomb JD et al (2011) Endogenous and diet-induced hypercholesterolemia in nonhuman primates: effects of age, adiposity, and diabetes on lipoprotein profiles. Metabolism 60:1165–1177
34. Hansen BC, Bodkin NL (1993) Primary prevention of diabetes mellitus by prevention of obesity in monkeys. Diabetes 42:1809–1814
35. Ortmeyer HK, Sajan MP, Miura A et al (2011) Insulin signaling and insulin sensitizing in muscle and liver of obese monkeys: peroxisome proliferator-activated receptor gamma agonist improves defective activation of atypical protein kinase C. Antioxid Redox Signal 14:207–219
36. Kemnitz JW, Elson DF, Roecker EB, et al (1994) Pioglitazone increases insulin sensitivity, reduces blood glucose, insulin, and lipid levels, and lowers blood pressure, in obese, insulin-resistant rhesus monkeys. Diabetes 43:204–211

Part IV

General Methodology

Chapter 12

Determination of Beta-Cell Function: Insulin Secretion of Isolated Islets

Michael Willenborg, Kirstin Schumacher, and Ingo Rustenbeck

Abstract

The kinetics of insulin secretion, not just the total amount, is of decisive relevance for the physiological regulation of glucose homeostasis. Thus to characterize the relevant features of the secretory response to an insulinotropic stimulus a method is needed which is able to resolve the temporal response pattern, in particular to distinguish the first phase from the second phase response. The perifusion of collagenase-isolated islets is a method which permits to register responses of near-physiological complexity with a preparation that can also be used for cell physiological and biochemical investigations on stimulus-secretion oupling.

Key words: Insulin secretion, Pancreatic islets, Beta cells, Collagenase digestion, Islet perifusion

1. Introduction

Research on the physiology and pathophysiology of insulin secretion requires the availability of isolated pancreatic islets and beta cells. This is not an easy task since the islet mass makes up only 1–2% of the surrounding exocrine tissue. Also, the islet itself is a heterogeneous mini-organ, consisting of several interacting cell types of which the beta cells make up about 70–80% (1, 2). So it may prove difficult to relate phenomena of insulin secretion to the underlying events in the beta cells, if they are studied in whole islet preparations. This is one of the reasons why the use of insulin secretory cell lines (sometimes euphemistically labeled as clonal beta cells) has become popular, even more so in the last decade because of their easy propensity for genetic manipulation. On the other hand, some animal models, such as the ob/ob mouse provide grossly hypertrophic islets containing up to 95% beta cells (3, 4). In both cases the question as to the physiological relevance of the observations has to be taken serious.

In the early days of insulin secretion research the rat was the preferred rodent species to study insulin secretion ex vivo. This was mainly due to the animal size (250 g vs. 25 g for a normal mouse) which permits perfused organ preparations, a very demanding task with mice (5). In fact the perfused pancreas is still the preparation which provides secretion measurements with the highest time resolution (6). The perifusion of isolated islets can be regarded as a reductionist variant of the perfused pancreas technique. It was only in the late 1960s, about 10 years after the invention of the insulin radioimmunoassay, that the collagenase digestion method was developed (7, 8), which permits the isolation of sufficiently large amounts of sufficiently pure endocrine tissue from the pancreas within a reasonable time (for an overview on the early history of beta cell research see (9)). To our knowledge there is no evidence that the collagenase digestion systematically distorts the response pattern as compared to studies using microdissected islets.

2. Materials

2.1. Buffer and Enzymes

1. Krebs-Ringer buffer (KR buffer): 115 mM NaCl, 20 mM $NaHCO_3$, 10 mM HEPES, 5 mM Glucose, 4.7 mM KCl, 2.56 mM $CaCl_2$, 1.2 mM KH_2PO_4, 1.2 mM $MgSO_4$, and 0.2% (w/v) albumin. To prepare a sterile KR buffer fill 13.44 g NaCl, 3.36 g $NaHCO_3$, 700.77 mg KCl, 752.74 mg $CaCl_2$ (dihydrate), 326.26 mg KH_2PO_4, 591.55 mg $MgSO_4$ (heptahydrate), 4.76 g HEPES, 1.98 g Glucose (monohydrate), and 4.0 g albumin (bovine serum albumin, fraction V) into a 2 L plastic beaker and dissolve it in 1.9 L aqua bidest. Adjust the pH value to 7.4 with 1 M NaOH, transfer the solution into a volumetric flask, rinse the plastic beaker once with 0.1 L aqua bidest and fill up the volume in the flask to 2.0 L. Afterwards 100 mL portions are filled into heat-sterilized Schott flasks using a sterile filtering device (Sartorius, Göttingen, Germany). These flasks are then stored at 4–6°C until needed. Immediately before the use the pH value should be checked, because it may increase with storage time. For the immediate use of freshly isolated islets the Krebs-Ringer buffer need not be sterile. If islets or beta cells are isolated with the intention to culture them a sterile preparation of the KR buffer is needed.

2. Collagenase: The use of collagenase specifically produced for islet isolation does not guarantee satisfactory results. The velocity and selectivity of the digestion has to be assessed with each new batch. Currently, we utilize NB 8 broad range collagenase (Serva, Heidelberg, Germany) specific activity 1.36 units/mg.

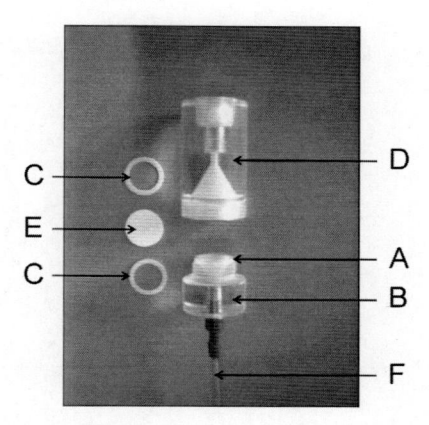

12 Determination of Beta-Cell Function: Insulin Secretion of Isolated Islets

Fig. 1. Assembly of the perifusion chamber. Place the filter support (**a**) into the lower half of the chamber (**b**), then one silicone gasket (**c**) each into the openings of the lower (**b**) and the upper half (**d**) Place the filter membrane (**e**) on the silicone gasket in the lower half and screw the upper on the lower half. The mixed cellulose ester membrane is quite delicate, care must be taken not to crumple or shear it when screwing both halves of the chamber together.

2.2. Equipment

1. Surgical equipment: 2 tweezers (one broad, one sharp), 1 micro Iris scissors (straight), 1 dissecting surgical scissors (curved), 1 medium-sized scissors (straight). These are carefully cleaned after each use, kept in a steel case, and are heat-sterilized before renewed use.

2. Stereomicroscope: The collection of the islets from the digest of the exocrine pancreas requires a stereomicroscope, having a second one is recommended for the collagenase injection method. There is a range available from all major manufacturers. Older models such as Zeiss Stemi from the 1980s are quite sufficient. Illumination is best done by a cold light source with glass fiber light guides (e.g., Schott KL 150 B or newer models).

3. Perifusion chamber: There is no commercially available perifusion chamber for batch perifusion of pancreatic islets. However, any scientific workshop should be able to produce a useful specimen. In the present design (Fig. 1) the islets are placed on a hydrophilic mixed cellulose ester membrane of a sufficiently large surface (Millipore SMWP 01300, 13 mm diameter, pore size 5.0 µm), so that each single islet is perifused by fresh medium. The filter is held in place by a perforated support disc and is firmly fixed by screwing the upper and the lower part of the perfusion chamber together.

4. Perifusion apparatus: The perifusion chamber may be placed in any environment that keeps a constant temperature of 37°C (such as a water bath), but it may be more convenient to use a thermostated housing (water-jacketed and attached to a circulation water bath, e.g., Haake F4291) that contains a reservoir for the perifusion media, a place for the peristaltic pump and a

place for the perifusion chamber. A detailed description was published years ago (10). It is imperative that the perifusion media are oxygen-saturated by bubbling with oxygen/carbon dioxide (95/5, v/v). This gas mixture should pass a gas-wash bottle before it is led into the perifusion medium. A peristaltic pump with a low pulsation is recommended (e.g., ismatec REGLO digital with 12 rollers, but older pumps like LKB Varioperpex with 6 rollers are also useful). The fraction collector should have a constant position of the drop outlet to minimize the distance between the perifusion chamber and the collection site (see Note 1).

2.3. Measurement of Insulin Content

Up to the 1990s, in-house prepared RIAs were mostly utilized for quantification. Meanwhile, a number of insulin ELISA- and RIA-kits are commercially available. RIAs based on ^{125}I-labeled insulin are still competitive as far as the sensitivity and dynamic range are concerned (e.g., rat insulin RIA kit by LINCO Research, St Charles, MI). If flexibility and/or lack of a radioisotope laboratory matter, ELISA is the method of choice. In the authors' laboratory the insulin ELISA supplied by Mercodia (Uppsala, Sweden) is used according to the manufacturer's protocol. It utilizes 96 microwell plates and thus the absorbance measurement requires a microplate reader (e.g., Wallac Victor, PerkinElmer, Waltham, MA). The calculation of the insulin content from the absorbance value can be done by any spreadsheet program, however the use of more dedicated programs such as Prism (GraphPad, La Jolla, CA) is more convenient.

3. Methods

3.1. Conventional Collagenase Digestion

1. The mouse is sacrificed by cervical dislocation. After sacrifice the abdominal fur is sprayed with 70% ethanol (see Note 2), then lifted with a tweezers an incised longitudinally by a fine scissors. Rectangular incisions placed halfways permit to separate the subcutaneous connective tissue from the abdominal musculature. When a sufficiently large area of musculature is free, the abdominal cavity is cut open and the intestine displaced so that the stomach and the duodenum become visible.

2. The pancreas is excised by a fine scissors along the major curvature of the stomach, then along the concavity of the duodenum and initial portion of the jejunum and finally the caudal part is removed from the spleen. The excised pancreas (or pieces of pancreas) is immediately immersed in ca. 3 mL ice-cold Krebs-Ringer buffer in a glass vial.

3. Adherent visceral fat is cut off and the pieces of clean pancreatic tissue are transferred into another glass vial containing 2 mL

KR buffer where they are minced into fine pieces by cutting with a scissors (sharp, straight) for about 5 min. The suspension of finely minced tissue is aspirated by a 1 mL Eppendorf pipette (the blue tip is cut ca 5 mm from the distal opening for easier aspiration) and transferred into a screw-cap glass vial containing 2 mg of collagenase (see Note 3).

4. After screwing the cap on the glass vial, it is firmly fixed in a shaking water bath set at 37°C and 328 strokes/min. After an incubation time of about 8–10 min (depending on the activity of the collagenase batch) the glass vial is removed, shaken vigorously by hand for ca. 30 s, and then filled with ice-cold Krebs-Ringer buffer to stop the digestion process. The suspension of islets and digested exocrine is allowed to settle, the supernatant carefully removed by suction and replaced by fresh KR buffer.

5. This suspension is poured into a black glass Petri dish and placed under a stereomicroscope (Fig. 2). Ideally, the islets should have that little of exocrine tissue attached that they can be collected by an Eppendorf pipette and placed in another Petri dish with fresh KR buffer (see Note 4). Finally, transfer the islets to a conical vessel. This permits to aspirate the entirety of the isolated islets in a small volume of buffer and to inject them into the perifusion chamber pre-filled with KR buffer (see Note 5).

3.2. Collagenase Digestion by Ductal Injection

1. Sacrifice and opening of the abdominal cavity are done as described above for the conventional collagenase digestion method. The small intestine is carefully displaced to the left until the bile duct leading from underneath the liver to the middle part of the duodenum becomes visible. The common orifice of the bile duct and the pancreatic duct, the Papilla Vateri can be recognized as a white spot at the outer wall of the duodenum.

2. A small vessel clamp is placed on the Papilla Vateri. It should be positioned slightly distal to the white spot to avoid clamping of the bile duct and thus prohibiting the injection of the collagenase solution (see Note 6).

3. Dissociate the bile duct gently from the surrounding connective tissue using the sharp tweezers and the small scissors to have it fully accessible for injection. Place the mouse under a stereomicroscope.

4. Put the cannula (Braun Sterican® 0.3 × 12 mm) on the 2 mL syringe (Braun Inject) filled with ice-cold collagenase solution and bend it for a more shallow injection angle. Put one branch of the tweezers below the bile duct to use it as a slide for the injection cannula (Fig. 3).

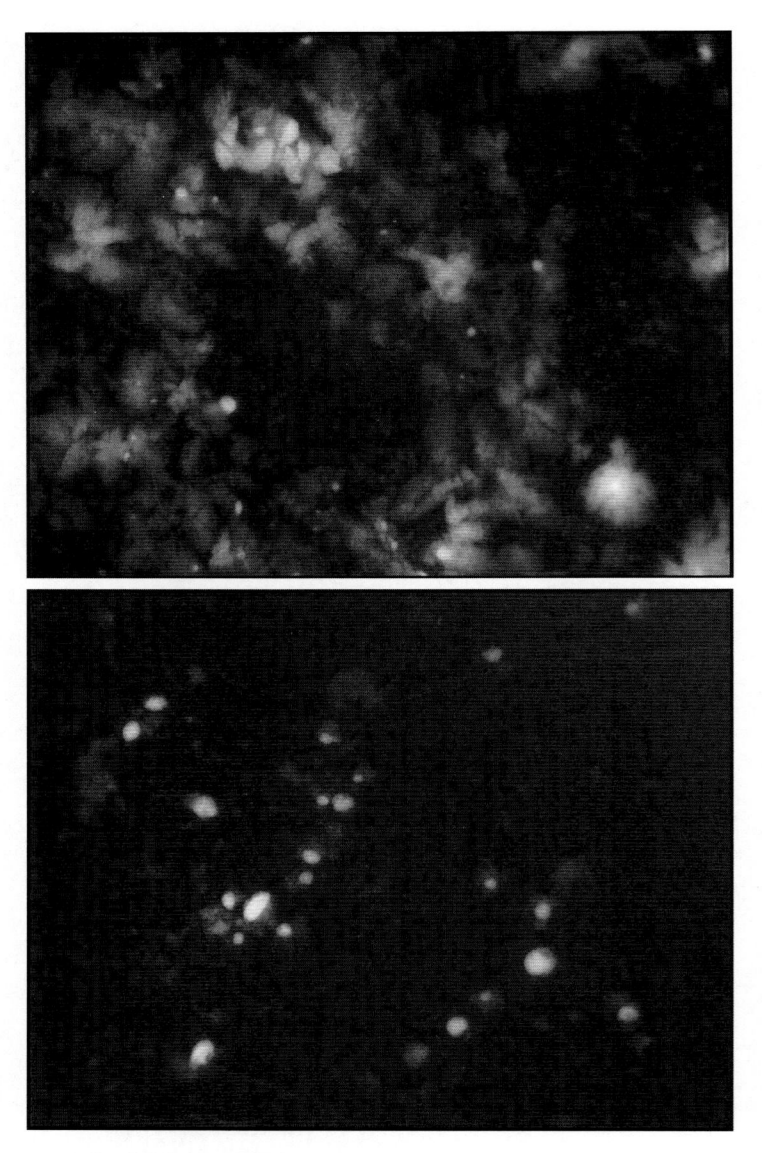

Fig. 2. View of the pancreatic preparation at different stages of collagenase digestion. The *upper* picture shows the result after 5 min of digestion of the conventionally prepared pancreas. All islets are still connected to exocrine tissue, the majority is surrounded by exocrine tissue. The *lower* picture shows islets that have been collected and placed in another Petri dish after a collagenase digestion of appropriate duration. Most of the cellular debris is only loosely attached to the islets. Occasionally, larger portions of exocrine tissue may be cut away by aid of a syringe needle. However, avoid lengthy manipulations.

5. Place the tip of the cannula in the lumen of the bile duct while slightly pressing the syringe piston (Fig. 3). When the access to the duct is established correctly, a swelling of the bile duct, and after injection of some more fluid, also of the entire pancreas can be observed.

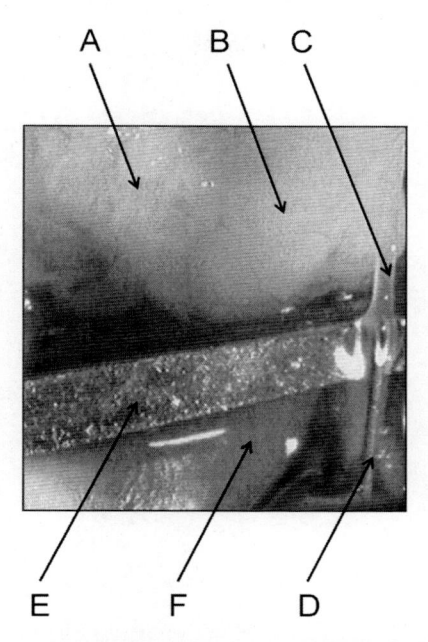

Fig. 3. View of the cannulated bile duct during collagenase injection (as seen in the craniocaudal direction). (a) denotes the head of the pancreas (recognizable by the lobular structure, since some collagenase solution has already been injected), (b) denotes the adjacent part of the duodenum and (c) the dilated bile duct filled with collagenase solution. For easier insertion of the injection cannula (d) a branch of the tweezers was used as a slide (e). Below the branch of the tweezers is the left lobe of the liver (f).

6. After injection of the total volume of the collagenase solution the entire pancreas should appear drastically swollen. Remove the vessel clamp and place the intestine to the right side so that the tail of the pancreas is accessible.

7. Seize it with a tweezers and dissociate it from the spleen with a second tweezers. Then the pancreas is separated as completely as possible from the stomach and duodenum and put into a 10 mL conic plastic tube (Sarstedt) (see Note 7).

8. Put the tube with the pancreas into a water bath set at 37°C and let it incubate for 9 min. Thereafter shake the tube vigorously by hand for 1 min. The preparation should now appear nearly homogeneous with no solid pieces of tissue recognizable.

9. Stop the digestion by filling up the tube with ice-cold KR buffer and shaking for a few seconds. Centrifuge at $300 \times g$ for 15 s, discard the supernatant and redisperse the sediment with 9 mL ice-cold KR buffer. Centrifuge again at $300 \times g$ for 15 s.

10. After redispersion of the sediment, the suspension is poured into a black glass Petri dish (100 mm) and placed under a stereomicroscope. The islets can be easily picked with an Eppendorf pipette and placed into another Petri dish containing fresh KR buffer. This procedure is repeated twice (see Note 8).

196 M. Willenborg et al.

3.3. Culture of Islets and MIN6 Pseudo-Islets

1. The freshly isolated islets can be used immediately for perifusion experiments (see Note 9) or can be kept in tissue culture depending on the type of experiment (see Note 10).

2. If the latter is intended the islets have to be washed several times in sterile cell culture medium under the clean bench before placing them in the cell culture incubator. Cell culture medium RPMI 1640 (Invitrogen) with 5 mM glucose (10 mM glucose for the first 3 h after isolation) and 10% FCS has proven to give satisfactory results with primary islets (see Note 11).

3. Insulin-secreting MIN6 cells (11), when growing in suspension, form aggregates of 3,000–5,000 cells which can be used like primary islets to study the secretion dynamics (12).

4. To promote the formation of MIN6 cell aggregates, hydrophobic dishes for suspension cell culture (Sarstedt, No. 83.1802.002) are used. Like monolayer MIN6 cells, pseudo-islets are cultured in DMEM medium (high glucose, 4.5 g/L) supplemented with 4 mM L-glutamine, 15% FCS, 50 μM 2-mercaptoethanol and penicillin/streptomycin (all obtainable from Invitrogen) at 37°C and 5% CO_2 and are harvested after 8 days (see Note 12).

3.4. Batch Perifusion of Islets

1. Switch on the immersion circulator and water bath at least 1 h prior to the perifusion experiment to allow complete equilibration of the temperature.

2. After final control of the pH value the perifusion media (KR buffer containing the respective insulin secretagogues) are placed in the water bath and bubbled with oxygen/carbon dioxide (95/5, v/v) for at least 20 min.

3. The perifusion media are then placed in a reservoir of the thermostated housing and continuously aerated with oxygen/carbon dioxide (95/5, v/v) to keep the oxygen tension constant.

4. Assembly of the perifusion chamber is done as explained in the legend to Fig. 1.

5. Place the assembly in a retort clamp and fill the entire chamber with KR buffer using a syringe attached to the lower tubing (Fig. 1f). Then aspirate 50 freshly isolated islets by an Eppendorf pipette and inject them into the opening of the upper half of the chamber. Let them settle on the filter membrane.

6. Attach the buffer-filled tubing from the peristaltic pump to the opening of the upper half, remove the syringe from the distal tube and tape assembly to the inner wall of the water-jacketed housing (see Note 13). Connect the distal, draining tube with the drop counter of the fraction collector.

7. Place as many glass vials (10 mL glass centrifuge tubes) into the fraction collector as required by the experimental protocol.

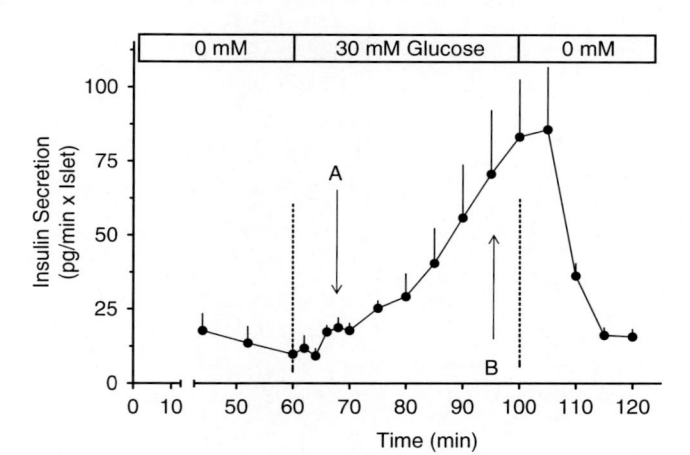

Fig. 4. Insulin secretion of freshly isolated perifused mouse islets. After 60 min of perifusion in the absence of glucose the glucose concentration is raised to a nearly maximal stimulatory value (30 mM). It is remarkable that under this condition the first phase is strongly reduced (**a**) which is followed by a steep ascending second phase (**b**). Data are means ± SEM of four independent experiments. This shows that the widely held belief that the mouse islet cannot produce an ascending second phase response is not well founded.

Start the pump (flow rate 1 mL/min) and switch the collector on. Sampling intervals (typically between 1 and 10 min) are set depending on the expected changes in secretion rate (Fig. 4).

8. At the end of the perifusion the content of each glass vial is vortex-mixed and 1 mL of each fraction is filled into an Eppendorf cup and kept frozen at −20°C until measurement of the insulin content.

9. The filter membrane with the attached islets is removed from the perifusion chamber and the chamber is then reassembled. To clean the system distilled water is pumped through for 30 min, then 70% ethanol for 15 min, and again distilled water for 15 min. Then the chamber is disassembled and wiped dry.

3.5. Insulin ELISA

1. Bring samples (stored at −20°C) and reagents of the insulin ELISA kit (stored at 2–8°C) to room temperature. Mix the thawed samples by vortex. Open the sealed package of the test kit containing the 96 well plate.

2. Pipette 10 μL of at least 5 calibrator concentrations (e.g., 0; 0.15; 0.4; 1.0; 5.5 μg/L) in duplicate into appropriate wells. Do the same with the perifusion samples. Add 100 μL enzyme conjugate solution using an 8-channel pipette (e.g., Eppendorf Xplorer).

3. Incubate on a plate shaker at 260 rpm for 2 h at room temperature.

4. To remove unbound enzyme the use of an automatic plate washer is convenient, but manual washing (by an 8-channel pipette) is

equally acceptable. In the latter case aspirate carefully all fluid from the wells and add 240 µL washing solution. Repeat five times. After the final aspiration turn the plate upside down on a piece of lab tissue paper.

5. Add 200 µL tetramethylbenzidine (TMB) into each well and incubate in the dark for 15 min at room temperature. Terminate by adding 50 µL of the stop solution to each well.

6. Place the plate into a microplate reader, activate the shaking function for 5 s, then read absorbance at 450 nm.

7. Set up a non-linear calibration function (second degree polynomial) from the mean values of the five calibrators and calculate the insulin content by regression. Calculate the secretory rate by taking into account the perifusion rate, the sampling intervals, and the number of islets. Express secretion as pg insulin per minute and per islet (see Notes 14 and 15).

4. Notes

1. The switch between the different perifusion media may be done simply by removing the tubing and placing it by hand into the vessel containing the next medium. To avoid air bubbles getting trapped in the tubing the pump has to be stopped and restarted, which may lead to artifactual transient increases of secretion. This can be avoided by use of a valve, placed between the reservoir of the perifusion media and the pump. A valve is necessary if fraction intervals of less than one min are intended (10).

2. The ethanol is intended to disinfect the skin but also to simply prevent hair of the fur to fall into the opened abdominal cavity and to contaminate it.

3. Fat seems to inhibit the collagenase activity and to decrease the selectivity of the digestion. The final collagenase concentration in the digestion step is 1.4 PZU/mL KR buffer.

4. With some experience about 50 islets can be collected from one NMRI mouse pancreas, requiring ca. 20 min collection time at the stereomicroscope. With this number of islets the different size of the islets does not matter, in paired comparisons of a small number of islets the size should be matched (13). The overall time from sacrifice until start of the experiment, regardless if this will be the perifusion or some other use of the isolated islets, is about 90 min.

5. The conventional collagenase digestion permits persons without much practical experience to isolate sufficient numbers of

viable pancreatic islets. Nevertheless, there are a number of variables in this procedure, which need to be adjusted individually. Considerable interindividual differences in islet collection efficacy both with respect to the number and the quality of the islets exist. From our experience the main causes of variability are the time required for the excision of the pancreas, the shaking by hand at the end of the collagenase incubation and the time required to collect the islets under the stereomicroscope.

6. However, placing the clamp at a too distal position also leads to a failed injection because the collagenase solution flows into the duodenum instead of flowing retrograde up the pancreatic duct.

7. Since the preparation of the pancreas may take place in a different location, e.g., an animal facility, the plastic tube should be kept on ice to prevent the beginning of the digestion during the transport to the laboratory where the islet collection takes place.

8. Repetition of this step is necessary because even with diluted collagenase the digestion proceeds visibly. This is also valid for the islet collection after conventional collagenase digestion. The main advantage of ductal injection method is the larger yield of islets. 100–200 islets can be isolated from one pancreas (14). However, the injection of the collagenase solution into the duct requires considerable training to yield consistent results.

9. In a number of publications it is stated that islets are routinely kept in culture for 1 or 2 days after isolation with the intention to let them recover from the stress of isolation. We have not yet obtained evidence that cultured islets are "better" than freshly isolated islets. Such a procedure may be appropriate if a close comparison of the secretion is intended with other parameters that are usually obtained from cultured islets or beta cells.

10. A specialized application is the simultaneous measurement of insulin secretion and cytosolic Ca^{2+} concentration using the fluorescent indicator Fura-2. For this purpose islets have to attach to a glass cover slip which can then be inserted into a perifusion chamber fixed on the stage of a fluorescence microscope. To achieve measurable secretion rates, three islets are placed in a drop of 30 µL on the middle of a 28 mm glass cover slip which has been coated with a mixture of 3.8 µL RPMI 1640 and 1.2 µL of rat tail collagen (type I from Sigma, 1 mg dissolved in 2 mL 0.2% acetate). The cover slip is contained in a 35 mm Petri dish. After attachment of the islets for 3 h 2.5 mL RPMI 1640 with 5 mM glucose are added and the islets stay in culture for up to 5 days until used for an experiment.

11. RPMI 1640 normally contains 10 mM glucose. RPMI without glucose can be obtained by special order. Glucose is then weighed in to give the desired concentration prior to sterile filtration.

12. When MIN6 cell pseudo-islets are used for perifusion experiments, at least 100 of these should be used to give basal secretion rates measurable by the standard insulin ELISA.

13. Sudden transient changes in the secretion rate which do not correlate with changes in the perifusion medium are mostly due to air bubbles. At the end of the perifusion the islets are firmly attached to the filter membrane by the pressure of the perifusion medium. It may not be easy to collect them all for further analysis.

14. Islet perifusion and quantification of immunoreactive insulin in the fractionated perifusate can currently be regarded as the gold standard in experimental diabetology. Neither the demonstration of increases in the cytosolic Ca^{2+} concentration (15) nor measurements of exocytosis at the single granule level (16) can substitute for this technique.

15. For those still interested in measuring the insulin release during a static incubation: Fill 20 mL Falcon tubes (one each per incubation) with 1.8 mL distilled water and warm in a waterbath set at 37°C. Aerate the water for 5 min with oxygen/carbon dioxide (95/5, v/v), then immediately close the tubes. Collect 15 islets per incubation and transfer in 200 µL KR buffer into a 1.5 mL Eppendorf cup. Place the cup into the Falcon tube and aerate it for 1 min. Close the Falcon tube and put it into a gently shaking water bath for 60 min to establish steady-state conditions. Then carefully remove the supernatant and replace it by 200 µL of pre-warmed test or control solution. Aerate again for 1 min and put the cup back into the Falcon tube. Close the tube and incubate in the shaking water bath for the intended time period. Thereafter collect aliquots for determination of the insulin content.

Acknowledgment

Help by Verena Lier-Glaubitz, Michael Belz, and Hany Ghaly is gratefully acknowledged. Work in the authors' lab was supported by grants from the Deutsche Forschungsgemeinschaft (DFG Ru 368/5-1), the Deutsche Diabetes Gesellschaft, and the Deutsche Diabetes Stiftung.

References

1. Jain R, Lammert E (2009) Cell-cell interactions in the endocrine pancreas. Diabetes Obes Metab 11(Suppl 4):159–167
2. Unger RH, Orci L (2010) Paracrinology of islets and the paracrinopathy of diabetes. Proc Natl Acad Sci U S A 107:16009–16012
3. Hamid M et al (2002) Comparison of the secretory properties of four insulin-secreting cell lines. Endocr Res 28:35–47
4. Hellman B (1965) Studies in obese-hyperglycemic mice. Ann NY Acad Sci 131:541–558
5. Lenzen S (1979) Insulin secretion by isolated perfused rat and mouse pancreas. Am J Physiol 236:E391–E400
6. Nesher R, Cerasi E (2002) Modeling phasic insulin release: immediate and time-dependent effects of glucose. Diabetes 51(Suppl 1):S53–S59
7. Moskalewski S (1965) Isolation and culture of the islets of Langerhans of the guinea pig. Gen Comp Endocrinol 44:342–353
8. Lacy PE, Kostianovsky M (1967) Method for the isolation of intact islets of Langerhans from the rat pancreas. Diabetes 16:35–39
9. Hellerström C (1994) Pancreatic B-cell research: origins, developments and future prospects. In: Flatt P, Lenzen S (eds) Frontiers of insulin secretion and pancreatic B-cell research. Smith-Gordon, London, pp 1–6
10. Panten U et al (1977) A versatile microperifusion system. Anal Biochem 82:317–326
11. Miyazaki J et al (1990) Establishment of a pancreatic beta cell line that retains glucose-inducible insulin secretion: special reference to expression of glucose transporter isoforms. Endocrinology 127:126–132
12. Hauge-Evans A et al (1999) Pancreatic beta-cell-to-beta-cell interactions are required for integrated responses to nutrient stimuli: enhanced Ca^{2+} and insulin secretory responses of MIN6 pseudoislets. Diabetes 48:1402–1408
13. Aizawa T et al (2001) Size-related and size-unrelated functional heterogeneity among pancreatic islets. Life Sci 69:2627–2639
14. Gotoh M et al (1987) Reproducible high yield of rat islets by stationary in vitro digestion following pancreatic ductal or portal venous collagenase injection. Transplantation 43:725–730
15. Hatlapatka K, Willenborg M, Rustenbeck I (2009) Plasma membrane depolarization as a determinant of the first phase of insulin secretion. Am J Physiol Endocrinol Metab 297: E315–E322
16. Hatlapatka K et al (2011) Bidirectional insulin granule turnover in the submembrane space during K^+ depolarization-induced secretion. Traffic 12:1166–1178

Chapter 13

Determination of Beta-Cell Function: Ion Channel Function in Beta Cells

Martina Düfer

Abstract

For the regulation of beta-cell function ion channels are of outstanding importance. Beta cells are specialized to convert changes in blood glucose concentration to an adequate secretory response. To achieve this, nutrient-induced alterations of electrical activity are directly coupled to changes in insulin release. Consequently, determination and analysis of ion channel activity are important tools for the characterization of beta-cell (patho)physiology and for the investigation of drugs that influence insulin release. With implementation of the patch-clamp technique it has become possible to analyze ion currents in beta cells under various conditions (e.g., in intact cells or independent of cell metabolism, as whole-cell currents or on a single channel level). In addition, this method enables to combine ion current recordings with determination of membrane potential and exocytosis. This chapter introduces the basic principles of different patch-clamp configurations and focuses on experimental protocols for ion channel recordings in beta cells.

Key words: Patch-clamp technique, Ion channel, Membrane potential, Single channel current, Perforated-patch, Cell-attached, Standard whole cell, Amphotericin B, Electrical activity, Oscillations

1. Introduction

Alterations in membrane conductance are a key event for regulation of insulin release. At resting conditions (glucose concentrations < 4–5 mM) the membrane potential (V_m) of beta cells is determined by the K$^+$ conductance of ATP-regulated K$^+$ channels (K$_{ATP}$ channels). A rise in glucose metabolism due to elevated glucose uptake elevates mitochondrial ATP generation. As a consequence the ATP/ADP ratio in vicinity of the K$_{ATP}$ channels increases thereby reducing the open probability of the K$_{ATP}$ channel. With the decrease in K$^+$ conductance an unidentified depolarizing current prevails leading to membrane depolarization. At a membrane potential of approximately –50 mV voltage-dependent Ca^{2+} channels

(Ca_v channels) open and Ca^{2+} action potentials appear (1–3). In contrast to rodents, in human beta cells action potentials at glucose concentrations below 10 mM (and thus at V_m negative to –45 mV) are mainly driven by Na^+ currents (4, 5). Action potential repolarization is determined by increasing outward current through voltage-dependent K^+ channels (K_v channels) and Ca^{2+}-regulated K^+ channels (K_{Ca} channels) (6–10).

Glucose-stimulated beta cells are characterized by an oscillatory electrical activity, i.e., rhythmical changes between periods with Ca^{2+} action potentials (bursts) and intervals where the plasma membrane is hyperpolarized below the threshold for Ca^{2+} action potentials (interbursts). The electrically silent interburst intervals are mediated by an increase in the open probability of K_{ATP} channels and K_{Ca} channels. Due to the delayed and slow onset of this current it is termed K_{slow} (8, 11–15). The length of burst phases increases with rising glucose concentrations (16). Therefore, besides determination of ion currents, calculation of the fraction of plateau phase (= percentage of time with action potentials, FOPP) is another parameter commonly used to investigate beta-cell function. Compounds that are expected to promote insulin release, e.g., K_{ATP} channel blockers, can be evaluated by their ability to shift the FOPP concentration-response curve of glucose to the left. Importantly, oscillations only occur in intact islets or larger cell clusters but not in single beta cells.

Further ion channels that also play a role for beta-cell regulation are e.g., channels of the transient receptor potential (TRP) family, volume-sensitive anion channels (VSACs) or hyperpolarization-activated, and cyclic nucleotide-gated (HCN) channels (17–22).

To determine the V_m of beta cells within intact islets measurements with sharp electrodes are the method of choice (16, 23). However, this procedure is not suited for detection of ion currents. By contrast, the patch-clamp technique allows combination of both, recording of V_m and ion currents, thereby providing manifold possibilities to investigate the significance of ion channels for beta-cell function. In brief, the cell membrane is clamped to a defined voltage protocol and the current response is measured (24–27). To get information about channel properties the cytosol of the beta cell is dialyzed by the pipette solution or, to investigate metabolism-dependent effects, the cell interior remains unaffected. The direct influence of compounds on single ion channels can be elucidated by tearing out a small piece of the membrane and exposing the inner or the outer surface of the membrane patch to diverse bath solutions (28). Variations in the patch-clamp protocol allow to differentiate between voltage-regulated and voltage-independent ion channels or to determine channel conductance, inactivation characteristics etc. Especially the K_{ATP} channel, the L-type Ca^{2+} channel and K_v channels have been extensively studied in rodent beta cells and insulin-secreting cell lines and lately there are also data available for human beta cells (1, 3, 6–10, 29–31). By switching from the voltage clamp to the current clamp mode ion channel recordings can be combined with measurement of V_m (12, 32).

2. Materials

2.1. Experimental Setup

1. Patch pipettes: Usually pipettes are pulled from borosilicate glass capillaries with filament. Wall thickness depends on the patch-clamp configuration: thin-wall capillaries (~0.2–0.4 mm) are commonly used for whole-cell experiments whereas thick-wall capillaries (~0.5–0.7 mm) have a higher signal-to-noise ratio and are preferred for single channel recordings. The pipettes are fabricated individually by a pipette puller. In brief, the glass capillary is heated, pulled apart in defined stages and finally broken by a hard pull, leading to two patch pipettes. The tip diameter (~1 μm) is varied by heat and mechanical force to achieve a resistance of approximately 3–5 MΩ for whole-cell recordings and 10–12 MΩ for excised or cell-attached patches. A final polishing step reduces the roughness of the tip and increases seal resistance. Conventional experiments with beta cells do not require any special treatment of the pipettes (coating etc.) (see Note 1).

2. Silver conductor: To conduct electric currents to the amplifier a chlorinated silver wire has to be dipped into the pipette solution. Make sure that there are no air bubbles between the tip of the patch pipette and the silver wire.

3. Bath electrodes: An Ag/AgCl electrode is necessary to set the zero current level. Usually a salt-filled agar bridge is used to stably place the electrode in the bath chamber. For preparation of the KCl/agar mixture 5% agar are dissolved in 3 M KCl. During heating, the solution has to be gently stirred to avoid formation of air bubbles. After preparation the mixture is filled by a syringe into small tubes as long as it is hot. Be careful not to fill the entire tube. The remaining space has to be backfilled with KCl. The agar bridge can be stored at 8°C in 3 M KCl solution. On the day of use exchange the KCl solution, put the Ag/AgCl electrode into the tube and fix it in the bath chamber. Be sure that the part filled with KCl is free of air bubbles.

4. Bath chamber and perifusion system: The perifusion system should allow a continuous exchange of thermostat-controlled bath solution (see Note 2).

5. Patch-clamp setup: Usually the bath chamber is positioned on an inverted microscope placed on an anti-vibration table. The holder of the patch pipette and the silver wire are connected to the patch-clamp headstage. The position of the pipette can be

altered manually and via a micromanipulator. The headstage is connected to the patch-clamp amplifier that is controlled by the respective software of the manufacturer.

6. CCD camera: A conventional CCD camera and a monitor are useful for positioning the pipette under visual control and for checking the quality of the cell during the experiment.

7. Oscilloscope: The conventional software programs mainly offer an oscilloscope window to monitor changes in current or voltage. Nevertheless, an external oscilloscope is recommended (see Note 3).

8. Faraday cage: The whole setup is shielded against electromagnetic waves by a faraday cage. It is very important to properly ground the whole equipment. At worst, noise precludes the read-out of current or V_m recordings (see Note 3).

2.2. Bath and Pipette Solutions

Composition of the solutions depends on (a) the patch-clamp configuration and (b) the ion channel of interest. Usually, the pipette solution is similar to the intracellular milieu and the bath solution matches the extracellular fluid (except for inside-out patches where the bath solution substitutes for the intracellular milieu).

In the following tables examples for bath and pipette solutions used in our laboratory are listed. To avoid hydrolysis solutions containing nucleotides should be freshly prepared or stored at −20°C and kept on ice during the day of use.

1. Options for bath solutions:

Bath solution for (mM)	Whole-cell, outside-out K⁺ current, V_m	Whole-cell Ca_v current	Inside-out K⁺ current
NaCl	140	115	–
KCl	5	–	130
TEA-Cl[a]	–	20	–
MgCl$_2$	1.2	1.2	–
CaCl$_2$	2.5	10	4
Glucose[b]	0.5	0.5	–
Tolbutamide	(0.1)[c]	0.1	–
EDTA	–	–	10
HEPES	10	10	10
pH	7.4 with NaOH	7.4 with NaOH	7.4 with KOH

[a]TEA-Cl (tetraethylammonium-chloride) is added to block K⁺ currents
[b]A low concentration of glucose in the bath solution is recommended to stabilize cellular integrity
[c]To block K_{ATP} channels in recordings of K_v currents

2. Options for pipette solutions:
   (a) *Standard whole-cell recordings.*

Pipette solution for (mM)	K⁺ current	Ca$_v$ current
KCl	130	–
HCl	–	58
CsCl[a]	–	50
N-methyl-D-glucamine	–	70
MgCl$_2$	4	4
CaCl$_2$	2	2
EGTA	10	10
Na$_2$ATP	0.65	3
HEPES	10	10
pH	7.15 with KOH	7.15 with CsOH

   [a]To block K⁺ currents

   (b) *Perforated-patch whole-cell recordings.*

Pipette solution for (mM)	K⁺ current, V_m	Ca$_v$ current
KCl	10	10
Cs$_2$SO$_4$	–	70
K$_2$SO$_4$	70	–
NaCl	10	10
MgCl$_2$	4	7
CaCl$_2$	2	–
EGTA	10	–
HEPES	10	10
Amphotericin B[a]	250 µg/mL	250 µg/mL
pH	7.15 with KOH	7.15 with NaOH

   [a]For preparation of amphotericin stock solution (see Note 4)

   (c) *Cell-attached and excised patch single channel recordings.*

Pipette solution for (mM)	K⁺ current
KCl	130
MgCl$_2$	1.2
CaCl$_2$	2
EGTA	10
HEPES	10
pH	7.4 with KOH

3. Methods

To determine ion currents with the patch-clamp technique a circuit feedback is used to set V_m of a cell to a desired command voltage (V_{com}). With the voltage clamped (*voltage clamp mode*) the membrane current is measured and converted to voltage that can be displayed on the oscilloscope. For registration of V_m the current is clamped to zero (*current clamp mode*). Depending on the question and the ion channel of interest different patch-clamp configurations, pipettes and bath solutions are used. Examples for solutions are listed in the Subheading 2.2.

The general procedure of seal formation and establishment of the most important configurations are described in the following.

3.1. Seal Formation and Electrical Access

1. Dispersed beta cells, clusters of cells or whole islets, either attached to plastic culture dishes or glass coverslips, are placed on the microscope stage and the perifusion is started. After wash-out of the culture medium (see Note 5) the experiment can start (see Note 2).

2. For patch-clamp recordings constitution of membrane surface and temperature of the bath solution are very important. Seal formation gets more difficult with sticky membranes and increasing temperature (see Note 6). The temperature for the determination of ion channels or V_m usually ranges from 22 to 26°C.

3. After putting the patch pipette into the bath solution the voltage offset (V_0) has to be compensated. Thereafter, the baseline of the current should be close to zero.

4. "Gigaseal" formation: A small piece of the plasma membrane (the membrane "patch") has to be tightly adhered ("sealed") to the pipette. The electrical resistance of this seal should be $\geq 10^9$ Ω (= gigaohm-seal, gigaseal) to ensure that the small patch below the pipette is, compared to other routes, a low resistance pathway and thus the favored way for current flow. For seal formation the patch pipette is carefully moved to the cell surface. Contact between pipette and plasma membrane is visible by a stepwise rise in resistance. At that point movement of the pipette is stopped and mild suction is applied to obtain a gigaseal (see Notes 7 and 8). When the gigaseal has been established, correct for capacitive spikes resulting from the stimulus test pulse with the fast compensation tool of the amplifier (see Notes 5, 9, and 10).

5. Getting electrical access to the beta cells:
   To measure single channel currents with intact cellular metabolism (*cell-attached mode*) no further manipulation of the cell

membrane has to be done after gigaseal formation. Electrical access to the whole cell can be achieved either by rupturing the membrane beneath the pipette by brief suction (*standard whole-cell configuration*) (see Note 11) or by permeabilization of the membrane patch with pore-forming polyene antimycotics (nystatin, amphotericin B) (*perforated-patch configuration*) (see Note 4). Membrane resistance can be determined by correction of capacitive transients with the slow compensation tool of the patch-clamp amplifier (see Notes 12 and 13).

6. For ion channel recordings the membrane of the beta cell is clamped to −70 or −80 mV in most protocols and currents are induced by individual voltage protocols depending on the ion channel that should be investigated (examples are given in Subheading 3.3) (see Note 14).

7. To control the quality of the experiment check series resistance, leak current and seal resistance during the recording (see Notes 11, 12, and 15).

8. Excised patches:
If the direct influence of drugs or substrates on single channels has to be investigated the patch pipette is quickly withdrawn and the patch is ripped off the membrane (*excised patch*) (see Notes 16–18).

3.2. Patch-Clamp Configurations

Figure 1 summarizes the procedures leading to different patch-clamp configurations.

1. Cell-attached and open cell-attached configuration.
In this patch configuration the pipette is kept on the surface of the cell. After gigaseal formation the membrane potential is

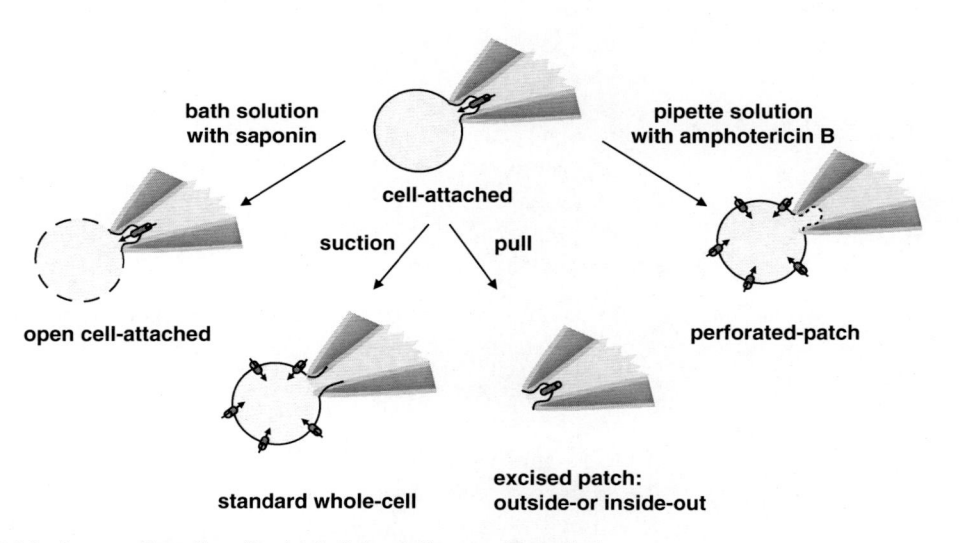

Fig. 1. Patch-clamp configurations (for detailed description see chapter 3.2).

controlled by the cell except for the small piece beneath the patch pipette. This configuration can be used for investigation of single channel properties in its "physiological" environment. It is very difficult to define the exact membrane potential in this mode.

If the composition of the cytosol should be manipulated by clamping the concentration of nucleotides or metabolites of low molecular weight the cells could be permeabilized by saponin or alpha-toxin. The pores are large enough for molecules <3 kD but exclude permeation of larger proteins (33, 34).

2. Perforated-patch configuration.
   This method is used to record V_m or whole-cell currents in beta cells with intact metabolism. Electrical access to the cell is achieved by pore-forming antibiotics. Pores are selective for cations but are not permeable for anions, glucose, enzymes, metabolites, nucleotides, etc. >300 D (see Notes 4, 12, 13, and 19).

3. Standard whole-cell configuration.
   In this configuration the cell is dialyzed with the pipette solution (see Note 11). Ion channel modulators that act from the cytosolic site can be applied via the patch pipette.

4. Excised patches: inside-out or outside-out configuration.
   In this mode single channel currents can be investigated without any influence of the cytosol. Depending on the part of the membrane facing the bath solution *inside-out* (cytosolic membrane surface exposed to the bath) or *outside-out* patches are formed (see Notes 16–18). Excised patches are frequently used, e.g., to test whether drugs or metabolites directly interact with K_{ATP} channels. Especially for analysis of ion channels with low single channel conductance (e.g., Ca_v channels (see Note 20), K_{Ca} channels of small or intermediate conductance) a very high seal resistance is necessary to minimize leak current and noise.

3.3. Voltage Protocols for Recordings of Ion Currents

Conventionally, cation fluxes from the extracellular to the intracellular space are illustrated by downward deflections and respective anion currents as upward deflections. Figure 2 shows some examples for voltage protocols and the resulting ion currents of murine beta cells.

1. Determination of currents in the whole-cell configuration: Cells are clamped to –70 mV.

   K_{ATP} currents are measured during 300 ms pulses to –60 and –80 mV at 15 s intervals.

   Voltage-activated K⁺ and Ca²⁺ currents, respectively, can be detected, e.g., by 50–150 ms voltage steps from –70 to 0 mV at 15 s intervals. Leak compensation prevents overlap with K_{ATP} current.

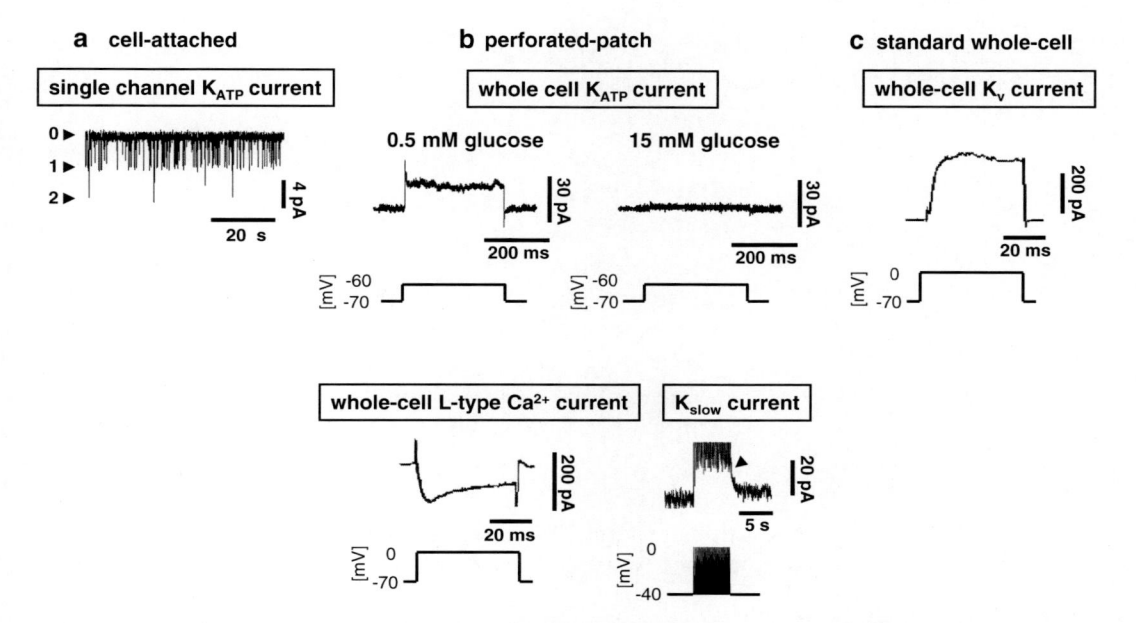

Fig. 2. (A) Recording of K_{ATP} channels in cell-attached patches. Arrowheads indicate simultaneous opening of 0, 1, or 2 K_{ATP} channels. (B) Registration of K_{ATP} (upper trace), Ca^{2+} (lower trace, left) and K_{slow} currents (lower trace, right) in the perforated-patch configuration. The arrowhead indicates maximal amplitude of K_{slow}. (C) Standard whole-cell current through K_v channels.

2. Determination of currents in excised patches:

   The voltage protocol for analysis of ion currents in excised patches depends on the composition of bath and pipette solution:

   If the concentration of the charge carrier is equal in bath and pipette solution no current is detectable after patch excision. Channel openings reoccur after clamping V_m to potentials positive or negative to 0 mV.

   For K_{ATP} channel recordings in the inside-out configuration, single channel openings are often recorded by clamping the patch to 50 mV (pipette positive vs. membrane). In this case, K^+ ions flow from pipette solution into bath solution and are therefore presented as inward currents.

3. Determination of K_{slow} currents:

   K_{slow} currents are composed of K_{ATP} and K_{Ca} currents that activate with increasing Ca^{2+} influx during the burst phase. The voltage protocol for activation of K_{slow} is designed to simulate a burst of Ca^{2+} action potentials:

   After a depolarizing step from –70 to –40 mV a train of 26 voltage ramps (–40 to 0 to –40 mV within 200 ms) is applied. This train of simulated Ca^{2+} action potentials is followed by a period of 10 s at –40 mV before stepping back to –70 mV (8, 14).

3.4. Characteristics of Ion Currents and V_m in Beta Cells

To identify beta cells in a preparation of islet cells several methods can be useful:

1. Glucose-dependence of V_m.

    In low glucose metabolically intact cells have a resting V_m of −70 to −80 mV.

    Elevating glucose concentration increases membrane depolarization. In rodent beta cells the threshold for Ca^{2+} action potentials is between 5 and 7 mM glucose. With suprathreshold glucose concentrations single beta cells respond with a continuous depolarization with Ca^{2+} action potentials on top of a plateau. Beta cells within large clusters or intact islets display oscillations. If oscillations occur in cell clusters the bursting pattern is more irregular compared to whole islets (see Note 21).

    Alpha cells are spontaneously active even in a very low glucose concentration (0.5 mM) (35). The effect of increasing glucose concentrations on V_m of alpha cells is not yet clear. With glucose concentrations above 10 mM hyperpolarization as well as depolarization of V_m have been described (36, 37).

2. Glucose-dependence of K_{ATP} channel activity.

    In contrast to beta cells, K_{ATP} current is much lower in alpha cells and the sensitivity to glucose or tolbutamide is clearly reduced (35).

3. Cell size.

    Combined analysis of immunohistochemistry and cell capacity has shown that membrane capacity (C_m) of alpha cells ranges from 3 to 5 pF, whereas C_m of insulin-positive cells is larger than 6 pF (38).

4. Na^+ current.

    In alpha cells a transient tetrodotoxin-sensitive inward current through voltage-activated Na^+ (Na_v) channels is induced by a 50 ms voltage step from −70 to 0 mV.

    In mouse beta cells Na_v channels are fully inactivated at resting V_m (39). Therefore, the voltage pulse only induces a sustained inward current that is sensitive to Ca_v channel blockers (38).

    Note: in human beta cells Na_v channels are not inactivated but contribute to the upstroke of glucose-induced action potentials (4).

5. Single-cell PCR.

    To make sure that the patch-clamped cell is really a beta cell the cytosol can be aspirated in the patch pipette after the experiment and tested for the presence of insulin mRNA by PCR.

4. Notes

1. Patch pipettes: to avoid damage or contamination of the pipette tip the pipettes should be pulled on the day of the experiment and kept in a closed box until use.

2. It is important to maintain a constant flow rate to avoid seal breaking due to variations in solution level. If perfusion is too fast you may lose the seal in response to up- and downturns during solution changes.

3. Electrical grounding is very important for recording of "good" data. To monitor noise or any other interference an external oscilloscope is very helpful. 50 Hz hum is one of the most typical problems arising from ground loops between the instruments. Another source of noise with higher frequencies ("digital noise") may be the monitor, oscilloscope, computer, or instrument power supplies. And finally, microscope, micromanipulator, as well as the perifusion system can induce noise. Usually, a metal bar with several holes for banana plugs to ground the equipment is installed at one side of the faraday cage. This is connected to the mains ground or to the signal ground of the patch-clamp amplifier by a copper wire. The instruments outside the faraday cage should be grounded to the same mains ground, e.g., via a power strip.

4. Handling of amphotericin B for perforated-patches: for the stock solution (50 mg/mL) use H_2O-free DMSO. After diluting with pipette buffer ultrasonicate the mixture to get a homogeneous suspension. If particle size is still too large you may filter the suspension prior to application (0.3 µm). Final concentrations range between 200 and 300 µg/mL amphotericin B. Solutions should be kept in the dark and be prepared freshly each day. The DMSO stock can be stored at −20°C for some days.

5. Protein-containing solutions: due to alterations in the membrane surface sealing is very difficult in the presence of albumin. Before starting an experiment wait until the medium (containing fetal calf serum or bovine serum albumin) is completely exchanged by bath solution. If albumin has to be present in the bath solution (e.g., to avoid that lipophilic drugs stick to the glass walls, tubes, etc.), use albumin-free buffer for seal formation and change thereafter.

6. Temperature: stability of the patch configurations is reduced with rising temperature due to increased membrane fluidity. Most experiments, including metabolism-dependent changes of ion currents, can be performed at 22–26°C. Note that temperature must be above 32°C for determination of exocytosis.

7. Gigaseal formation: for a beginner defining the right speed to place the patch pipette on the cell surface will be a challenge. If the pipette is dropped too fast the membrane will be damaged, if it is too slow the seal resistance will not reach the gigaohm range. The easiest way to track the first contact between cell surface and pipette is to look on the current response induced by the test pulse. A stepwise decrease and a concomitant increase in resistance (approx. 1 MΩ) indicate that the pipette tip has touched the membrane. At that point stop the movement of the pipette and start a gentle suction.

8. Time for seal formation: best results are achieved if seal formation occurs immediately after touching the plasma membrane. If much underpressure has to be applied larger parts of the membrane are sucked into the pipette. This can negatively influence exchange of intracellular factors beneath the pipette tip or falsify calculation of series resistance.

9. Good gigaseals range from 1.5–4 GΩ. Low resistance seals increase the leakage current and thus the current noise.

10. Sometimes seal formation can be accelerated by application of 10 mV hyperpolarizing voltage steps after touching membrane surface.

11. In the standard whole-cell configuration series resistance should be <20 MΩ. After rupturing of the membrane cytosolic compounds are diluted and replaced by the pipette solution, e.g., a steady increase in K_{ATP} current indicates wash-out of ATP. Wait before an experiment until series resistance and current response are stable.

12. For determination of ion currents in the perforated-patch mode series resistance should be between 20 and 30 MΩ. Lower series resistance indicates that the membrane patch below the pipette has been disrupted, higher resistance leads to underestimation of the current and indicates inadequate electrical access. Breaking from the perforated-patch into the whole-cell configuration is accompanied by wash-out of nucleotides, therefore, a fast and drastic increase in K_{ATP} current together with a sudden drop in series resistance is a reliable marker for membrane damage.

13. The process of amphotericin B- or nystatin-induced pore-forming is indicated by a constant decline of series resistance. Electrical access is usually obtained within 10–15 min after sealing. If the time for patch perforation is very long either the concentration of the antibiotic can be elevated or the tip diameter of the pipette can be enlarged. But note that this also increases the risk for breaking into the whole-cell mode.

14. To avoid unintentional membrane depolarization V_{com} should be fitted to the expected value (e.g., the resting V_m) or the

program should be switched to the current clamp mode soon after seal formation.

15. Ensure that your setup (micromanipulator, headstage, pipette holder, etc.) is stable. Pipette drift is not so much a problem for excised patches but can reduce the stability of all patch-clamp configurations with attached cells.

16. Channel rundown: a phenomenon frequently observed in single channel recordings of K_{ATP} currents is the time-dependent reduction of channel openings, the so-called rundown. Channel activity in excised inside-out patches can be restored by short pulses of Mg-ATP ("refreshing").

17. Inside-out patches are usually started in bath solutions representing the extracellular milieu to avoid K^+-induced depolarization of the membrane. After patch excision the solution is switched to buffers with high K^+ concentration.

18. Outside-out patches can be identified by the lack of K_{ATP} channel inhibition after addition of Mg-ATP to the bath solution.

19. For experiments in the perforated-patch configuration starting at a stimulatory glucose concentration has the advantage that intact beta cells can be identified by the occurrence of Ca^{2+} action potentials. Formation of a gigaseal may become more difficult at very low glucose concentrations (<3 mM) especially after a longer perifusion time.

20. Ca^{2+} currents: to increase the amplitude of currents through Ca_v channels Ba^{2+} can be used instead of Ca^{2+}. Note that inactivation of L-type Ca^{2+} channels is clearly reduced with Ba^{2+} as charge carrier (29, 40).

21. Oscillations of V_m in patch-clamped beta cells are often irregular hampering evaluation of experiments with respect to burst frequency or FOPP. More regular burst pattern can be achieved by rising extracellular Ca^{2+} concentration to 10 mM.

References

1. Ashcroft FM, Rorsman P (1989) Electrophysiology of the pancreatic beta-cell. Prog Biophys Mol Biol 54:87–143
2. Henquin JC, Nenquin M, Ravier MA et al (2009) Shortcomings of current models of glucose-induced insulin secretion. Diabetes Obes Metab Suppl 4:168–179
3. Drews G, Krippeit-Drews P, Düfer M (2010) Electrophysiology of islet cells. In: Islam MS (ed) Adv Exp Med Biol 654, Springer, pp 115–163
4. Pressel DM, Misler S (1990) Sodium channels contribute to action potential generation in canine and human pancreatic islet B cells. J Membr Biol 116:273–280
5. Braun M, Ramracheya R, Bengtsson M et al (2008) Voltage-gated ion channels in human pancreatic beta-cells: electrophysiological characterization and role in insulin secretion. Diabetes 57:1618–1628
6. Smith PA, Bokvist K, Arkhammar P et al (1990) Delayed rectifying and calcium-activated K^+ channels and their significance for action potential repolarization in mouse pancreatic beta-cells. J Gen Physiol 95:1041–1059

7. Henquin JC (1990) Role of voltage- and Ca^{2+}-dependent K^+ channels in the control of glucose-induced electrical activity in pancreatic B-cells. Pflügers Arch 416:568–572
8. Düfer M, Gier B, Wolpers D et al (2009) SK4 channels are involved in the regulation of glucose homeostasis and pancreatic beta-cell function. Diabetes 58:1835–1843
9. Düfer M, Neye Y, Hörth K et al (2011) BK channels affect glucose homeostasis and cell viability of murine pancreatic beta cells. Diabetologia 54:423–432
10. Houamed KM, Sweet IR, Satin LS (2010) BK channels mediate a novel ionic mechanism that regulates glucose-dependent electrical activity and insulin secretion in mouse pancreatic β-cells. J Physiol 588:3511–3523
11. Rolland JF, Henquin JC, Gilon P (2002) Feedback control of the ATP-sensitive K^+ current by cytosolic Ca^{2+} contributes to oscillations of the membrane potential in pancreatic beta-cells. Diabetes 51:376–384
12. Smith PA, Ashcroft FM, Rorsman P (1990) Simultaneous recordings of glucose dependent electrical activity and ATP-regulated K^+-currents in isolated mouse pancreatic beta-cells. FEBS Lett 261:187–190
13. Krippeit-Drews P, Düfer M, Drews G (2000) Parallel oscillations of intracellular calcium activity and mitochondrial membrane potential in mouse pancreatic B-cells. Biochem Biophys Res Commun 267:179–183
14. Kanno T, Rorsman P, Göpel SO (2002) Glucose-dependent regulation of rhythmic action potential firing in pancreatic beta-cells by K_{ATP}-channel modulation. J Physiol 545:501–507
15. Zhang M, Houamed K, Kupershmidt S et al (2005) Pharmacological properties and functional role of Kslow current in mouse pancreatic beta-cells: SK channels contribute to Kslow tail current and modulate insulin secretion. J Gen Physiol 126:353–363
16. Meissner HP, Schmelz H (1974) Membrane potential of beta-cells in pancreatic islets. Pflügers Arch 351:195–206
17. Islam MS (2011) TRP channels of islets. In: Islam MS (ed) Adv Exp Med Biol 704, Springer, 811–830
18. Togashi K, Hara Y, Tominaga T et al (2006) TRPM2 activation by cyclic ADP-ribose at body temperature is involved in insulin secretion. EMBO J 25:1804–1815
19. Wagner TF, Loch S, Lambert S et al (2008) Transient receptor potential M3 channels are ionotropic steroid receptors in pancreatic beta cells. Nat Cell Biol 10:1421–1430
20. Britsch S, Krippeit-Drews P, Gregor M et al (1994) Effects of osmotic changes in extracellular solution on electrical activity of mouse pancreatic B-cells. Biochem Biophys Res Commun 204:641–645
21. Best L (1999) Cell-attached recordings of the volume-sensitive anion channel in rat pancreatic beta-cells. Biochim Biophys Acta 1419:248–256
22. El-Kholy W, MacDonald PE, Fox JM et al (2007) Hyperpolarization-activated cyclic nucleotide-gated channels in pancreatic beta-cells. Mol Endocrinol 21:753–764
23. Meissner P (1990) Membrane potential measurements in pancreatic beta cells with intracellular microelectrodes. Methods Enzymol 192:235–246
24. Sakmann B, Neher E (1983) Single channel recording. Plenum Press, New York
25. Cook DL, Hales CN (1984) Intracellular ATP directly blocks K^+ channels in pancreatic B-cells. Nature 311:271–273
26. Findlay I, Dunne MJ (1985) Voltage-activated Ca^{2+} currents in insulin-secreting cells. FEBS Lett 189:281–285
27. Rorsman P, Bokvist K, Ämmälä C et al (1994) Ion channels, electrical activity and insulin secretion. Diabetes Metab 20:138–145
28. Houamed K, Fu J, Roe MW et al (2004) Electrophysiology of the pancreatic beta-cell. In: LeRoith D et al (eds) Diabetes mellitus: a fundamental and clinical text, 3rd edn. Lippincott, Williams and Wilkins, Philadelphia
29. Plant TD (1988) Properties and calcium-dependent inactivation of calcium currents in cultured mouse pancreatic B-cells. J Physiol 404:731–747
30. MacDonald PE, Wheeler MB (2003) Voltage-dependent K^+ channels in pancreatic beta cells: role, regulation and potential as therapeutic targets. Diabetologia 46:1046–1062
31. Jacobson DA, Mendez F, Thompson M et al (2010) Calcium-activated and voltage-gated potassium channels of the pancreatic islet impart distinct and complementary roles during secretagogue induced electrical responses. J Physiol 588:3525–3537
32. Düfer M, Krippeit-Drews P, Drews G (2002) Inhibition of mitochondrial function affects cellular Ca^{2+} handling in pancreatic B-cells. Pflügers Arch 444:236–243
33. Tarasov AI, Girard CA, Ashcroft FM (2006) ATP sensitivity of the ATP-sensitive K^+ channel in intact and permeabilized pancreatic beta-cells. Diabetes 55:2446–2454
34. Schulze DU, Düfer M, Wieringa B et al (2007) An adenylate kinase is involved in K_{ATP} channel

regulation of mouse pancreatic beta cells. Diabetologia 50:2126–2134
35. Quoix N, Cheng-Xue R, Mattart L et al (2009) Glucose and pharmacological modulators of ATP-sensitive K$^+$ channels control $(Ca^{2+})_c$ by different mechanisms in isolated mouse alpha-cells. Diabetes 58:412–421
36. Gromada J, Ma X, Høy M et al (2004) ATP-sensitive K$^+$ channel-dependent regulation of glucagon release and electrical activity by glucose in wild-type and SUR1$^{-/-}$ mouse alpha-cells. Diabetes 53(Suppl 3):S181–S189
37. Manning Fox JE, Gyulkhandanyan AV, Satin LS et al (2006) Oscillatory membrane potential response to glucose in islet beta-cells: a comparison of islet-cell electrical activity in mouse and rat. Endocrinology 147:4655–4663
38. Barg S, Galvanovskis J, Göpel SO et al (2000) Tight coupling between electrical activity and exocytosis in mouse glucagon-secreting alpha-cells. Diabetes 49:1500–1510
39. Plant TD (1988) Na$^+$ currents in cultured mouse pancreatic B-cells. Pflügers Arch 411:429–435
40. Rorsman P, Ashcroft FM, Trube G (1988) Single Ca channel currents in mouse pancreatic B-cells. Pflügers Arch 412:597–603

Chapter 14

Measurement of Glucose Homeostasis In Vivo: Glucose and Insulin Tolerance Tests

Francesco Beguinot and Cecilia Nigro

Abstract

The feasibility of investigating glucose tolerance and insulin action and secretion in vivo in mouse models has provided major insights into both type 2 diabetes pathogenesis and the identification of novel strategies to treat this common disorder. When initial studies provide evidence for altered levels of insulin and/or glucose in the animal blood, a number of well-characterized tests can be adopted to estimate glucose homeostasis and insulin action and secretion in vivo. These tests include model assessments, glucose and insulin sensitivity studies, and glucose clamps. None of them can be considered appropriate under all circumstances and there is significant variation in their complexity, technical ease, and invasiveness. Thus, while the euglycaemic hyperinsulinemic clamp represents the gold standard for measuring in vivo insulin action, less labor-intensive as well as invasive techinques are usually considered as the initial approach to evaluate glucose homeostasis. This section focuses on glucose and insulin tolerance tests. The clamp technique is described in Chapter 15.

Key words: Type 2 diabetes, Insulin resistance, Insulin sensitivity, Mouse phenotyping, Insulin secretion

1. Introduction

Insulin represents the major regulator of glucose homeostasis (1). The postprandial rise in plasma insulin enables appropriate disposal of blood glucose in the absorptive state, while the fall in plasma insulin contributes to maintaining euglycemia in the post-absorptive state and during starvation (2). In all mammals, these normal fluctuations in insulin levels are dependent upon the ability of pancreatic beta-cells to respond to changes in plasma glucose levels by modulating insulin secretion (3).

Type 2 diabetes is the most common abnormality of glucose homeostasis and the most frequent endocrine disorder (4). Current evidence indicates that, in the years preceeding type 2 diabetes

Major pathophysiological abnormalities
leading to impaired glucose tolerance

- Impaired insulin secretion
- Impaired glucose production
- Impaired glucose disposal
- Altered glucose tolerance

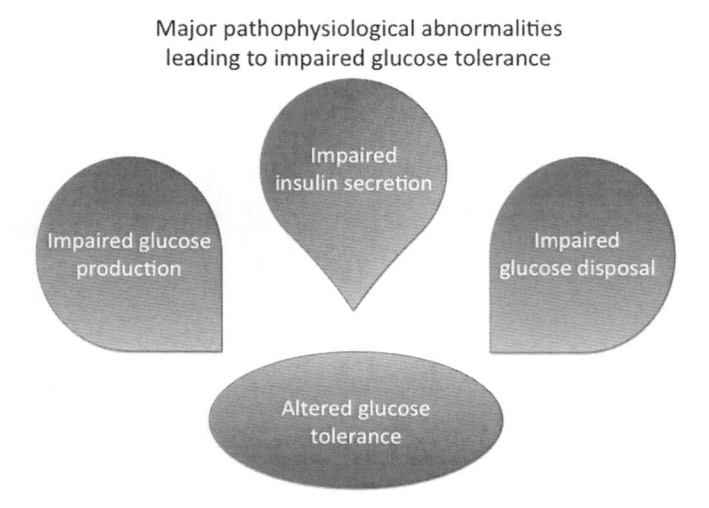

Fig. 1. Major alterations appearing in the natural history of type 2 diabetes.

onset, a progressive deterioration of insulin sensitivity in liver and peripheral tissues and of beta-cell insulin secretion occurs (Fig. 1). This leads to increasingly abnormal glucose tolerance and, finally, to type 2 diabetes (5). How these abnormalities are generated and have become established remain ultimately unclear, but tremendous interest to solve this problem has accumulated also due to the epidemic diffusion of type 2 diabetes. This circumstance has strengthened the motivation to adopt the convenient mouse model for dissecting the genetic and the molecular causes of type 2 diabetes.

In mice as in humans, derangement in glucose homeostasis is often suspected on the bases of elevated plasma insulin or glucose levels. These abnormalities can be further investigated in the mouse by methodologies similar to those commonly used in humans, including measurements of fasting and post-load glucose and insulin levels, glucose and insulin sensitivity tests, and the more invasive clamps (Table 1). These different approaches correlate quite well and may enable both an accurate characterization of glucose tolerance, i.e., the ability to rescue basal glycemia upon a load, and identification of major reasons for derangement in glucose homeostasis.

An important and general consideration when assessing glucose tolerance, plasma insulin, or glucose concentrations in mice (as well as in humans) is that the conditions under which these variables are measured must be carefully taken into account, as they are affected by a number of physiological and environmental factors in addition to pathological situations. These include physical activity levels, the time of the day and stress. For example, stress-induced increase in catecholamines and cortisol levels can enhance liver glucose production and affect the assessment of glucose tolerance (6). Also, mice usually exhibit higher cortisol levels in the evening, leading to increased glucose production. Finally, as for

Table 1
Basic methods used to assess insulin sensitivity and glucose tolerance

Test	Sample	Method
FPG and FPI	One 50 μL blood sample	Overnight or 4 h fasting glucose and insulin measurements
OGTT	Eight 3 μL blood samples	Overnight fast and glucose measurement after oral glucose load
IPGTT	Eight 3 μL blood samples	Overnight fast and glucose measurements after I.P. glucose load
IPITT	Six 3 μL blood samples	Overnight fast and glucose measurements after I.P. glucose load

FPG fasting plasma glucose; *FPI* fasting plasma insulin; *OGTT* oral glucose tolerance test; *IPGTT* intraperitoneal glucose tolerance test; *IPITT* intraperitoneal insulin tolerance test; *I.P.* intraperitoneal

many other tests used in the endocrinological assessment of the mouse phenotype, the validity of results obtained is largely dependent on methods of animal husbandry. Adequate experience of the personnel performing the tests is key to reduce the anxiety levels of the mice both before and during the experiments. Reference values for metabolite and hormone levels in many mouse strains are available through the Jackson Laboratories website (http://www.jacksonlaboratory.com).

2. Materials

2.1. Detection of Blood Glucose Concentrations

1. Blood glucose monitor and associated test strips for glucose measurement (e.g., Accu-Check Active, Roche Diagnostics).
2. Low and high-level glucose control solutions (e.g., Accu-Check Active glucose control solutions, Roche Diagnostics; low concentration: 50 mg/dL, reference range 42–72 mg/dL, and high concentration: 300 mg/dL, reference range 290–328 mg/dL).
3. Scalpel blade.

2.2. Detection of Insulin Concentration

1. Mouse serum or plasma.
2. Microtiter plate shaker.
3. Microtiter plate washer.

2.3. Oral Glucose Tolerance Test

1. 20% (w/v) aqueous glucose solution.
2. Animal scale.
3. Blood glucose monitor and test strips for glucose measurement (e.g., Accu-Check Active, Roche Diagnostics).
4. Scalpel blade.
5. 1-mL syringe (e.g., Terumo) and 22-G ball-tip needle (e.g., Popper and Sons).
6. Timer.

2.4. Intraperitoneal Insulin Tolerance Test

1. Animal scale.
2. Blood glucose monitor and test strips for glucose measurement (e.g., Accu-Check Active, Roche Diagnostics).
3. Fast-acting insulin solution.
4. Scalpel blade.
5. 1-mL syringe (e.g., Terumo) and 25-G × 5/8-in. Needles (e.g., Terumo).
6. Timer.

Also:
4. Plate reader with 450 nm reading capability.
5. Ultrasensitive Mouse Insulin ELISA kit (e.g., Mercodia).

3. Methods

3.1. Determination of Glycemia by Glucose Monitor

Blood glucose concentration is often the first parameter to be determined when defining the metabolic phenotype, as abnormalities are indicative of alterations in glucose homeostasis. Blood glucose can be assayed on plasma or serum samples, which is usually achieved by enzymatic methods using either hexokinase or glucose oxidase. Whether performed manually or automatically, this approach is specially useful when samples are to be frozen and/or analyzed at a later point in time. Alternatively, glucose concentration can be conveniently determined on whole blood using the portable glucose monitors designed for human diabetes self-control. These devices are inexpensive, easy to use, and provide fast and reliable results from very small volumes of blood. The protocol below describes the use of the Accu-Chek Active blood glucose monitor from Roche Diagnostics. Other widely used monitors include the HemoCue Glucose (HemoCue), BD Logic Blood Glucose Monitor (BD), Precision Xtra (Abbott), and One Touch Ultra (LifeScan).

1. Calibrate the blood glucose monitor as described in the manufacturer's user manual of the device, and repeat calibration each time a new box of test strips is used (see Note 1).

2. Using the low and the high-level glucose control solutions, execute a performance check on the monitor as described in the manufacturer's user manual of the device. This routine should be repeated each time a new box of test strips is used, or if uncertain of the monitor performance. Use the same lot of test strips for one experiment as intra-lot variations can occur (see Note 1).

3. Insert a new test strip in the device.

4. Draw an approximately 3 µL blood drop from a mouse by notching the lateral tail vein 1–2 cm from the tip using a scalpel blade and apply the drop to the test strip by touching the strip directly to the bleeding tail wound.

5. Read and record the test result (see Note 2).

6. Facilitate blood clotting by applying gentle mechanical pressure to the tail wound and return the mouse in its cage.

3.2. Determination of Insulinemia by ELISA

For measuring the plasma insulin concentration, we recommend the use of the Ultrasensitive Mouse Insulin ELISA by Mecordia. The assay is based on a solid-phase direct sandwich ELISA and adopts two monoclonal antibodies against separate epitopes of the insulin molecule. Sample insulin is immobilized by the first antibody bound to the assay well, followed by labeling with peroxidase-conjugated antibodies. The bound insulin is then revealed colorimetrically. Other commercially available ELISA kits for measuring insulin in small volumes include the Linko Research kit.

1. Pipet calibrator 0 (25 µL) into each well of a 96-well microtiter plate coated with mouse insulin antibody.

2. Pipet calibrators (5 µL) and mouse serum or plasma (5 µL) into duplicate wells of the antibody-coated microtiter plate (see Note 3).

3. Add 50 µL of antibody-enzyme conjugate reagent to each well (the reagent is prepared by diluting the concentrated antibody-enzyme conjugate provided with the commercial kit as specified in the manufacturer's instructions).

4. Incubate on a shaker for 2 h at room temperature 18–25°C.

5. Aspirate the reaction volume, add 350 µL of wash buffer to each well and aspirate completely. Repeat this procedure five more times. The wash buffer is prepared by diluting the concentrated wash buffer provided with the commercial kit as specified in the kit manufacturer's instructions.

6. After the last wash, invert the plate and tap firmly against absorbent paper.

7. Add 200 µL of TMB substrate reagent (provided with the kit) to each well (light-sensitive reagent).

8. Incubate 30 min at room temperature.
9. Add 50 µL stop solution.
10. Place the plate on the shaker for about 10 s to enable adequate mixing of substrate and stop reagents.
11. Measure the absorbance at 450 nm and compute results according to the kit manufacturer's instructions (for manual calculation, plot the calibrators on a log-log or log-in paper and read the insulin concentrations for each sample from the curve).
12. If the insulin concentration exceeds the value of the highest calibrator, dilute the sample tenfold with 0.9% NaCl and repeat the analysis.

3.3. Oral Glucose Tolerance Test

The oral glucose tolerance test (OGTT) enables an estimate of the clearance of a standard bolus of glucose. At variance from the intraperitoneal glucose tolerance test (IPGTT) described in Subheading 3.4, the OGTT is based on orally administered glucose, so that its clearance is also determined by intestinal factors. Animals tested by OGTT are starved for 14–16 h, followed by glucose administration by gavage and blood or plasma glucose measurement through the following 3 h. The oral gavage techniques are fully described in ref. (7). In each experimental setting, two trained persons should cooperate with one of them only performing the gavage in the entire group of animals. In order to achieve interpretable results, it is advisable that no more than 16 mice are treated in each experimental setting. Accordingly, accurate experimental design to divide the animal group is necessary.

1. Fast mice for 14–16 h (overnight) with constant access to drinking water.
2. On the following day, at 8:00 a.m., place each mouse in a fresh cage with access to water and identify each cage with the mouse number.
3. Record the weight of each mouse.
4. Calculate and record the volume of the 20% glucose solution required for oral gavaging of 2 g of glucose/kg (oral injection volume 10 µL/g body weight).
5. Prepare strips for glucose measurements, record sheets, and a 1 mL syringe for each animal containing the calculated glucose to be gavaged. One ball-tip needle can be used through the entire experiment, switching it between the different syringes upon fast external rinsing with 70% ethanol and water.
6. Calibrate the blood glucose monitor as described in Subheading 3.1.
7. Determine the basal glucose concentration in each mouse (T_0) by removing one mouse at a time, placing it on the top of its

cage and drawing blood from the lateral vein of the tail as previously outlined in Subheading 3.1. Place the blood sample on the test strip of the glucose monitor, read and record the result. Facilitate blood clotting on the tail incision as previously described and return the mouse in its cage.

8. After the basal glucose concentrations has been determined in all mice, perform gavaging and administer the glucose load to each mouse, maintaining a 30–60 s interval between animals, depending on the size of the experimental group. Start the timer upon the first mouse that has been gavaged. It takes at least 30 s for an experienced investigator to perform gavaging and blood glucose determination (see Note 4).

9. At T_{15}, measure the blood glucose again, starting with the first mouse gavaged and maintaining the same time interval until all of the mice in the experimental group have been assesed. To enable rebleeding, remove the clot from the incision and massage the tail as needed to enable sufficient blood flow.

10. Repeat this procedure at T_{30}, T_{60}, T_{90}, T_{120}, T_{150}, T_{180} (see Note 5).

11. At the end of the experiment, return mice in their original cages and make sure that none of them is bleeding. Also, make sure that food and drinking water are available for the animals again.

12. Data are usually plotted as glucose values vs. time. Statistical treatment of the data can be simplified by calculating, for each mouse, areas under the curves as in ref. (8).

3.4. Intraperitoneal Glucose Tolerance Test

The IPGTT measures the clearance of an intraperitoneally injected glucose load by tissues. Compared to the OGTT, IPGTT does not address the intestinal phase of glucose absorption and is, therefore, a less physiological test. The procedure is very similar to that used for OGTT with the exception that the glucose load is injected intraperitoneally rather than by gavaging (see Note 6). Accordingly, materials and methods will not be outlined again. Please refer to Subheading 3.3 for details (see Note 7). Same as for oral administration, a 2 g glucose/kg load should be used, with an intraperitoneal injection volume of 10 μL/g body weight. The same considerations on timing and group size apply to IPGTT and to OGTT (see Subheading 3.3).

3.5. Intraperioneal Insulin Tolerance Test

The intraperitoneal insulin tolerance test (IPITT) measures glucose levels upon administration of a standard insulin bolus, providing an estimate of the insulin sensitivity of the animal. Animals are fasted for 14–16 h and subjected to intraperitoneal insulin loading. Blood glucose levels are measured at different time points through the following 90 min.

As for glucose tolerance studies, experimental design of IPITT studies must take into serious consideration the size of the experimental sample. Again, it is advisable that no more than 16 animals are examined during the same experimental setup with two trained personnel units each of which is attributed specific roles in the experiment. To minimize technical variation, insulin should be injected by the same unit of personnel to all of the mice.

1. Fast mice for 14–16 h (overnight) with constant access to drinking water.
2. On the following day, at 8:00 a.m., place each mouse in a fresh cage with access to water and identify each cage with the mouse number.
3. Record the weight of each mouse.
4. Calculate and record the volume of insulin solution required for an intraperitoneal injection of 0.5 IU/kg in an injection volume of 3.6 μL/g body weight.
5. Prepare the 1 mL insulin syringes and 25-G×5/8-in. needles with the calculated volumes for each animal in the experiment. Prepare experiment record sheets and test strips for glucose measurement (see Note 8).
6. Calibrate the glucose monitor with the standard strip.
7. Determine the basal glucose levels in each mouse by removing one mouse at a time from its cage, placing it on the top of the cage and drawing blood from the lateral vein of the tail as outlined in Subheading 3.1. Facilitate blood cloting as described under in Subheading 3.1.
8. Inject insulin intraperitoneally in each mouse at 30–60 s interval between animals, depending on the size of the experimetal group. Start the timer when the first mouse is injected (see Note 9).
9. At T_{15}, determine blood glucose again, starting with the first mouse injected and using the same interval adopted for injection, until all the mice in the experimental group have been measured. To restart bleeding, gently remove the clot from the incision and massage the tail as needed to increase the blood flow.
10. Repeat the above sequence at T_{30}, T_{60}, and T_{90} after insulin injection. If at any time during implementation of the protocol, blood glucose falls below 36 mg/dL, the value must be confirmed. If confirmed, the mouse must be rescued by injecting 0.5–1.0 g glucose/kg from a 20% glucose solution as hypoglycemia might be otherwise lethal (see Note 10).
11. Data are usually presented by plotting glucose values vs. time. If mice significantly differ in their basal glucose levels, plotting % of basal value vs. time may represent a valid alternative.

12. Calculation of areas under the curve may provide additional information, especially if the initial and the late phases (the last 90–60 min, when counterregulatory hormones start playing a major role) are analyzed separately.

4. Notes

1. The small size of the blood volume of a normal mouse requires high sensitivity of all of the procedures adopted to assay circulating metabolites. This requirement is particularly strict in the case of glucose as the accomplishment of several metabolic tests needs repeated sampling over short periods of time.

2. For very low (<2 mM) or very high glucose levels (reported upper limit for the Accu-Check monitor is 33.3 mM), use of alternative methods to confirm readings is highly advisable.

3. Fasting insulin levels in many mouse strains are close to the sensitivity limit of most commercially available kits (0.2 μg/L for the Mercodia kit). Attention must be paid to the storage conditions of the serum/plasma samples and their freeze-thaw cycles. Also, the upper level detection limits of many commercial kits (7 μg/L for the Mercodia kit) are relatively low compared to the insulin levels which may be achieved in certain experimental conditions. This circumstance may require adequate dilution of the samples and retest.

4. Correct oral gavaging is essential and must be performed by experienced personnel to avoid tracheal instead of esophagus gavaging.

5. After the load (T_{15}), blood glucose is expected to increase 1.5–2-fold, followed by a slow return toward the basal values. However, in insulin-resistant states, peak glucose concentration is usually higher and returns slowly to the basal values. The kinetics of blood glucose excursion resembles that occurring during IPGTT, although glucose peak is usually reached later, it is somewhat more blunt and the return toward the basal condition is slower. During all tolerance tests, changes in glucose and insulin levels are dynamic. Therefore, the number of animals used in each experimental group must be small enough to precisely respect the scheduled timetable, particularly during the initial phases of the study where the most rapid changes occur (typically, the T_0 to T_{30} in the glucose tolerance tests).

6. An important technical concern, specially with obese mice, is that the glucose solution may end up to be injected in the adipose depots, slowing absorption. This circumstance may offer reasons for even greater concern when animals with large

difference in the amount of fat tissue are compared. Since direct possibilities to clarify this issue are scarce, efforts must be devoted at the time of data analysis to identify unresponsive animals.

7. Initial glucose peaks during IPGTT should be at least twofold higher than baseline levels but can be even tenfold higher depending on the particular experimental setup, including the mouse genetic background. When insulin is measured in addition to glucose, values usually follow the changes in glycemia. On the other hand, a significant increase in peak glucose (T_0–T_{30}) may be indicative of defective beta-cell function.

8. For some mouse strains, the insulin dose recommended in the above protocol may be too high and result in severe, even lethal hypoglycemia. Since this circumstance is somewhat unpredictable, it is advisable that a preliminary test with a small number of mice is implemented to assess the insulin sensitivity of the particular mouse strain under study. From a practical perspective, it is also advisable that only freshly prepared insulin solutions are used, as this will prevent excessive binding to the test tube walls and the syringe.

9. As in the case of IPGTT, adiposity may create reasons for concern when data from IPITT are to be analyzed, specially if study groups differ significantly for abdominal fat (see under Protocol 4).

10. Upon insulin injection, blood glucose typically falls from the basal levels until T_{30}, after which it tends to stabilize and slowly returns toward basal levels. Slower recovery from hypoglycemia may indicate failure of the counter-regulatory system and or impaired glucose production.

References

1. Pickup JC, Williams G (2005) Textbook of diabetes: selected chapters, 3rd edn. Blackwell Publishing, Oxford
2. Saltiel AR, Kahn CR (2001) Insulin signalling and the regulation of glucose and lipid metabolism. Nature 414:799–806
3. Andrali SS, Sampley ML, Vanderford NL et al (2008) Glucose regulation of insulin gene expression in pancreatic beta-cells. Biochem J 415(1):1–10
4. Sicree R, Shaw J, Zimmet (2009) The global burden: diabetes and impaired glucose tolerance. Diabetes Atlas, IDF. 4. International Diabetes Federation, Brussels
5. Cavaghan MK, Ehrmann DA et al (2000) Interaction between insulin resistance and insulin secretion in the development of glucose intolerance. J Clin Invest 106:329–333
6. Vranic M, Miles P, Rastogi K et al (1991) Effect of stress on glucoregulation in physiology and diabetes. Adv Exp Med Biol 291:161–183
7. Hedrich H (ed) (2004) The laboratory mouse. Elsevier Academic Press, London
8. Heikkinen S, Argmann CA, Champy MF et al (2007) Evaluation of glucose homeostasis. Curr Protoc Mol Biol Chapter 29:Unit 29B.3

Chapter 15

Measurement of Glucose Homeostasis In Vivo: Combination of Tracers and Clamp Techniques

Masakazu Shiota

Abstract

A tracer technique referred to as "pancreatic-blood glucose clamp" allows assessment in response to a change in blood glucose, insulin, and/or glucagon of whole body glucose disposal, endogenous glucose production, specific tissue/organ glucose uptake and storage, and insulin secretion. This technique is currently considered the optimal method for measurement of insulin sensitivity and glucose effectiveness. We describe here, for use in conscious-unrestrained mice and rats, the pancreatic-blood glucose clamp technique and its associated methods; which include catheterization of blood vessels; a clamp of plasma insulin, glucagon, and glucose; analyses of metabolites and tracers; and calculations.

Key words: Glucose-tracers, Catheterization, Pancreatic-blood glucose clamp, Hyperinsulinemic-euglycemic, Glucose clamp, Hyperglycemic, Insulin sensitivity, Glucose effectiveness

Abbreviations

Ci	Curie(s)
h	Hours
I.D.	Inner diameter
ip	Intraperitoneal injection
min	Minutes
O.D.	Outer diameter
U	Unit(s)
v/v	Volume/volume
w/v	Weight/volume

1. Introduction

To evaluate sensitivity/responsiveness of glucose metabolism to changes in glucose and insulin concentrations, one measures the degree of rise or fall of blood glucose levels in response to a glucose or insulin load; an index of glucose or insulin tolerance, respectively. While glucose and insulin tolerance tests are widely used for their simplicities and conveniences, they fail to isolate effects on glucose metabolism to changes solely in glucose or insulin concentration, since changes in one will alter the level of the other. A technique that is able to dissect individual contributions of glucose or insulin is commonly referred to as the "pancreatic-blood glucose clamp." This technique allows one to independently alter plasma levels of glucose, glucagon, or insulin by inhibiting endogenous secretion of glucagon and insulin and infusing glucose, glucagon, and insulin at rates required to maintain these agents at desired levels. The sensitivity/responsiveness of glucose metabolism to insulin and glucose is evaluated as changes in glucose uptake/utilization and glucose production rates, which are measured using glucose-tracers. A variation of the "pancreatic-blood glucose clamp" is the so called glucose clamp, which is a technique that evaluates the effectiveness of altered glucose levels to evoke insulin and glucagon secretion from the pancreas. Herein, we provide the methods for these clamp techniques and associated surgeries that were developed by us for mice (1–5) and rats (6–13) and used to assess insulin sensitivity and glucose effectiveness in conscious nonrestricted rodents.

2. Materials

2.1. Anesthesia for Catheterization Surgery

1. Chemical anesthesia: Pentobarbital sodium (Nembutal), 70 mg/kg intraperitoneal (ip) injection for normal mice, 50 mg/kg ip injection for normal rats (see Note 1).
2. Gas anesthesia: Isoflurane with anesthesia system, which includes a vaporizer, an oxygen cylinder, an evacuation system, and a rodent circuit set with mask.

2.2. Equipment for Surgery

1. Operating table and board.
2. Scissors: dissection and fine.
3. Forceps: dissection and fine.
4. Needle holder scissors.
5. Atraumatic forceps to retract tissue.
6. Ruler.

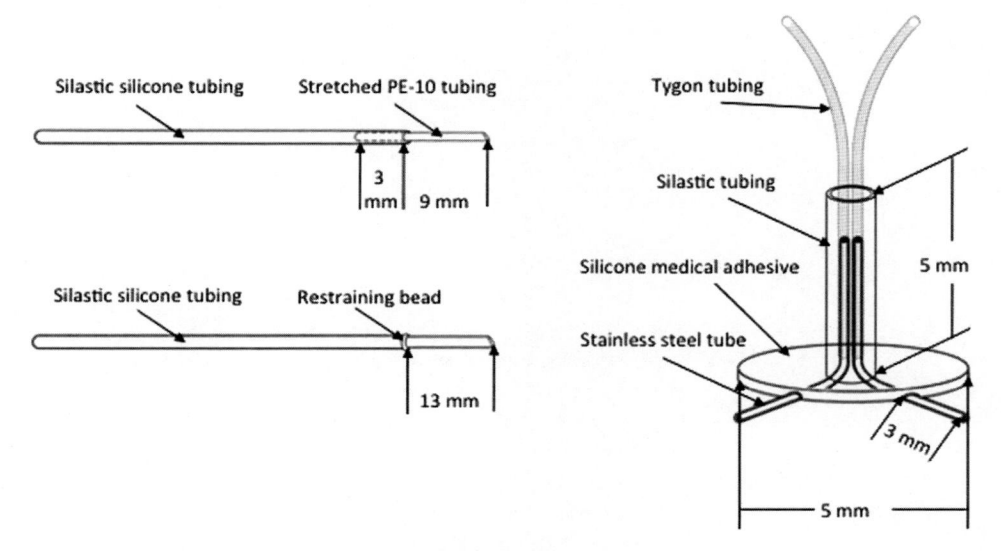

Fig. 1. Indwelling catheters and catheter holder for surgery of mice.

7. Razor blade.
8. Micro clips.
9. Stainless steel pipetting needle: 20 gauge and 38.1 mm length for mice, 14 gauge and 101.6 mm length for rats.
10. Suture: Silk (6-0 for rats and 7-0 for mice), Absorbable (4-0 for rats and 6-0 for mice), Nylon (4-0 for rats and 6-0 for mice).

2.3. Mouse Catheters

1. Arterial catheter (Silastic silicone laboratory tubing (0.3 mm I.D. and 0.63 mm O.D.) and Intramedic polyethylene tubing (PE-10: 0.28 mm I.D. and 0.61 mm O.D.)) (Fig. 1): PE-10 tubing is currently the smallest size of commercially available polyethylene tubing, but is still too thick for a mouse carotid artery. The PE-10 polyethylene tubing needs to be stretched by hand to reduce its size by ~40%. The tip of one end of a precut piece of stretched PE-10 tubing is inserted approximately 3 mm into Silastic silicone tubing, while the other end is beveled to an angle of 50–60° at the time of surgery. The length of the stretched PE-10 tubing from the pointed end to the base of the Silastic tubing is 9 mm, which coincides with the length needed to reach the aortic arch of an average-sized normal 30 g mouse, although the length of this tubing needs to be adjusted in parallel with body length, not body weight (see Note 2).
2. Jugular vein catheter (Silastic silicone laboratory tubing (0.3 mm I.D. and 0.63 mm O.D. and 0.51 mm I.D. and 0.94 mm O.D.)) (Fig. 1): The Silastic tubing of 0.51 mm I.D.

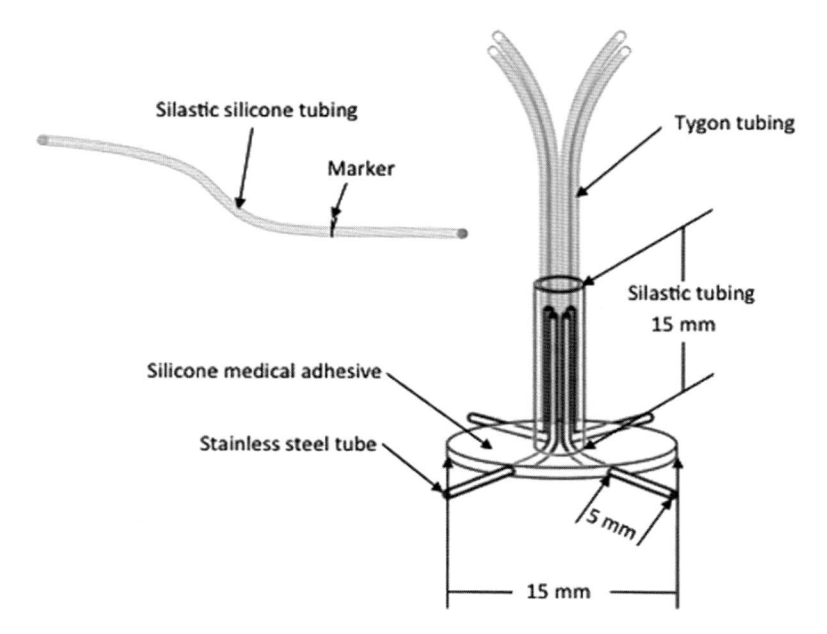

Fig. 2. Indwelling catheters and catheter holder for surgery of rats.

and 94 mm O.D. is cut to a length of 1 mm to be used as a restraining bead. The Silastic tubing of 0.3 mm I.D. and 0.63 mm O.D. is cut to a length of 6 cm and is inserted through the lumen of the restraining bead.

3. Catheter holder (Fig. 1): Two stainless steel tubes (27 gauge) are cut to a length of 12 mm and their edges are made smooth using a fine file. A 90° bend in the middle of each stainless steel tube is made, then 30 mm of Tygon tubing (0.25 mm I.D. and 0.76 mm O.D.) is attached to one end of each bent tube and then inserted through the lumen of a 5 mm piece of Silastic tubing (1.01 mm I.D. and 2.16 mm O.D.) until the bend of the stainless steel tube is reached; thus bundling the two tubes together (see Fig. 1). These connections are sealed by placing in a 5 mm diameter disc of silicone medical adhesive for 24 h allowing the other end of each steel tube to extend 3 mm from the adhesive disc.

2.4. Rat Catheters

1. Varying lengths of Silastic silicone tubing (0.51 mm I.D. and 0.94 mm O.D.) are used in rats as catheters for the carotid artery (10 cm), the jugular vein (10 cm), ileal vein (20 cm), and portal vein (25 cm) (Fig. 2). Based on the body length of a normal 300 g rat, put a marker using 7-0 silk suture on the Silastic tubing at 25 mm from the tip for the carotid artery and 30 mm for the jugular vein.

2. Catheter holder (Fig. 2): Four stainless steel tubes (22 gauge) are cut to a length of 30 mm and their edges are made smooth

using a fine file. A 90° bend in the middle of each stainless steel tube is made, then 40 mm of Tygon tubing (0.51 mm I.D. and 1.53 mm O.D) is attached to one end of each bent tube and then inserted through the lumen of a 10 mm piece of Silastic tubing (2.7 mm I.D. and 4.9 mm O.D.) until the bend of the stainless steel tube is reached; thus bundling the four tubes together (see Fig. 2). These connections are sealed by placing in a 15 mm diameter disc of silicone medical adhesive for 24 h allowing the other end of each steel tube to extend 5 mm from the adhesive disc.

2.5. Clamp Reagent Preparation

1. [3-^{3}H]-glucose and [^{14}C]-2-deoxyglucose infusate: [3-^{3}H]-glucose and [^{14}C]-2-deoxyglucose are stored in 95% ethanol to prevent bacterial contamination. To avoid infusing ethanol into an animal, the volume of solution that contains the required amount of [3-^{3}H]-glucose and [^{14}C]-2-deoxyglucose is dispensed and the ethanol is removed by evaporation under air. The dried [3-^{3}H]-glucose and [^{14}C]-2-deoxyglucose are reconstituted with saline.

2. Mouse and rat serum: Blood is collected from a 24-h fasted normal mouse or rat, allowed to coagulate (~5 min), and then centrifuged at $1,800 \times g$ for 15 min at 4°C. The serum is separated and stored at −80°C until needed.

3. Insulin and glucagon: Insulin and glucagon are dissolved in saline that contains mouse or rat serum at 3% (v/v).

4. Somatostatin: Somatostatin is dissolved in saline that contains mouse or rat serum at 3% (v/v).

5. 50% (w/v) Glucose.

6. 222 mM $Ba(OH)_2$ and 222 mM $ZnSO_4$.

7. 20 U/mL Heparin in saline.

2.6. Clamp Equipment

1. Metabolic cage.
2. Infusion pumps.
3. 500 µL capacity centrifuge tubes: Aliquot heparin into the bottom of each tube; 50 mU for a mouse study and 400 mU for a rat study.
4. Syringes for blood sampling: 300 µL insulin syringe for a mouse study and 1 mL syringe with blunted needle (22 gauge) for a rat study.
5. Syringes for infusion.
6. "Y" shape tubing connector: 27 gauge stainless steel for a mouse, 22 gauge stainless steel for a rat.
7. Micro-Renathane tubing: 0.30 mm I.D. and 0.64 mm O.D. for a mouse, 0.64 mm I.D. and 1.02 mm O.D. for a rat.

3. Methods

3.1. Mouse Surgery

3.1.1. Catheterization of Common Carotid Artery (Fig. 3)

1. The anesthetized mouse is placed on its abdomen and body length is measured from tip of nose to base of tail. The anesthetized mouse is then placed on its back with its head towards the operator.
2. The skin is incised approximately 5 mm up from the pectoral muscle. The carotid artery lies on the sternohyoid muscle, which is covered by the omohyoid muscle. The omohyoid muscle is gently separated from the sternohyoid muscle. The carotid artery is exposed and the adjacent vagus nerve is carefully separated from the artery.
3. A piece of doubled thread (7-0 silk suture) is passed under the artery and cut into two pieces. The anterior thread is tied tightly, as anteriorly as possible, to occlude the artery; as the first half-hitch knot of thread is formed. A loose posterior ligature is positioned several millimeters away. A small clamp is placed on the most distal posterior portion of the carotid artery to stop the flow of blood.
4. A small incision using fine scissors is made a few millimeters below the anterior ligature.
5. The tip of the catheter is inserted into the artery and pushed to the small clamp. While holding the inserted catheter along with the arterial wall with forceps, remove the small clamp. Now push the stretched PE-10 catheter forward towards the heart to reach the aortic arch (see Fig. 5); a distance of 9 mm based on the body length of a normal 30 g mouse.

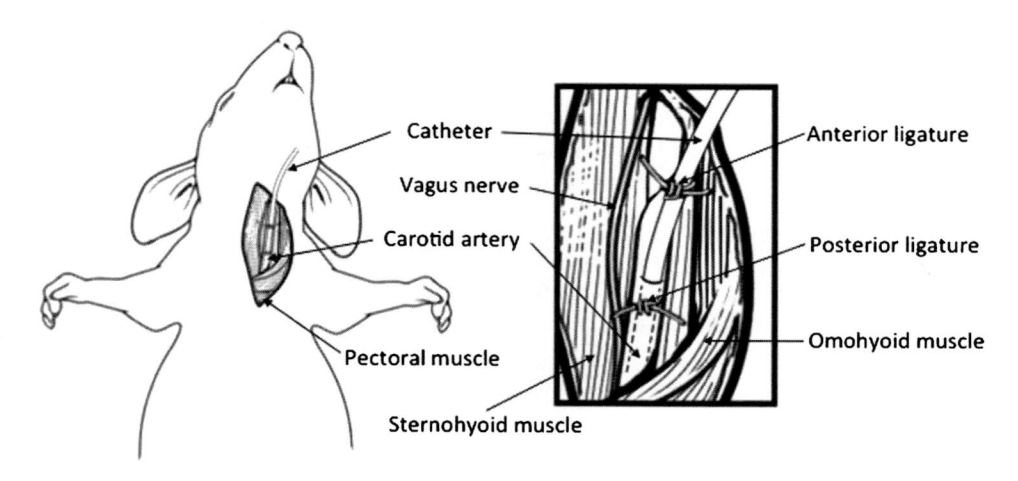

Fig. 3. Placement of catheter into carotid artery.

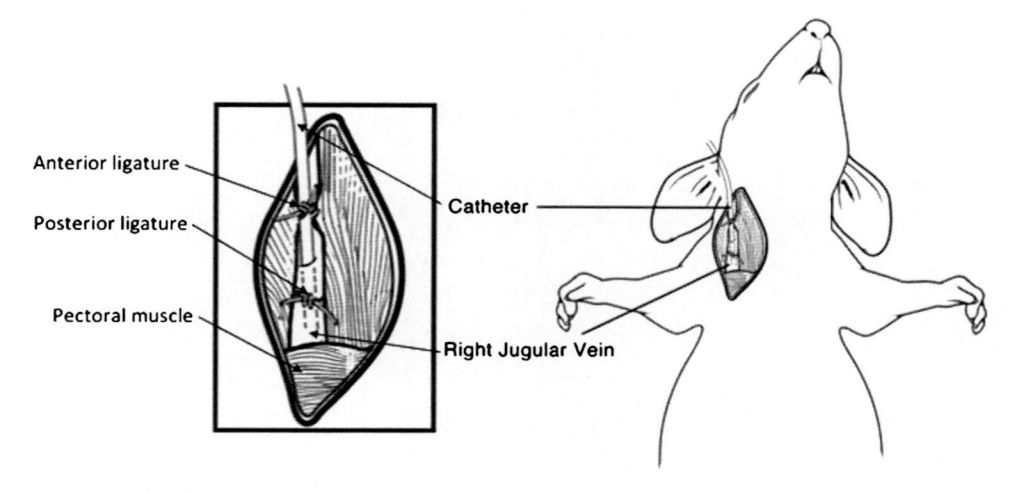

Fig. 4. Placement of catheter into jugular vein.

6. The catheter is flushed with 200 U/mL of heparin in saline and a suitable stainless steel pin is inserted into the end of the catheter.

7. The catheter is then anchored into place with the posterior ligature and the ends of the previously made anterior ligature.

3.1.2. Catheterization of Jugular Vein (Fig. 4)

1. The anesthetized mouse remains on its back with its head towards the operator.
2. Approximately 3 mm of the jugular vein, up to the pectoral muscle, is gently cleaned of fat and connective tissue by blunt dissection.
3. A piece of doubled thread (7-0 silk suture) is passed under the vein and cut into two pieces. The anterior thread is tied tightly to occlude the vein as the first half-hitch knot of thread is formed.
4. The vein is semi-transected with fine scissors between the two threads a few millimeters below the anterior ligature.
5. The tip of the catheter is inserted into the vein, pushing forwards towards the heart until the restraining bead to reach the superior vena cava (see Fig. 5); a distance of 11~12 mm based on body length of a normal 30 g mouse. The correct positioning of the catheter is tested by gauging the ease with which blood can be withdrawn.
6. After testing the position of the catheter, the catheter is flushed with 200 U/mL of heparin in saline and a suitable stainless steel pin is inserted into the end of the catheter.
7. The catheter is then anchored into place with the posterior ligature and the ends of the previously made anterior ligature.

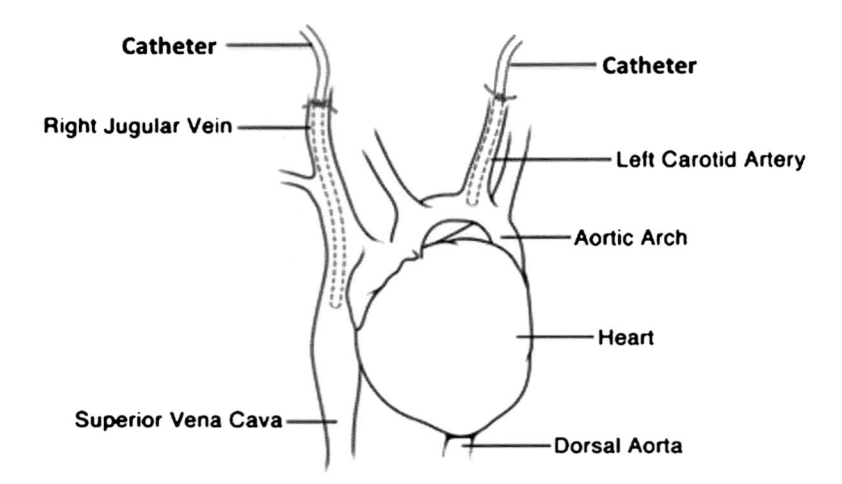

Fig. 5. Position of carotid artery catheter within the descending limb of the aortic arch and position of jugular vein catheter within the superior vena cava.

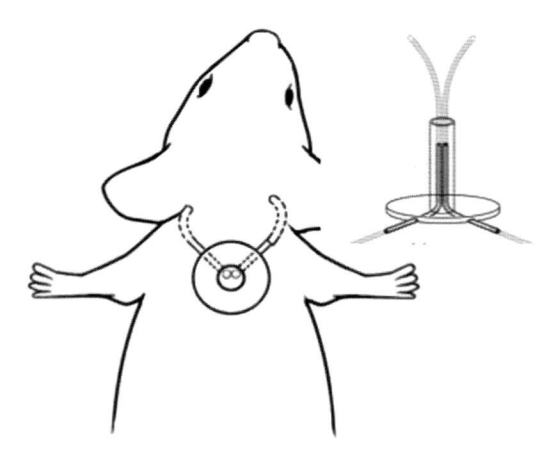

Fig. 6. Placement of catheter holder to secure catheters as they exit from the back of a mouse.

3.1.3. Fix Catheters to Exit from the Back of the Mouse (Fig. 6)

1. Place the mouse on its abdomen and make an interscapular incision of the skin of about 5 mm in length.
2. Insert a stainless steel pipetting needle (18 gauge) through the interscapular incision under the skin to the arterial catheter incision.
3. Slide the arterial catheter into the stainless steel pipetting needle and pull the needle back under the skin and out through the interscapular incision. The arterial catheter's exit and access site is now from the back of the mouse in the interscapular region.
4. Do same process for the jugular vein catheter.
5. The incisions made at carotid artery and jugular vein are closed using 6-0 nylon.

6. Clamp the catheter using a mini clip, cut at an appropriate position, slide the stainless steel tube of the catheter holder into the catheter, and ligate the catheters and stainless steel tubing using 6-0 silk suture.

7. The interscapular incision is closed over the catheter holder via two-layer fashion, first connective tissue with absorbable 6-0 suture then skin with 6-0 nylon suture, permitting the Tygon tubing exodus through the skin.

3.2. Rat Surgery

3.2.1. Catheterization of the Common Carotid Artery (Fig. 3)

1. The anesthetized rat is placed on its back with its head towards the operator.

2. The skin is incised approximately 20 mm up from the pectoral muscle. The carotid artery lies on the sternohyoid muscle which is covered by the omohyoid muscle. The omohyoid muscle is gently separated from the sternohyoid muscle. The carotid artery is exposed and the adjacent vagus nerve is carefully separated from the artery.

3. A piece of doubled thread (6-0 silk suture) is passed under the artery and cut into two pieces. The anterior thread is tied tightly, as anteriorly as possible, to occlude the artery; as the first half-hitch knot of thread is formed. A loose posterior ligature is positioned several millimeters away. A small clamp is placed on the most distal posterior portion of the carotid artery to stop the flow of blood.

4. A small incision is made using fine scissors a few millimeters below the anterior ligature.

5. The tip of the catheter is inserted into the artery and pushed to the small clamp. While holding the inserted catheter along with the vessel wall with forceps, remove the small clamp. Now push the catheter forward towards the heart to reach the aortic arch (see Fig. 5); a distance of 25 mm based on the body length of a normal 300 g rat.

6. After testing catheter position, the catheter is flushed with 200 U/mL of heparin in saline and a suitable stainless steel pin is inserted into the end of the catheter.

7. The catheter is then anchored into place with the posterior ligature and the ends of the previously made anterior ligature.

3.2.2. Catheterization of the Jugular Vein (Fig. 4)

1. The anesthetized rat remains on its back with its head towards the operator.

2. Approximately 10 mm of the jugular vein, up from the pectoral muscle, is gently cleaned of fat and connective tissue by blunt dissection.

3. A piece of doubled thread (6-0 silk suture) is passed under the vein and cut into two pieces. The anterior thread is tied tightly to occlude the vein; as the first half-hitch knot of thread is formed.

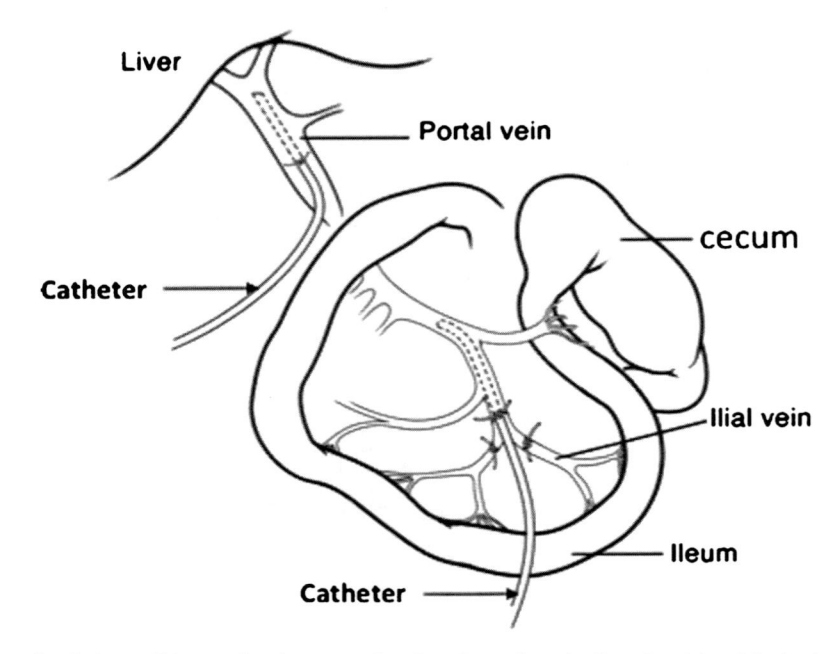

Fig. 7. Position of catheters within portal and mesenteric veins after catheterization of portal and ileal veins.

4. The vein is placed under light tension and then semi-transected with fine scissors between the two ligatures.
5. The tip of the catheter is inserted into the vein, pushing forwards towards the heart to reach the superior vena cava (see Fig. 5); a distance of 30 mm based on body length of a normal 300 g rat. The correct positioning of the catheter is tested by gauging the ease with which blood can be withdrawn.
6. After testing the position of the catheter, the catheter is flushed with 200 U/mL of heparin in saline and a suitable stainless steel pin is inserted into the end of the catheter.
7. The catheter is then anchored into place with the posterior ligature and the ends of the previously made anterior ligature.

3.2.3. Catheterization of Portal and Ileal Veins (Fig. 7)

1. With the anesthetized rat on its back, a middle incision is made into the abdominal cavity from just above the urethral opening to about three-quarters of the way up the abdomen.
2. Open the abdominal wall using atraumatic forceps.
3. Expose the portal vein by relocating the intestine to the left side of the animal using a cotton pad.
4. Holding a 22 gauge needle between fingers and the vessel wall with forceps, insert the 22 gauge needle into the portal vein. Then pull the needle out of the portal vein, while simultaneously inserting the tip of the catheter through the hole made by the needle. Push the tip of the catheter close to the liver and fix the catheter to the portal vein wall.

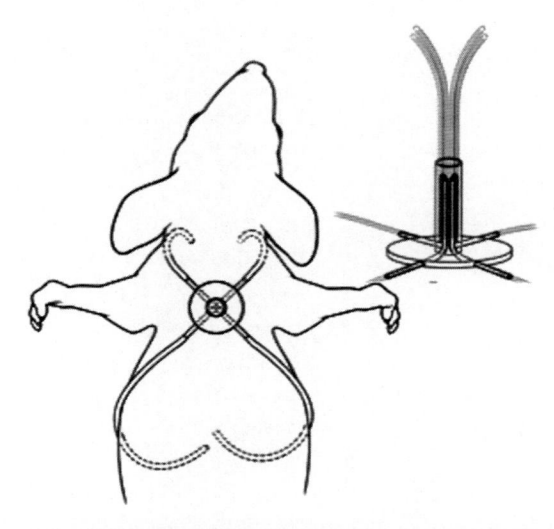

Fig. 8. Placement of catheter holder to secure catheters as they exit from the back of a rat.

5. Place the catheter so it runs along the vena cava and replace the intestine to its normal position.
6. The cecum and ileum are pulled out and laid on saline-moistened cotton. Find the vein region shaped like a "Y" and ligate the two branches of the vein using 6-0 silk suture. A loose ligature is positioned in the trunk part of the vein.
7. Cut an end of the catheter to form a sharp tip and fill the catheter with 200 U/mL of heparin in saline.
8. Push on the trunk of the vein with a small cotton ball to prevent bleeding and cut the joint part of the vein using fine scissors.
9. Insert tip of catheter into newly created hole and push it into the mesenteric vein. Ligate the catheter to the vein gently.
10. Anchor the catheters to the abdominal wall using 4-0 silk suture and close abdominal wall using 4-0 absorbable suture with the catheters exiting the abdomen but remaining under the skin.

3.2.4. Fix Catheters to Exit from the Back of the Rat (Fig. 8)

1. Place rat on its abdomen and make an interscapular ~2 cm cut of the skin.
2. Insert stainless steel pipetting needle (14 gauge) through this cut and under the skin from interscapular region to the incision made for the arterial catheter.
3. Slide the catheter into the needle and pull the needle back and out from under the skin. The catheter should now exit from the back of the animal.

4. Do the same process for the jugular vein, ileal vein, and portal vein catheters.
5. The incisions made at carotid artery, jugular vein, and in abdomen are closed using 4-0 nylon.
6. Clamp the catheter using a mini clip, cut at an appropriate position, slide the stainless steel tube of the catheter holder into the catheter, and ligate the catheters with the stainless steel tubing using 6-0 silk suture.
7. The interscapular incision is closed over the catheter holder via two-layer fashion, first connective tissue with absorbable 4-0 suture then skin with 4-0 nylon suture, permitting the Tygon tubing exodus through the skin.

3.3. Setup of Animals (see Note 3)

3.3.1. Mouse Setup (Fig. 9)

Weigh mouse, suck up any coagulation in the catheters, and fill the catheters with clean heparinized saline (10 U heparin/mL saline). The mouse is transferred to a metabolic cage without food, but with bedding in the cage to reduce stress. Just before tracer infusion, catheters of the mouse are connected to micro-Renathane tubing (0.3 mm I.D., 0.64 mm O.D.) for infusing tracer and glucose and for collecting blood.

3.3.2. Rat Setup (Fig. 10)

Weigh rat, suck up any coagulation in the catheters, and fill the catheters with clean heparinized saline (10 U heparin/mL saline). The rat is transferred to a metabolic cage without food, but with bedding in the cage to reduce stress. If urine needs to be collected,

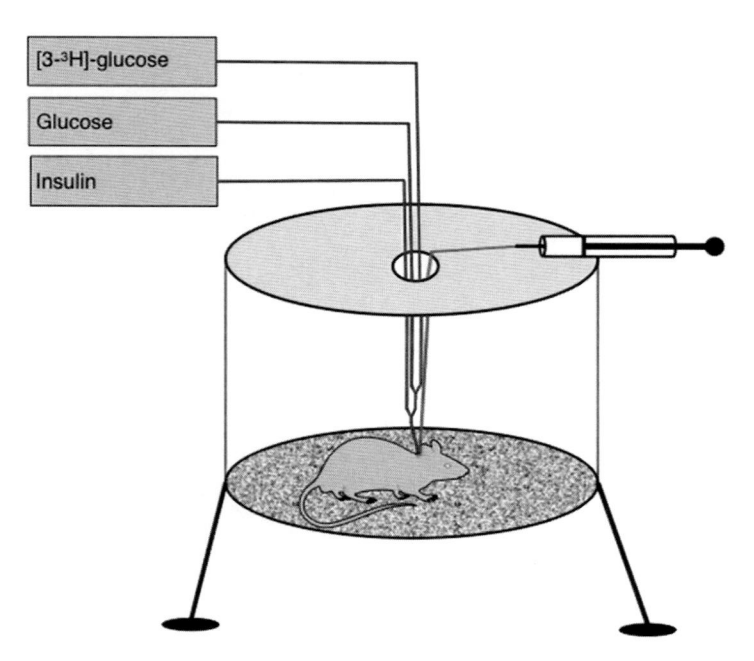

Fig. 9. Mouse setup in metabolic cage for a clamp study.

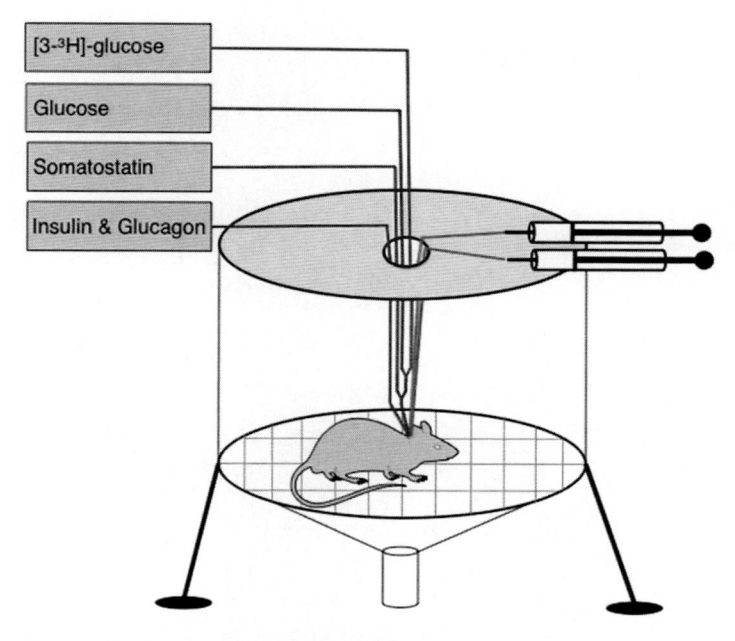

Fig. 10. Rat setup in metabolic cage for a clamp study.

place rat on a wire mesh rather than bedding as shown in Fig. 10. Just before tracer infusion, catheters of the rat are connected to the micro-Renathane tubing (0.64 mm I.D., 1.02 mm O.D.) for infusing tracer and glucose and for collecting blood.

3.4. Clamp Studies

3.4.1. Mouse Pancreatic-Blood Glucose Clamp (Hyperinsulinemic-Euglycemic Clamp, Fig. 11)

Mice are fasted for 2–3 h prior to a clamp study to ensure postfeeding glucose absorption is complete. A typical study protocol consists of a 60-min tracer equilibration period (–90 to –30 min), a 30-min basal period (–30 to 0 min), and a 120-min test period (0–120 min) (see Note 4). At the start of the equilibration period, a 300 µCi/kg bolus of [3-^{3}H]-glucose is given through the jugular vein catheter followed by a continuous infusion of [3-^{3}H]-glucose at 3 µCi/kg/min (see Note 5). The equilibration period should be 60 min to allow complete equilibration between infused tracer and body glucose. A basal period of 30–60 min is used to measure glucose flux under a non-treated condition.

During the test period, a group of mice are kept without additional treatment and are designated as the basal group. In a second group of mice, a clamp group, insulin is infused into the systemic circulation through the jugular vein catheter. Plasma glucose levels are maintained at basal levels by infusing a 25% glucose solution at a variable rate. After 90 min into the clamp period, [^{14}C]-2-deoxyglucose (450 µCi/kg) is infused into the systemic circulation as a bolus through the carotid arterial catheter. To maintain blood glucose at the desired level during the clamp period, blood glucose levels are monitored every 5–10 min, which requires 1–5 µL of blood (dependent upon glucometer) to be dropped onto a test strip of a

		Measured parameters		Total volume of Collected blood
Symbol	Blood Glucose	Plasma Glucose and Tracers	Plasma Insulin	
↑	1~5			1~5
↑	1~5	20		21~25
↑	1~5	20	20	41~45

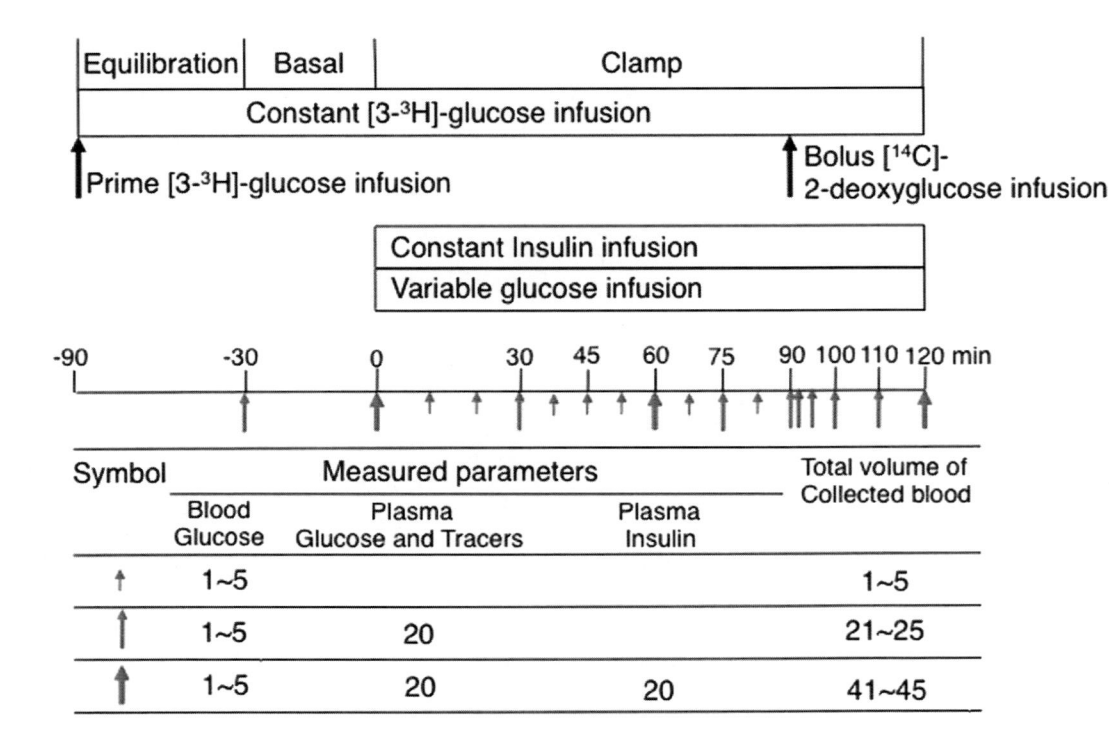

Fig. 11. A typical protocol for a hyperinsulinemic-euglycemic clamp for mice.

handheld glucose meter. To measure plasma glucose and tracer radioactivities, 10 µL plasma is required. Therefore, 20 µL of blood is collected through the arterial catheter every 15 min during the basal and test period prior to [^{14}C]-2-deoxyglucose infusion; then at 2, 5, 10, 20, and 30 min after [^{14}C]-2-deoxyglucose infusion. To measure plasma insulin, 5 µL plasma is required for a single assay. Therefore, 20 µL of blood is sampled from the arterial catheters every 60 min during the basal and test periods. A typical time schedule of blood sampling for measurement of parameters is shown in Fig. 11.

Collected blood is immediately transferred to a heparinized tube (500 µL capacity). Whole blood is immediately centrifuged at 18,000×g for 2 min to separate plasma. Blood cells are suspended in saline and centrifuged at 18,000×g for 10 s. The supernatant is removed and discarded. Blood cells are reconstituted with saline and given back to the test animal after blood sampling at 0, 30, 60, and 90 min during the clamp study. Immediately after the last blood sampling at 120 min, the animal is anesthetized with an intravenous infusion of sodium pentobarbital (60 mg/kg) and a laparotomy is performed. Typically, the left lobe of the liver, as well as skeletal muscle (vastus lateralis, gastrocnemius, and soleus), is frozen in situ using Wollenberger tongs precooled in liquid nitrogen.

	Equilibration	Basal	Clamp		

Constant [3-³H]-glucose infusion

↑ Prime [3-³H]-glucose infusion

↑ Bolus [¹⁴C]-2-deoxyglucose infusion

Constant somatostatin infusion
Constant Insulin infusion
Constant glucagon infusion
Variable glucose infusion

-150   -60 -30   0   30 45   60   75   90 100 110 120 min

Symbol	Measured parameters			Total volume of Collected blood
	Blood Glucose	Plasma Glucose and Tracers	Plasma Insulin and Glucagon	
↑	1~5			1~5
↑	1~5	50		51~55
↑	1~5	50	150	201~205

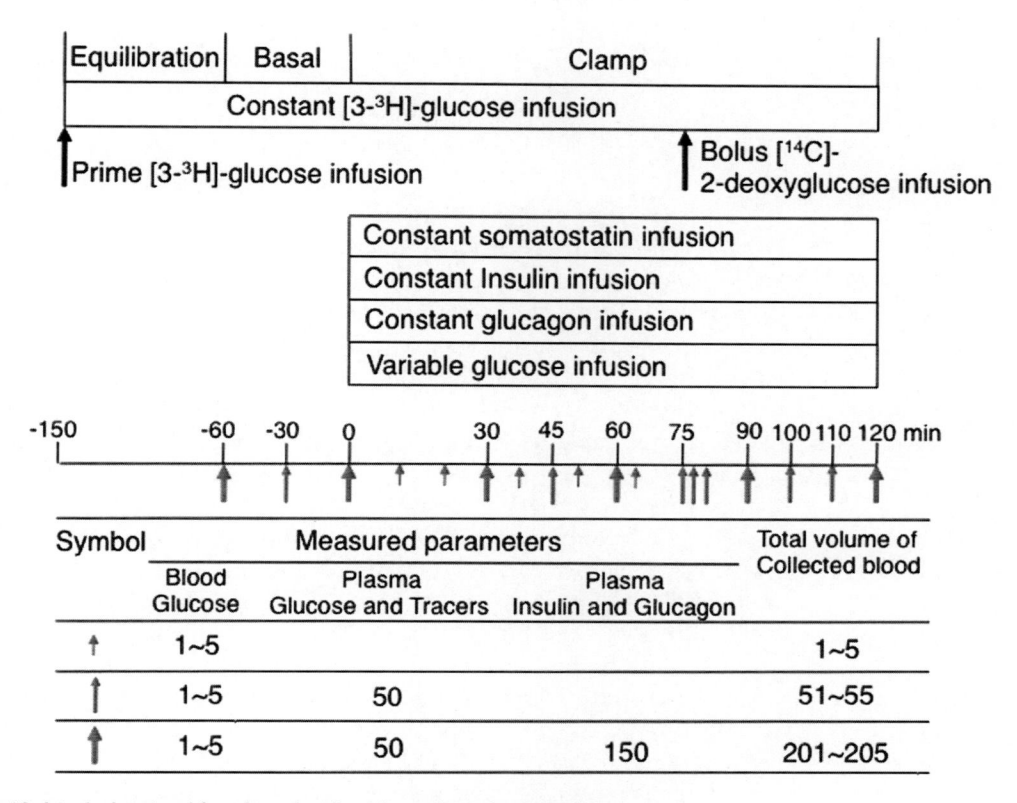

Fig. 12. A typical protocol for a hyperinsulinemic-euglycemic clamp for rats.

3.4.2. Rat Pancreatic-Blood Glucose Clamp (Hyperinsulinemic-Euglycemic Clamp, Fig. 12)

Rats are fasted for at least 4 h, typically 6, prior to a study to ensure post-feeding glucose absorption is complete. A typical study protocol consists of a tracer equilibration period, a basal period, and a clamp test period (see Note 4). At the start of the equilibration period, a 60 μCi/kg bolus of [3-³H]-glucose is given through the jugular vein catheter followed by a continuous infusion of [3-³H]-glucose at 0.6 μCi/kg/min (see Note 5). To complete the equilibration between infused tracer and body glucose, the equilibration period should be 90 min. A basal period of 30–60 min is used to measure glucose flux under a non-treated condition.

During the test period, a group of animals are kept without additional treatment and are designated as the basal group. In a second group of animals, a clamp group, somatostatin is infused through the jugular vein catheter. The infusion rate of 2–10 μg/kg/min in normal rats needs to be empirically adjusted so as to inhibit endogenous insulin and glucagon secretion (see Note 6). Insulin and glucagon are infused into the hepatic portal system through the ileal vein catheter (see Note 7). For a 6-h fasted normal rat, insulin and glucagon are infused at 1.2 mU/kg/min and

2.6 ng/kg/min, respectively, to maintain basal levels of these hormones (insulin at ~0.8 ng/mL and glucagon at ~50 pg/mL). If these hormones are infused into the systemic circulation through the jugular vein, insulin should be infused at ~0.8 mU/kg/min and glucagon at 2.6 ng/kg/min to maintain basal blood glucose levels without glucose infusion.

When a hyperinsulinemic clamp is performed, plasma insulin levels are raised by linearly increasing the insulin infusion rate (see Note 8). Plasma glucose levels are maintained at a desired level by adjusting the infusion rate of a 50% glucose solution (see Note 9). Constant plasma [3-^{3}H]-glucose-specific activity is maintained during the test period by altering the infusion rate of [3-^{3}H]-glucose. At 45 min prior to the end of the test period, [^{14}C]-2-deoxyglucose (150 μCi/kg) is infused into systemic circulation as a bolus through the carotid arterial catheter.

Total volume of blood sampled during a clamp study should be kept below 10% of total blood volume of the animal. Total blood volume is approximately 6–7% of body weight (~20 mL for a 300 g normal rat). To maintain blood glucose at the desired level, blood glucose levels are measured every 5–10 min during the clamp period, which requires 1~5 μL of blood (dependent upon glucometer) to be dropped onto a test strip of a handheld glucose meter. To measure plasma glucose and tracer radioactivities, 25 μL plasma is required. Therefore, 50 μL of blood is taken through the arterial catheter every 15 min during the basal period and prior to [^{14}C]-2-deoxyglucose infusion during the test period; then at 2, 5, 15, 30, and 45 min after [^{14}C]-2-deoxyglucose infusion. To measure plasma insulin and glucagon, 5 and 50 μL plasma are required for a single assay of insulin and glucagon, respectively. Therefore, 150 μL of blood is sampled from the arterial and portal catheters every 30 min during the basal and test periods. A typical time schedule of blood sampling for measurement of parameters is shown in Fig. 12.

Collected blood is immediately transferred to a heparinized tube (500 μL capacity). At each sampling time, whole blood is immediately centrifuged at 18,000×g for 2 min to separate plasma. Blood cells are suspended in saline and centrifuged at 18,000×g for 10 s. The supernatant is removed and discarded. Blood cells are reconstituted with saline and given back to the test animal after the blood sampling at 0, 30, 60, and 90 min during a clamp study. Right after the last blood sampling at 120 min, the animal is anesthetized with an infusion of sodium pentobarbital (40 mg/kg) into systemic circulation through the arterial catheter and a laparotomy is performed. Typically, the left lobe of the liver, as well as skeletal muscle (vastus lateralis, gastrocnemius, and soleus), is frozen in situ using Wollenberger tongs precooled in liquid nitrogen. This procedure takes less than 20 s from the point of successful anesthesia.

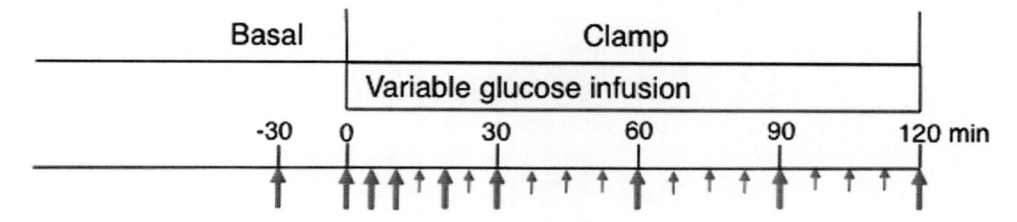

For mouse

Symbol	Measured parameters		Total volume of Collected blood
	Blood Glucose	Plasma Insulin	
↑	1~5		1~5
⇑	1~5	25	26~30

For rat

Symbol	Measured parameters		Total volume of Collected blood
	Blood Glucose	Plasma Insulin, glucagon and C-peptide	
↑	1~5		1~5
⇑	1~5	250	251~255

Fig. 13. A typical protocol for a hyperglycemic clamp for mice or rats.

3.4.3. Mouse or Rat Glucose Clamp (Hyperglycemic Clamp, Fig. 13)

Animals are fasted for 6 h prior to the clamp study. The protocol consists of a 30-min basal period (−30 to 0 min) and a 120-min test period (0–120 min) (see Note 10). During the test period, plasma glucose levels are raised and maintained at the desired level by infusing a 50% glucose solution at a variable rate. Blood samples are taken from the arterial catheter using a 1 mL syringe and transferred immediately to a 500 µL heparinized centrifuge tube. Blood glucose levels are monitored using a handheld glucose meter. At each sampling time, whole blood is immediately centrifuged at $18,000 \times g$ for 2 min to separate plasma. Blood cells are suspended in saline, centrifuged at $18,000 \times g$ for 10 s, and supernatant removed. Blood cells are reconstituted with saline and given back to the test animal after blood sampling at 0, 5, 10, 20, 30, 60, 90, and 120 min during the clamp study.

3.5. Analyses

3.5.1. Measurement of Tracer ((3-³H)-Glucose) in Infusate and Plasma

Preparation of plasma and infusate:

1. Preparation of Infusate: (3-^{3}H)-glucose infusate (20 µL) is mixed with 5 mL of saturated bensoic acid solution (3 g/L) that contains 5 mM glucose, and then 25 µL of this mixture is transferred into a 500 µL centrifuge tube followed by the addition of 125 µL of 222 mM $Ba(OH)_2$ and 125 µL of 222 mM $ZnSO_4$.

2. Preparation of Plasma: Immediately after obtaining a blood sample from an animal, it is placed into a heparin containing 500 μL centrifuge tube, blood is centrifuged at 3,000×g for 2 min to collect plasma. Of this plasma, an aliquot of 25 μL is transferred into a new 500 μL centrifuge tube, deproteinized by adding 125 μL of 222 mM Ba(OH)$_2$ and 125 μL of 222 mM ZnSO$_4$ solutions, kept on ice for 1 h and centrifuged at 3,000×g for 10 min. The supernatant is stored at −80°C.

Plasma glucose determination using a standard 96-well plate:

1. Buffer: 1 mL of ATP (280 mg) and NaHCO$_3$ (280 mg) in water, 96 mL of 200 mM Tris–HCl (pH 7.4), 2 mL of 500 mM MgCl$_2$, NADP (200 mg), Hexokinase (250 U), Glucose-6-phospate dehydrogenase (250 Unit).

2. Glucose Standard: Make 0, 3, 5, 7, 10, 15, 20, 25, and 30 mM glucose solutions by dissolving the appropriate amount of glucose into a 4% albumin solution. An aliquot of 25 μL of each glucose standard is transferred into a 500 μL centrifuge tube, then deproteinized by adding 125 μL of 222 mM Ba(OH)$_2$ and 125 μL of 222 mM ZnSO$_4$ solutions, keep on ice for 1 h, and centrifuged at 3,000×g for 10 min. These supernatants of the glucose standards are stored at −80°C.

3. Assay Procedure: Set microplate reader to read absorbance at 340 nm. Assay in a 96-well plate a mixture of sample (10 μL) and buffer (200 μL). Incubate plate at room temperature for 15 min. Read absorbance.

Radioactivity of plasma [3-^{3}H]-glucose and [^{14}C]-2-deoxyglucose:

1. Transfer 50 μL for mice and 100 μL for rats of deproteinized plasma into a scintillation vial and dry in a vacuum oven.

2. Add 1 mL water and dissolve the precipitate completely.

3. Add 10 mL scintillation solution, mix well and count radioactivity.

3.5.2. Measurement of Tissue Phosphorylated (^{14}C)-2-Deoxy-Glucose and Incorporation of (3-^{3}H)-Glucose and (^{14}C)-2-Deoxy-Glucose into Glycogen

Reagents and solutions:

1. 30% (w/v) Potassium hydroxide.
2. Acetate buffer (0.2 M, pH 4.8).
3. Amyloglucosidase solution: Dissolve 10 mg of lyophilized enzyme preparation (50 U/mg protein) in 50 mL acetate buffer.
4. Triethanolamine/magnesium buffer (0.3 M TEA/4 mM MgSO$_4$, pH 7.6).
5. ATP/NADP/G6PDH/TEA buffer: Dissolve 60 mg of ATP·Na$_2$H$_2$·3H$_2$O and 80 mg of β-NADP in 99 mL of 0.3 M TEA/4 mM MgSO$_4$ buffer and add 200 U of glucose-6-phosphate dehydrogenase.

Tissue preparation:

1. In a 15 mL centrifuge tube, add 3 mL of 30% KOH and place it in a boiling water bath.
2. Weigh tissue (0.2–0.4 g for liver, 0.5–1.0 g for muscle), add tissue to tube in boiling water bath, and heat for 15–20 min.

Measurement of tissue phosphorylated [^{14}C]-2-deoxyglucose (14):

1. Digested tissue solution (1 mL from Tissue preparation step 2) is transferred into a new tube and neutralized with the addition of 1 mL of 1 M HCl.
2. Neutralized solution (0.2 mL) is added to 1 mL of 6% HClO$_4$ and a second aliquot of neutralized solution (0.2 mL) is added to 0.5 mL of 222 mM Ba(OH)$_2$ and 0.5 mL of 222 mM ZnSO$_4$.
3. After centrifugation at $20,000 \times g$ for 5 min, 1 mL of each HClO$_4$ and Ba(OH)$_2$/ZnSO$_4$ supernatants are used for the determination of radioisotope content after the addition of 10 mL of scintillation solution.
4. The difference between [^{14}C]-radioactivity in HClO$_4$ and Ba(OH)$_2$/ZnSO$_4$ supernatants represents the sum of the content of [^{14}C]-2-deoxyglucose-6-phosphate, [^{14}C]-2-deoxyglucose-1-phosphate, UDP-[^{14}C]-2-deoxyglucose, and [^{14}C]-2-deoxyglucose in glycogen.

Measurement of glycogen content and incorporation of [3-^{3}H]-glucose and [^{14}C]-2-deoxyglucose into glycogen:

1. Digested tissue solution (1 mL from Tissue preparation step 2) is added to 2 mL of 100% ethanol, mixed well, and kept at 4°C overnight.
2. The next day this mixture is centrifuged at $18,000 \times g$ for 30 min and the supernatant is discarded.
3. The centrifuge tube with the precipitant is placed into boiling water for 10 min to evaporate any remaining ethanol.
4. The tube is then placed at room temperature; 1 mL of water is added to dissolve the precipitant.
5. To the dissolved precipitant, add 2 mL of 100% ethanol, mix well, and incubate on ice for 2 h.
6. Centrifuge at $18,000 \times g$ for 30 min and discard the supernatant.
7. The centrifuge tube with the precipitant is placed into boiling water for 10 min to evaporate any remaining ethanol.
8. Repeat the process of steps 4–7.
9. Add 2 mL of water to dissolve precipitant and call this "glycogen solution."

10. Mix 0.2 mL of glycogen solution and 1.8 mL of amyloglucosidase solution in a centrifuge tube. Incubate at 40°C with shaking for 2 h.

11. Use 1 mL of this digested glycogen solution to determine radioisotope content after addition of 10 mL of scintillation solution.

3.5.3. Glucose Incorporation into Glycogen

1. Transfer 0.5 mL of "glycogen solution" (Subheading 3.5.2, step 9) into a scintillation vial and dry it in a vacuum oven.
2. Add 0.5 mL water and dissolve the precipitant completely.
3. Add 10 mL scintillation solution, mix well, and count the radioactivity.
4. Calculation:

$$\mu\text{mol glucose per g tissue} = \frac{\text{Radioactivity(dpm)}}{[3\text{-}^3\text{H}]\text{SA in plasma glucose}} \times \frac{4}{0.5} \times \frac{1}{\text{tissue weight(g)}}$$

3.5.4. Tissue Glucose Assay (Use Cuvettes, 4 mL Capacity)

1. Sample size assayed is 50 µL of digested glycogen solution if derived from liver or 200 µL if derived from skeletal muscle.
2. Add ATP/NADP/G6PDH/TEA buffer (2 mL), mix, and after 5 min read the first absorbance (A_1) at 340 nm. Then add 2 Units of hexokinase, mix, and after 10 min read the second absorbance (A_2) at 340 nm.
3. Calculations:

$$\mu\text{mol glucose per g liver} = \frac{A_2 - A_1}{6.23} \times \frac{(2 + 0.05 + 0.005)}{0.05} \times 4 \times \frac{1}{\text{tissue weight(g)}}$$

$$\mu\text{mol glucose per g muscle} = \frac{A_2 - A_1}{6.23} \times \frac{(2 + 0.2 + 0.005)}{0.2} \times 4 \times \frac{1}{\text{tissue weight(g)}}$$

3.5.5. Calculation of Glucose Appearance, Glucose Disappearance, and Endogenous Glucose Production Rates

1. Rate of glucose appearance: The measured rates of [3-^{3}H]-glucose are used to estimate the unlabeled glucose appearance ([3-^{3}H]Ra) as calculated using the Steele's equation (15), which is based on a one-pool model and on the initial assumption of instant mixing of glucose in its entire space. The equation is written as follows:

$$[3\text{-}^3\text{H}]\,\text{Ra} = \frac{[3\text{-}^3\text{H}]\,\text{GI}*(0.5V_\text{D}(PG_1 + PG_2)/2 \times ([3\text{-}^3\text{H}]\text{SA-PG}_2[3\text{-}^3\text{H}]\text{SA-PG}_1)/(t_2\text{-}t_1))}{([3\text{-}^3\text{H}]\text{SA} - PG_2 + [3\text{-}^3\text{H}]\text{SA} - PG_1)/2}$$

Where [3-³H]GI* is the infusion rate of [3-³H]-glucose, PG_1 and PG_2 are plasma glucose concentrations at time t_1 and t_2, [3-³H]SA-PG_1 and [3-³H]SA-PG_2 are [3-³H] specific activities of plasma glucose at times t_1 and t_2, V_D is the glucose distribution volume (mL/kg), and $0.5V_D(PG_1 + PG_2)/2$ is the effective fraction of glucose pool.

2. Rate of glucose disappearance: Unlabeled glucose disappearance rates are determined from [3-³H]-glucose disappearance ([3-³H]Rd) according to Steele's equation as:

$$[3\text{-}^3\text{H}]Rd = [3\text{-}^3\text{H}]Ra - 0.5V_D[(PG_2 - PG_1)/(t_2 - t_1)]$$

3. Rate of endogenous glucose production: Endogenous glucose production rate is determined as the difference between [3-³H]Ra and exogenous glucose infusion rates (see Note 11).

3.5.6. Measurement of Glucose Uptake in Different Tissues In Vivo Using 2-Deoxy-Glucose (see Note 12)

The quantity of glucose used per unit time (Ri) (14):

$$Ri = \frac{[^{14}C]\tau}{LC \int_0^t (C_B^* / C_B) dt}$$

Where LC is a lumped constant that is a correction factor for the discrimination against 2-deoxyglycose by the glucose transporter and phosphorylation pathways, C_B^* is the blood 2-deoxyglucose expressed in terms of radioactivity, and C_B is blood glucose concentration. LC was reported to be 0.95 for soleus muscle, 1.05 for extensor digitorum longus muscle, 0.86 for epitrochlearis muscle, and 0.61 for adipose tissue (14).

3.6. Summary

In this chapter, we describe the catheterization techniques and clamp methods which we developed and use to assess insulin and glucose sensitivity in mice and rats. These methods can be used to assess the sensitivity to other hormones (e.g., glucagon) and metabolites. The methods for mice were transferred to the Mouse Metabolic Phenotype Center of Vanderbilt University. This Center assists investigators with clamp studies and they have reported valuable suggestions based on their experiences (16, 17). The combined insights, descriptions, and methods of these clamp techniques should provide guidance to both new and experienced investigators.

4. Notes

1. For obese and/or diabetic mice and rats, use a slightly (~10%) lower dose of chemical anesthesia for catheterization surgery.
2. After surgically placing this catheter and allowing 4–5 days of recovery from the surgery, if infusion of a solution into the

catheter is possible but one cannot draw blood, then in future surgeries extend the catheter length (9 mm) by 0.5–1 mm. Likewise, if the mouse is expected to lose body weight (a measure of normal growth) that will not be regained after surgery, then insert a catheter that is 0.5–1 mm shorter than 9 mm.

3. Mice and rats are housed with a set light/dark cycle, usually 12 h light/12 h dark, which is the primary synchronizing agent for many of the animal's circadian rhythms. Feeding behavior exhibits circadian rhythm, as rats and mice eat ~70–80% of their total daily food intake during the dark cycle (18–20). The circadian rhythm of food intake causes a fluctuation of hepatic glycogen content, hepatic glucose production rate, and the relative contribution of glycogenolysis and gluconeogenesis to total hepatic glucose production. Hepatic glycogen content of rats and mice fed ad libitum is higher early morning; after which, glycogen content decreases progressively to ~10% of these levels. As glycogen content decreases, the relative contribution of glycogenolysis to hepatic glucose production decreases while the contribution of gluconeogenesis increases. With a longer fast, hepatic glucose production and glucose disappearance rates are decreased. Therefore, depending on the objective of the study, the time of day and length of fasting relative to the light/dark cycle should be fixed.

4. This clamp method is performed to evaluate the sensitivity/responsiveness of glucose metabolism to insulin action and glucose effectiveness. Therefore, one should measure glucose disappearance and infusion rates as an index of whole body glucose disposal rate. As an index of liver sensitivity to insulin and/or glucose effectiveness, endogenous glucose production rate and liver glycogen synthesis rate from plasma glucose are measured. Glucose uptake and glycogen synthesis in muscle and adipose tissue is measured as an index of insulin sensitivity and/or glucose effectiveness of these tissues. To evaluate the sensitivity to insulin, plasma insulin levels are raised while blood glucose levels are maintained at basal by infusing glucose to compensate for any increase in glucose disposal. An alternative, to evaluate the effectiveness of glucose mass (blood glucose concentration), blood glucose levels are raised while plasma insulin levels are kept at basal.

5. The volume of plasma needed to measure plasma glucose concentration, tracer radioactivity, glucose turnover rate, and glycogen synthesis needs to be considered in order to determine the appropriate infusion rate of $[3-^3H]$-glucose and the bolus infusion dose of $[^{14}C]$-2-deoxyglucose. If plasma glucose concentration and the glucose turnover rate are constant, the radioactivity in plasma is linearly correlated with tracer infusion rate. Alternatively, if tracer infusion rate is constant, the radioactivity

of plasma [3-^{3}H]-glucose is inversely correlated with the glucose turnover rate. For example, the glucose turnover rate relative to body weight is approximately two times higher in normal mice than in normal rats. Therefore, approximately two times higher infusion rate of [3-^{3}H]-glucose is needed to obtain the same levels of tracer radioactivity in mice than in rats.

6. Efficacy of somatostatin is variable with each lot prepared and with different animal models; therefore, the efficacy needs to be checked with each lot and animal model studied.

7. Physiologically, insulin secreted from the pancreas flows into the portal vein and through the liver before reaching systemic circulation. Liver is the major organ responsible for clearing insulin with approximately 50% of first pass insulin taken up by the liver. As a result, insulin concentration in the portal vein is 2~2.5 times higher than that of systemic circulation, as measured in dogs (21, 22) and rats (7). Therefore, when insulin is infused through the portal vein, an insulin gradient is created between the portal vein and hepatic artery, with arterial plasma insulin being 60% lower. If insulin is infused into the systemic circulation, it fails to create this physiological insulin gradient. Instead, insulin concentration in the arterial plasma is slightly higher than that of the portal vein; thereby, the impact of insulin on hepatic glucose metabolism may be lower with systemic infusion.

8. Plasma insulin concentration and insulin clearance rate are quite different among animal models. For example, models of obese and/or type 2 diabetes have higher plasma insulin levels and lower insulin clearance rates relative to plasma insulin levels. Therefore, insulin infusion rates need to be adjusted to accommodate these differences among animal models.

9. Metabolism of glucose by liver is profoundly affected by circulating levels of glucose and by the route of glucose delivery. With physiological glucose ingestion after a meal, absorbed glucose enters into the blood circulation through the portal vein, which causes a negative arterial-portal glucose gradient. The presence of a negative arterial-portal glucose gradient, portal glucose signal has been reported to promote hepatic glucose uptake (23, 24). Therefore, the relative importance of different organs for disposal of a glucose load may differ between systemic and portal delivery. If one wishes to measure the effect of glucose via this portal glucose signal, then the glucose should be infused into the portal vein. If one wishes to measure only the effect of circulating levels of glucose, glucose should be infused into the systemic circulation via the jugular vein catheter.

10. Hyperglycemic clamp technique, which is not accompanied by pancreatic clamp, is used to evaluate glucose effectiveness on pancreatic insulin secretion in vivo.

11. During hyperinsulinemic hyperglycemic clamps in normal rats, one may obtain a negative value for endogenous glucose production. This discrepancy is due to the paradox that tracer-derived glucose disposal rates are less than the exogenous glucose infusion rates. The tracer-derived glucose disposal rate can be equal to but never less than the exogenous glucose infusion rate because the tracer-derived glucose disposal rate represents total glucose flux. This discrepancy, however, is reported by numerous investigators and the potential mechanism was extensively discussed by Argoud et al. (25) and Bell et al. (26). The precise mechanism has yet to be determined.

12. As natural glucose does, uptake of 2-deoxyglucose is mediated by a glucose transporter and phosphorylated by hexokinase. The resulting 2-deoxyglucose-6-phosphate is incorporated into glycogen (27). On the other hand, since 2-deoxyglucose-6-phosphate is not isomerized by hexose-6-phosphate isomerase, 2-deoxyglucose cannot be metabolized further in the glycolytic pathway. Therefore, if the hydrolysis of 2-deoxyglucose-6-phosphate by glucose-6-phosphatase is negligible, it accumulates within cells as 2-deoxyglucose-6-phosphate, 2-deoxyglucose-1-phosphate, UDP-2-deoxyglucose, and glycogen. Thus, to obtain the most accurate measure of the rate of glucose uptake into tissues, it is necessary to add the rate of glucose uptake (as determined by accumulation of 2-deoxyglucose products within the tissue) to the rate of incorporation of 2-deoxyglucose into glycogen (27).

Acknowledgements

I deeply thank Dr. Richard L. Printz, Ph.D., (Department of Molecular Physiology and Biophysics, Vanderbilt University School of Medicine, Nashville, Tennessee, U.S.A.) for his assistance in preparation of this Chapter and Mr. Dominic Doyle, M.A., (Creative Services, Vanderbilt University Medical Center, Nashville, Tennessee, U.S.A.) for his assistance with illustrations for ures.

References

1. Niswender KD, Shiota M, Postic C et al (1997) Effects of increased glucokinase gene copy number on glucose homeostasis and hepatic glucose metabolism. J Biol Chem 272: 22570–22575
2. Postic C, Shiota M, Niswender KD et al (1999) Dual roles for glucokinase in glucose homeostasis as determined by liver and pancreatic beta cell-specific gene knock-outs using Cre recombinase. J Biol Chem 274:305–315
3. She P, Burgess SC, Shiota M et al (2003) Mechanisms by which liver-specific PEPCK knockout mice preserve euglycemia during starvation. Diabetes 52:1649–1654
4. She P, Shiota M, Shelton KD et al (2000) Phosphoenolpyruvate carboxykinase is necessary for the integration of hepatic energy metabolism. Mol Cell Biol 20:6508–6517
5. Uno K, Katagiri H, Yamada T et al (2006) Neuronal pathway from the liver modulates

energy expenditure and systemic insulin sensitivity. Science 312:1656–1659
6. An J, Muoio DM, Shiota M et al (2004) Hepatic expression of malonyl-CoA decarboxylase reverses muscle, liver and whole-animal insulin resistance. Nat Med 10:268–274
7. Chu CA, Fujimoto Y, Igawa K et al (2004) Rapid translocation of hepatic glucokinase in response to intraduodenal glucose infusion and changes in plasma glucose and insulin in conscious rats. Am J Physiol Gastrointest Liver Physiol 286:G627–G634
8. Fujimoto Y, Donahue EP, Shiota M (2004) Defect in glucokinase translocation in Zucker diabetic fatty rats. Am J Physiol Endocrinol Metab 287:E414–E423
9. Fujimoto Y, Torres TP, Donahue EP et al (2006) Glucose toxicity is responsible for the development of impaired regulation of endogenous glucose production and hepatic glucokinase in Zucker diabetic fatty rats. Diabetes 55: 2479–2490
10. Nagle CA, An J, Shiota M et al (2007) Hepatic overexpression of glycerol-sn-3-phosphate acyltransferase 1 in rats causes insulin resistance. J Biol Chem 282:14807–14815
11. Shin JS, Torres TP, Catlin RL et al (2007) A defect in glucose-induced dissociation of glucokinase from the regulatory protein in Zucker diabetic fatty rats in the early stage of diabetes. Am J Physiol Regul Integr Comp Physiol 292:R1381–R1390
12. Torres TP, Catlin RL, Chan R et al (2009) Restoration of hepatic glucokinase expression corrects hepatic glucose flux and normalizes plasma glucose in zucker diabetic fatty rats. Diabetes 58:78–86
13. Torres TP, Fujimoto Y, Donahue EP et al (2011) Defective glycogenesis contributes toward the inability to suppress hepatic glucose production in response to hyperglycemia and hyperinsulinemia in zucker diabetic fatty rats. Diabetes 60:2225–2233
14. Ferre P, Leturque A, Burnol AF et al (1985) A method to quantify glucose utilization in vivo in skeletal muscle and white adipose tissue of the anaesthetized rat. Biochem J 228:103–110
15. Steele R (1959) Influences of glucose loading and of injected insulin on hepatic glucose output. Ann N Y Acad Sci 82:420–430
16. Ayala JE, Samuel VT, Morton GJ et al (2010) Standard operating procedures for describing and performing metabolic tests of glucose homeostasis in mice. Dis Model Mech 3: 525–534
17. McGuinness OP, Ayala JE, Laughlin MR et al (2009) NIH experiment in centralized mouse phenotyping: the Vanderbilt experience and recommendations for evaluating glucose homeostasis in the mouse. Am J Physiol Endocrinol Metab 297:E849–E855
18. Mathews CE, Wickwire K, Flatt WP et al (2000) Attenuation of circadian rhythms of food intake and respiration in aging diabetes-prone BHE/Cdb rats. Am J Physiol Regul Integr Comp Physiol 279:R230–R238
19. Possidente B, Birnbaum S (1979) Circadian rhythms for food and water consumption in the mouse, Mus musculus. Physiol Behav 22: 657–660
20. ter Haar MB (1972) Circadian and estrual rhythms in food intake in the rat. Horm Behav 3:213–219
21. Shiota M, Galassetti P, Monohan M et al (1998) Small amounts of fructose markedly augment net hepatic glucose uptake in the conscious dog. Diabetes 47:867–873
22. Torres TP, Sasaki N, Donahue EP et al (2011) Impact of a glycogen phosphorylase inhibitor and metformin on basal and glucagon-stimulated hepatic glucose flux in conscious dogs. J Pharmacol Exp Ther 337:610–620
23. Galassetti P, Shiota M, Zinker BA et al (1998) A negative arterial-portal venous glucose gradient decreases skeletal muscle glucose uptake. Am J Physiol 275:E101–E111
24. Pagliassotti MJ, Cherrington AD (1992) Regulation of net hepatic glucose uptake in vivo. Annu Rev Physiol 54:847–860
25. Argoud GM, Schade DS, Eaton RP (1987) Underestimation of hepatic glucose production by radioactive and stable tracers. Am J Physiol 252:E606–E615
26. Bell PM, Firth RG, Rizza RA (1986) Assessment of insulin action in insulin-dependent diabetes mellitus using (6(14)C) glucose, (3(3)H)glucose, and (2(3)H)glucose. Differences in the apparent pattern of insulin resistance depending on the isotope used. J Clin Invest 78:1479–1486
27. Colwell DR, Higgins JA, Denyer GS (1996) Incorporation of 2-deoxy-D-glucose into glycogen. Implications for measurement of tissue-specific glucose uptake and utilisation. Int J Biochem Cell Biol 28:115–121

Chapter 16

Measurement of Insulin Sensitivity in Skeletal Muscle In Vitro

Henrike Sell, Jørgen Jensen, and Juergen Eckel

Abstract

Glucose disposal in skeletal muscle is a major target for insulin action and assessment of insulin-regulated glucose uptake under in vitro conditions allows the direct determination of insulin sensitivity in this organ. For this purpose, a variety of muscle preparations from different parts of the body can be used. We describe here a detailed protocol for using epitrochlearis muscle strips and additionally for using primary skeletal muscle cells.

Key words: Glucose uptake, Muscle strips, Skeletal muscle cells

1. Introduction

Skeletal muscle is the largest organ in the body and responsible for the vast majority of glucose disposal, involving either oxidation or storage in the form of glycogen (1). This process is tightly controlled by insulin involving a highly complex signaling cascade that finally leads to translocation of the glucose transporter GLUT4 to the plasma membrane, enhanced glucose uptake and oxidation and stimulation of glycogen synthesis. In the intact organism, glucose disposal is a highly complex process involving the interplay between different organs and in vivo insulin sensitivity is determined using the hyperglycemic–euglycemic clamp (2). In vitro, insulin sensitivity is defined as the half-maximal concentration of the hormone required to achieve a certain response, mostly glucose transport or glycogen synthesis. Insulin resistance, which is the hallmark of obesity and the metabolic syndrome (3) comprises a reduced insulin sensitivity and/ or a reduced maximal response. In many in vitro studies related to muscle insulin resistance, single high insulin doses have been used.

We recommend to perform dose–response experiments in muscle cells to get a more complete picture of the underlying mechanisms that determine muscle insulin sensitivity. For muscles studied in vitro, insulin sensitivity can be evaluated with an insulin concentration around EC_{50} combined with a concentration stimulating glucose uptake maximally (4) to reduce the number of animals used.

As outlined above, insulin stimulates a cascade of signaling molecules including the insulin receptor, insulin receptor substrates, and a variety of downstream kinases, all involved in the divergent actions of this hormone. The serine/threonine kinase PKB/Akt plays a key role in this process and the phosphorylation of this enzyme is used in a large number of studies to monitor insulin sensitivity in different tissues (5). Although Akt plays a pivotal role in mediating glucose transport and activation of glycogen synthesis, the direct measurement of these final metabolic readouts should be considered as the "gold standard" of in vitro analysis of insulin sensitivity. This is due to a number of observations that Akt activity and these final metabolic events do not always correlate, most likely resulting from additional, potentially crosstalking signaling pathways (6).

Muscles dissected from different parts of the body from both rodents and other animals have been extensively used for measuring muscle insulin sensitivity in vitro. We present here a detailed protocol for preparation of *epitrochlearis* muscle from rats and its use for measuring glucose uptake and glycogen synthesis. This muscle preparation can also be electrically stimulated (7), thus insulin sensitivity and contractile activity can be monitored under the same controlled conditions. This method is ideal when working with a certain animal model, however, the limited viability excludes long term studies. For this purpose, muscle cell lines or primary muscle cells are much more suitable. We describe here the use of primary human skeletal muscle and present a detailed protocol for measuring glucose uptake.

2. Materials

2.1. Muscles In Vitro

The buffers are made from deionized water and chemicals of analytical grades. The buffer used contains bicarbonate, and the concentrations of salts and ions described by Krebs-Henseleit in 1932 (8). The buffer is gassed with 5% CO_2 and 95% O_2 and glucose and pyruvate, BSA and HEPES are added. We recommend ^{3}H-2-deoxyglucose as tracer for estimation of glucose uptake after correction of extracellular space with ^{14}C-mannitol (see Note 1).

1. Stock solutions I and II can be prepared in advance. Stock solution I contains: 1.16 M NaCl, 46 mM KCl, 11.6 mM KH_2PO_4, and 253 mM $NaHCO_3$ (see Note 2). Stock solution

II contains: 25 mM $CaCl_2$ and 11.6 mM $MgSO_4$. Stock solutions are stored at 4°C.

2. Prepare the following buffer at the day when experiments take place. The experimentation buffer contains (e.g., 500 mL): 50 mL Stock I, 50 mL Stock II, and 400 mL H_2O. Gas the buffer for 30 min with 5% CO_2/95% O_2 at room temperature (see Note 3). Add 0.1% BSA, glucose (5.5 mM), pyruvate (2 mM), and HEPES (5 mM) and adjust pH to 7.4 (see Note 4). Seal the modified Krebs-Henseleit buffer (KHB_M) and put on ice.

3. Add 9.25 kBq/mL (0.25 µCi/mL) ^{3}H-2-deoxyglucose and 3.7 kBq/mL (0.1 µCi/mL) ^{14}C-mannitol (see Note 5). Prepare adequate volumes of ^{3}H-2-deoxyglucose containing uptake buffer so that specific activity can be counted in triplicates. Divide the ^{3}H-2-deoxyglucose containing uptake buffer in volumes needed for different insulin concentrations.

4. Insulin is diluted to concentrations 1,000-fold higher than the desired concentrations in the experiments. (see Note 6). Add insulin in desired concentrations to the ^{3}H-2-deoxyglucose uptake buffers.

2.2. Skeletal Muscle Cells

1. The following media are required for primary skeletal muscle cell culture. Skeletal muscle growth medium: alpha-MEM/F12 containing 7.78 mM glucose, 10 µg/mL insulin, 5% FCS, 50 µg/mL fetuin, 10 ng/mL epidermal growth factor, 1 ng/mL fibroblast growth factor, 0.4 µg/mL dexamethasone, 20 U/mL peniciline, 20 µg/mL streptomycin, 50 ng/mL amphoterecin b, pH 7.4.

   Skeletal muscle differentiation medium: alpha-MEM containing 5.56 mM glucose, 20 U/mL peniciline, 20 µg/mL streptomycin, 50 ng/mL amphoterecin b, pH 7.4

2. Prepare an insulin solution of 100 µM in 5 mM HCl. Store at −20°C.

3. Dissolve 5 mg cytochalasin B in 417 µL ethanol under a hood and immediately transfer to 416.5 mL PBS to obtain a 0.25 µM solution. Storage is possible at 4°C for up to a month.

4. Prepare 1 M NaOH solution. Concentrated acetic acid is used to neutralize NaOH after dissolving the cells. Adjust the volume of acetic acid to completely neutralize NaOH.

5. Radioactive L-glucose and D-glucose solutions should be prepared immediately prior to their use. L-glucose serves as a measure of nonspecific uptake and as a background measurement that should be repeated on each experimental day. Deoxy-D-glucose is not metabolized and its accumulation in the cells upon insulin stimulation is measured in this assay. Prepare a solution of L-^{14}C-glucose at a concentration of 185 kBq/mL (5 µCi/mL) diluted in differentiation medium. Calculate 50 µL/probe and 100 µL for controls. Prepare a solution of 2-deoxy-D-^{14}C-glucose at a

oncentration of 185 kBq/mL (5 µCi/mL) diluted in differentiation medium. Calculate 50 µL/probe and 100 µL for controls.

6. Prepare scintillation vials containing 10 mL of a scintillation cocktail (e.g., AquaSafe 300 from Zinsser Analytic) for each probe, duplicates of the two radioactive glucose solutions and two blanks.

7. Insulin can be diluted in differentiation medium for immediate use.

3. Methods

3.1. Glucose Uptake in Isolated Muscle

Various muscles are used for measurement of insulin sensitivity in vitro from mice and rats. Incubated muscles receive oxygen and nutrients from the medium and the two limiting factors are the size of the muscles (diffusion distance) and the temperature. The solubility of oxygen in the buffer decreases by increased temperature and the metabolic rate increases in the muscles. The preferred muscle is the *epitrochlearis* muscle from rats below 150 g. The *epitrochlearis* muscle is a thin flat muscle with a diffusion distance below 0.5 mm for all muscle fibers (see Note 7). Temperatures at or below 30°C are suggested (see Note 8). Indeed other muscles can be used. The diaphragm was initially used; the muscle is thin and viable but a bit unhandy and may differ from other muscles because of continuous activity. Intact *soleus* and *extensor digitorum longus* (EDL) muscles can be incubated intact from rats of 60–80 g. *Soleus* and EDL can easily be split into two strips from rats below 150 g. From larger rats, strips with diameter below 1 mm can be obtained for studies. From mice, *soleus*, EDL, and *epitrochlearis* can be dissected for in vitro measurements of insulin sensitivity. We recommend that muscles are incubated on holders at their resting length. However, *epitrochlearis* muscle can be incubated floating in buffer.

1. Muscles are dissected, preincubated for 30 min prior to measurement of 2-deoxyglucose uptake during 30 min with different concentrations of insulin.

2. Dissect muscles with minimal stretching while kept moisture.

3. Pre-warm (while gassing) KHB_M for 3–5 min and incubate dissected muscles for 30 min at 30°C allowing recovery from dissection (see Note 9).

4. Move muscles to pre-warmed ^{3}H-2-deoxyglucose uptake buffers with different insulin concentrations and incubate for 30 min at 30°C while gassing with 5% CO_2/95% O_2. After 30 min, remove muscles from holders and blot on filter paper to remove excess buffer and freeze in liquid nitrogen.

5. Weigh muscles and dissolve in 1 M KOH for 20 min at 70°C and count radioactivity (see Note 10).

6. Calculate ^{3}H-2-deoxyglucose uptake after correction of extracellular space with ^{14}C-mannitol.

7. Muscles can be contracted in vitro prior to analysis of insulin sensitivity (Fig. 1). Alternatively, rats can be exercised in vivo and muscles removed immediately for measurements of insulin sensitivity in vitro as described above.

Full dose response curves with 5–7 insulin concentration require a large number of rats. Insulin sensitivity can be evaluated with a single insulin concentration around EC_{50} together with a concentration stimulating glucose uptake maximally (e.g., 10,000 U/mL). Be aware that insulin sensitivity decreases substantially by increasing weight from 100 to 200 g in Wistar rats.

3.2. Glucose Uptake in Human Myotubes in Cell Culture

Glucose uptake can be measured in both primary skeletal muscle myotubes and in muscle cell lines. C2C12 mouse myoblasts and L6 rat myoblast are widely used. The protocols used for these cell lines vary in some aspects from this protocol but the overall procedure is similar.

Another rapid quantitative assay complementary to glucose uptake is the quantification of cell surface GLUT4 containing a myc-tag (9).

1. Human myoblasts are seeded at a density of about 100,000 cells/sixwell cavity and grown in skeletal muscle growth medium to confluence with medium change every 2–3 days. Upon confluence, medium is changed to skeletal muscle cells differentiation medium with medium change every 2–3 days. After 5–7 days of differentiation, myogenic markers, insulin receptor, and GLUT4 expression are increased to their maximum and cells can be used for glucose uptake experiments or analysis of insulin signaling.

2. In order not to stress the cells, any change of medium should be avoided directly before the glucose uptake experiment (see Note 11). Overnight treatment of myotubes with the compound or protein of interest is ideal. All calculations are based on a presumed volume of 1 mL used in each sixwell cavity. Measurement in triplicates is useful—one sixwell dish is sufficient for three basal and three insulin-stimulated samples.

3. As the handling of each sixwell dish is time consuming at certain steps, the experiment should be started with a time delay for each dish. Up to eight dishes can be used one after another and started every 3 min.

4. Prior to glucose uptake, myotubes are stimulated with insulin. Dilute the insulin stock solution to 10 μM and add 10 μL to each cavity. Incubate the cells for exactly 30 min at 37°C and 5% CO_2.

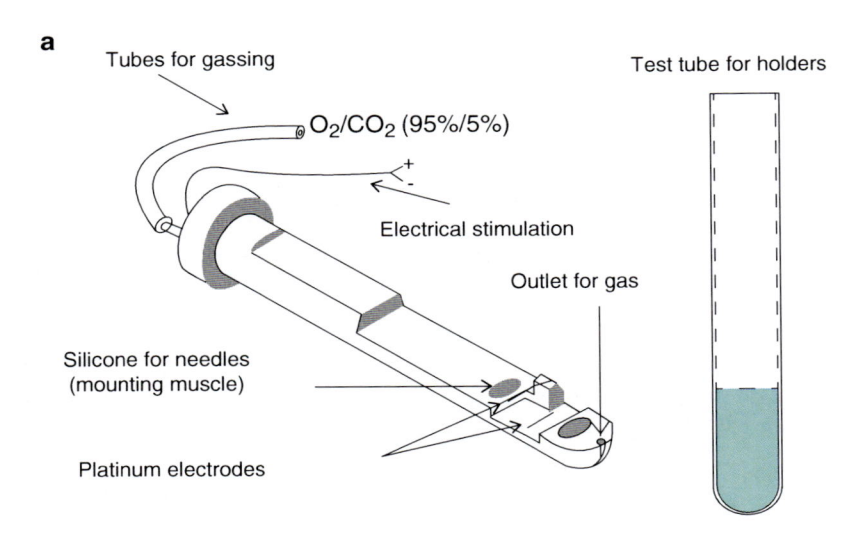

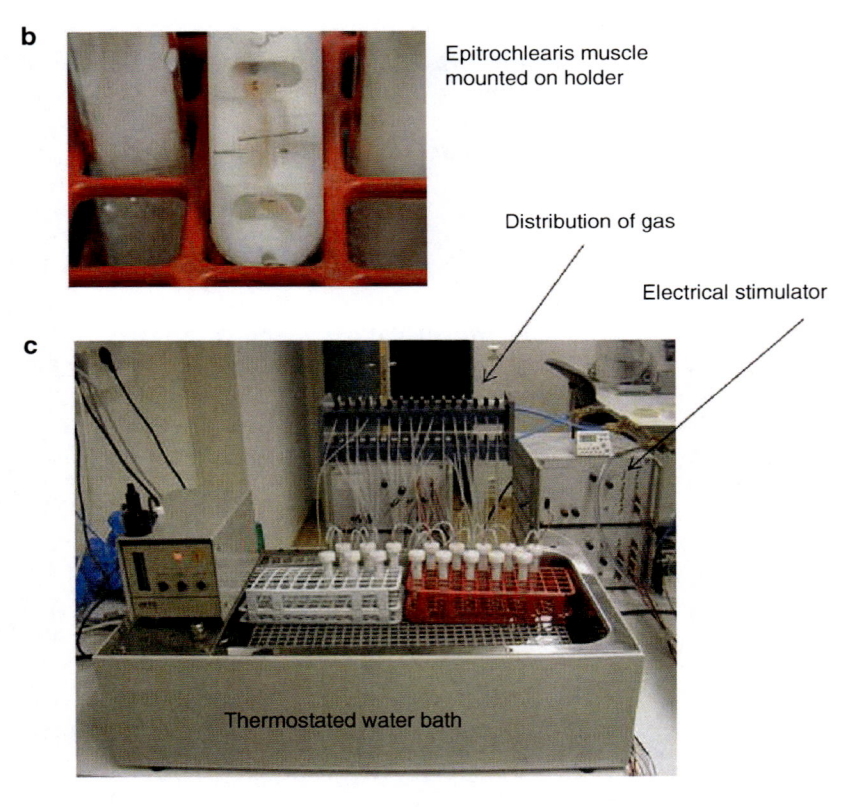

Fig. 1. Laboratory setup for in vitro studies with skeletal muscles. (**a**) Schematic drawing of apparatus (holders) for muscle contraction in vitro. Muscles can be mounted by needles at their resting length within 30 s after dissection. (**b**) Picture showing epitrochlearis muscles mounted and incubated. The buffer is gassed continuously during experiment; see bobble just above the muscle. (**c**) Complete setup for in vitro studies with skeletal muscles in the laboratory in Oslo. The system is easily handled and allows incubating a substantial number; two persons can incubate 48–72 muscles/day. The system was developed in 1995 by JJ and has been extensively used in many experiments. (Copyright, Jørgen Jensen, Oslo).

5. Add 50 µL of radioactive glucose (L-glucose or deoxy-D-glucose) per cavity and incubate the cells for 2 h at 37°C and 5% CO_2.

6. Put each sixwell dish on ice and remove all liquid from the cells. Immediately wash with 1 mL of cytochalasin B per cavity twice.

7. Add 1 mL NaOH per cavity for dissolving the cells and incubate for 30 min at 37°C. Neutralize afterwards with the appropriate volume of acetic acid. Neutralization should be performed carefully by gently shaking the plates and waiting until sparkling is discontinued.

8. Transfer each sample completely into a scintillation vial. Transfer 50 µL of each original radioactive glucose solution into a scintillation vial. All samples should be shaked vigorously to mix both liquids. Prior to measurement, the probes should rest for at least 2 h.

9. Measure the probes in the appropriate scintillation counter (for example LS6000 or LS6500 from Beckman Coulter). The counting time for each probe should be adjusted to minimize the counting error to be lower than 3% (normally 10–30 min are sufficient). Reading can be done in cpm (counts/min) or dpm (disintegration/min). Values for L-glucose are averaged and used as a background to be subtracted from all sample values (see Notes 12–14).

10. The measurement of the original radioactive glucose solutions can serve to calculate the absolute amount of glucose incorporated into the cells. Counts can be converted to moles of glucose taken up.

4. Notes

1. Insulin sensitivity can also be evaluated by measurement of glycogen synthesis with ^{14}C-glucose. This method is reliable but it must be considered that glycogen synthase may limit rate of glycogen synthesis rather than glucose uptake (10). Glucose transport can be measured with ^{3}H-3-O-methylglucose and ^{14}C-mannitol to correct for extracellular space. Glucose transport using 3-O-methylglucose shall be performed over 10 min as 3-O-methylglucose is not phosphorylated and reverse transport limits sensitivity. This method is less sensitive than ^{3}H-2-deoxyglucose uptake and ^{14}C-glycogen synthesis and is not recommended unless specific questions are addressed.

2. Krebs and Henseleit originally suggested all components to be prepared in six separate buffers.
3. Make, e.g., 100 mL extra buffer to check that pH ~7.4.
4. Other buffers can be used.
5. Ethanol can be evaporated, storage solution for radio-labeled glucose analogues if preferred.
6. Of convenience, we normally use the insulin Actrapid from Novo Nordisk (Denmark), which can be stored in fridge.
7. Methodological considerations and viability of epitrochlearis has been discusssed by Wallberg-Henriksson (11).
8. For more information about effects of temperature and diffusion distance on viability see (12).
9. *Epitrochlearis* muscles are stretched during dissection and lactate content is doubled immediately after dissection. After 20 min of incubation, lactate concentration is comparable to resting muscles in vivo.
10. Muscles can with advantage be freeze dried before weighing. Water content increases from ~75 to ~80% during incubation; mainly due to increased extracellular space (7).
11. Glucose uptake in skeletal muscle cells can also be performed in Krebs-Ringer-buffer. In this case, cells should be preincubated in this buffer for 2.5 h.
12. Instead of using L-glucose, deoxy-D-glucose uptake can also be measured in the presence of cytochalasin B to account for nonspecific glucose uptake which can be subtracted from each determination to obtain specific uptake.
13. Counts can also be normalized to the protein concentration of lysates.
14. Insulin-stimulated glucose uptake is dependent on the skeletal muscle cell donor and might vary. Normally, insulin induces a 1.5- to 2.5-fold glucose uptake compared to basal (13).

Acknowledgments

HS is supported by DFG SE 1922/2-1. JJ research has been supported by grants from Novo Nordisk Foundation. JE and JJ are supported by participation in COST BM0602 (Network supported by European Community). JE is supported by the Commission of the European Communities (collaborative project ADAPT, contract number HEALTH-F2-2008-201100).

References

1. Jornayvaz FR, Samuel VT, Shulman GI (2010) The role of muscle insulin resistance in the pathogenesis of atherogenic dyslipidemia and nonalcoholic fatty liver disease associated with the metabolic syndrome. Annu Rev Nutr 30:273–90
2. DeFronzo RA, Tobin JD, Andres R (1979) Glucose clamp technique: a method for quantifying insulin secretion and resistance. Am J Physiol 237:E214–23
3. Eckardt K, Taube A, Eckel J (2011) Obesity-associated insulin resistance in skeletal muscle: Role of lipid accumulation and physical inactivity. Rev Endocr Metab Disord 12:163–72
4. Buren J, Lai YC, Lundgren M et al (2008) Insulin action and signalling in fat and muscle from dexamethasone-treated rats. Arch Biochem Biophys 474:91–101
5. Schultze SM, Jensen J, Hemmings BA et al (2011) Promiscuous affairs of PKB/AKT isoforms in metabolism. Arch Physiol Biochem 117:70–7
6. Zierath JR, Krook A, Wallberg-Henriksson H (2000) Insulin action and insulin resistance in human skeletal muscle. Diabetologia 43:821–35
7. Aslesen R, Jensen J (1998) Effects of epinephrine on glucose metabolism in contracting rat skeletal muscles. Am J Physiol 275:E448–56
8. Krebs AH, Henseleit K (1932) Untersuchungen über die Harnstoffbildung im Tierkörper. Hoppe-Seyler's Z Physiol Chem 210:33–66
9. Wang Q, Khayat Z, Kishi K et al (1998) GLUT4 translocation by insulin in intact muscle cells: detection by a fast and quantitative assay. FEBS Lett 427:193–7
10. Jensen J, Jebens E, Brennesvik EO et al (2006) Muscle glycogen inharmoniously regulates glycogen synthase activity, glucose uptake, and proximal insulin signaling. Am J Physiol Endocrinol Metab 290:E154–E162
11. Wallberg-Henriksson H (1987) Glucose transport into skeletal muscle. Influence of contractile activity, insulin, catecholamines and diabetes mellitus. Acta Physiol Scand Suppl 564:1–80
12. Segal SS, Faulkner JA (1985) Temperature-dependent physiological stability of rat skeletal muscle in vitro. Am J Physiol 248:C265–70
13. Sell H, Laurencikiene J, Taube A et al (2009) Chemerin is a novel adipocyte-derived factor inducing insulin resistance in primary human skeletal muscle cells. Diabetes 58:2731–40

Chapter 17

Beta-Cell Autoimmunity

Yannick F. Fuchs, Kerstin Adler, and Ezio Bonifacio

Abstract

Beta cell destruction in autoimmune diabetes is accompanied by the presence of autoantibodies and autoreactive T cells against beta cell antigens. Autoantibodies to insulin are predictive of future diabetes in man and in the non-obese diabetic mouse model. Furthermore, the detection of peripheral autoreactive CD8+ T cells in this mouse model is indicative of beta cell killing and correlates with the development of diabetes. We describe two protocols that are helpful for the detection of beta-cell autoimmunity in mice. The first protocol describes the detection of insulin-specific autoantibodies using a radio-binding assay. The other is a general CD8+ T cell ELISpot protocol for the detection of peptide-specific responses of CD8+ T cells from secondary lymphoid organs or pancreatic islets.

Key words: Autoimmune diabetes, Insulin autoantibodies, Radio-binding assay, CD8+ T cell, ELISpot, Beta-cell autoimmunity

1. Introduction

Type 1 diabetes (T1D) is an autoimmune disease in which insulin-producing pancreatic beta cells are attacked by the immune system. Components of the adaptive immune system play a fundamental role in this self-directed immune response. Autoantibodies directed against beta cell-specific targets are produced by B lymphocytes and their detection has become a reliable prognostic marker to determine the risk of humans to develop T1D (1–4). Autoreactive T cells infiltrating the islets recognize their target autoantigen via their T cell receptor and mediate the momentous beta cell destruction leading to insulin dependency.

Autoantibodies to islet antigens are a characteristic feature of preclinical T1D (5). The major antigen targets of these autoantibodies so far identified in man are insulin, glutamic acid decarboxylase (GAD), IA-2, and Zinc transporter 8 (ZnT8). Insulin is also a target of autoantibodies in the non-obese diabetic (NOD) mouse model (6), and the early presence of insulin autoantibodies can be predictive of future diabetes in the NOD mouse (4). More than a decade ago, the First International Workshop on Lessons From Animal Models for Human Type 1 Diabetes (7) identified insulin but not GAD or IA-2 as specific autoantigens of humoral autoimmunity in NOD mice. Two years later, a second murine autoantibody workshop concluded a remarkable inter-laboratory concordance for radio-binding assays to identify insulin autoantibodies in NOD mice (8). This supports the findings for human serum specimens, concluding that radio-binding assays are the most sensitive and specific assays for the detection of insulin autoantibodies (9). Recently, improved nonradioactive assay methods have been developed and may substitute the current radio-binding assays for the detection of insulin autoantibodies in mouse models (10) and potentially man.

With respect to T cells, $CD8^+$ cytotoxic T lymphocytes play a major role in beta cell killing (11, 12). $CD8^+$ T cells recognize autoantigenic peptides presented on MHC class I and key for the detection of autoantigen-specific $CD8^+$ T cell responses is the knowledge of autoantigenic peptides presented on these MHC molecules. Direct labeling for detection of autoantigen-specific $CD8^+$ T cells is possible and referred, but requires the production of MHC class I multimers loaded with the adequate autoantigenic peptide for each T cell specificity tested. Therefore, functional $CD8^+$ T cells assays that involve the co-cultivation of $CD8^+$ T cells with antigen presenting cells (APCs) loaded with autoantigenic peptides are often used to detect specific $CD8^+$ T cell responses. These include assays that determine $CD8^+$ T cell-mediated specific lysis of APCs (13, 14), measure intracellular staining of effector cytokines in $CD8^+$ T cells (15, 16) or ELISpot assays that allow for the detection of secreted cytokines after peptide stimulation (17). We will describe a simple and robust ELISpot protocol that can be used for various applications and has been successfully used with $CD8^+$ T cells from secondary lymphoid organs and pancreatic islets.

2. Materials

2.1. Detection of Insulin Autoantibodies

1. Assay buffer TBT: 50 mM Tris, pH 8.0, 1% Tween 20. Pour approximately 900 mL double-distilled water into a 1 L graduated cylinder. Weigh 6 g Tris and transfer to the cylinder. Measure 10 mL Tween 20 and add to the cylinder. Mix and adjust pH with HCl (see Note 1). Make up to 1 L using double-distilled water. Mix and store at 4°C. Prepare 1 L assay buffer per 100 assay tubes (corresponds to 25 samples).

2. Assay tubes: 5 mL round bottom polystyrene tubes.

3. Radio-labeled Antigen: ^{125}I-labeled lyophilized Tyr^{14}A (^{125}I) insulin (Sanofi-Aventis, Frankfurt, Germany; specific activity

13.43 GBq/mg; 0.128 nmol/L). Re-suspend lyophilized insulin with 2 mL double-distilled water containing 5% BSA to prepare a stock solution of 10 µCi/mL (see Note 2). Calculate and dilute 1.5 µL of this stock solution into 25 µL assay buffer for each tube to be included into the assay (see Note 3).

4. Non-radio-labeled antigen for competition: human insulin (e.g., Insuman Rapid, Sanofi-Aventis, Frankfurt, Germany). Dissolve the human insulin in assay buffer to obtain a solution of 8 U human insulin per mL.

5. Protein-A/Protein G Sepharose for immune precipitation: Protein A-Sepharose CL-4B (GE Healthcare), and GammaBind Plus Sepharose (GE Healthcare).

6. Calibrators: one insulin autoantibody negative serum from C57BL/6 mice as negative control (a pool from several mice can be used), one insulin autoantibody positive serum, which can be a pool of serum samples from female NOD mice. The calibrators should be of sufficient volume to use for the duration of planned experiments.

7. Assay quality control samples. Two samples representing low positive and moderate positive IAA concentrations are advised. All calibrators and quality control samples should be appropriately stored (e.g., –20°C) in small aliquots (e.g., 100 µL) in sealed tubes samples.

8. Multistep pipette.

9. Liquid dispenser capable of dispensing 1.8 mL.

10. Swinging bucket bench centrifuge with tube carriers.

11. Gamma counter.

2.2. Detection of Peptide Responsiveness of CD8+ T Cells

1. General material

   Sterile 35% ethanol.

   Sterile and pyrogen-free PBS (PBS-PF) for washing and dilution prior cellular assay.

   PBS for washing after cellular assay.

   Double-distilled H_2O.

   Multichannel pipette (e.g., 30–300 µL) and/or multistep pipette.

   Squirt bottle with wide spout for washing.

   Sterile, pyrogen-free liquid reservoirs.

   Plastic seals for 96-well plates.

   Non-fuzzing tissues.

   CO_2-incubator (37°C, 100% humidity, 5% CO_2).

   Swinging bucket bench centrifuge with tube carriers.

   Immunospot image analyzer for spot counting.

2. Cells and media

Cells of interest:

Use T cell depleted splenocytes as APCs (see Note 4) and CD8+ T cells isolated from organs of interest and processed to the desired purity using magnetic bead enrichment and/or cell sorting (see Note 5).

Culture media for cells:

RPMI 1640 containing 10% FBS, 100 U/mL penicillin, 100 μg/mL streptomycin, 10 μM nonessential amino acids, 10 mM HEPES, 1 mM Na-pyruvate, 50 μM β-mercaptoethanol, 2 mM L-glutamine.

Peptides and stimuli:

Synthesized peptides of interest dissolved in appropriate solvent (e.g., DMSO, PBS depending on the peptide composition). Positive control stimulus (e.g., anti-CD3/anti-CD28/anti-CD137 mouse T-activator Dynabeads (Invitrogen)) (see Note 6).

3. ELISpot material

ELISpot plate: PVDF membrane-bottomed 96-well plates MSIPS4510 (Millipore).

ELISpot anti-IFNγ coating and detection antibody pair for mouse IFNγ (Ucytech, CT65510) diluted in distilled sterile H_2O according to the manufacturers' recommendations and stored in aliquots at −80°C until use.

Blocking buffer: Blocking stock solution B (Ucytech, CT362) stored in aliquots at 4°C and diluted 1:10 in sterile PBS-PF before use.

PBS containing 10% heat inactivated FCS (PBS 10).

PBS containing 0.5% heat inactivated FCS (PBS 0.5).

Staining components: Sigma ExtrAvidin-AP (Sigma); SigmaFast NBT-BCIP tablets (Sigma).

3. Methods

3.1. Detection of Insulin Autoantibodies by Radio-Binding Assay

Insulin autoantibodies in murine blood specimens are measured by binding to ^{125}I-labeled insulin in a protein A/G radio-binding assay as originally developed by Williams et al. (18), optimized by Naserke et al. (19), and further modified for murine samples by minor modifications (20). The assay is represented as laboratory B in the animal models of diabetes workshop (7).

Measurements should be performed on coded samples that are operator-blinded. Each step of the assay is conducted on wet ice.

1. All assays must include the calibrators and quality control sera.
2. All samples are tested in duplicate with and without excess cold insulin competition. Therefore, prepare four assay tubes per sample.
3. Day 1. For each calibrator, control, and test sample, add 2.5 µL of sample (serum or plasma) to each of the four tubes.
4. Using multistep pipettes, add 25 µL assay buffer to all tubes designated for no competition (i.e., two of the four tubes per sample) and add 25 µL non-radio-labeled insulin (8 U/mL in assay buffer) to the tubes designated for excess cold insulin competition.
5. Add 25 µL pre-diluted radio-labeled insulin in assay buffer to all tubes and seal all tubes with parafilm. Keep the remaining pre-diluted radio-labeled insulin for measurement of total counts.
6. Centrifuge assay tubes for 30 s at $500 \times g$ in a swing bucket centrifuge at 4°C to bring all contents to the bottom. Shake tubes briefly on a horizontal shaker at 1,000 rpm.
7. Incubate assay tubes for 66–72 h at 4°C.
8. Day 3 (around 48 h after setting up the assay). Prepare the Protein-A sepharose calculating 2 mg of Sepharose per 60 µL assay buffer for each tube of the assay. Mix the Sepharose with a rotating wheel or similar apparatus for 15 min. Store it overnight at 4°C. On the next morning (day 4), add GammaBind Plus Sepharose (6 µL for each tube of the assay) to the Protein-A Sepharose solution. Wash the Sepharose beads by centrifugation for 5 min at $500 \times g$ in a swing bucket centrifuge at 4°C. Discard the supernatant and add fresh assay buffer. Repeat this step twice. Finally add assay buffer so that 50 µL of solution will contain 2 mg pre-swollen Protein A-Sepharose CL-4B and 6 µL pre-swollen GammaBind Plus Sepharose.
9. Add 50 µL of the pre-swollen Protein A-Sepharose CL-4B and GammaBind Plus Sepharose mix to each tube.
10. Incubate tubes for 1 h at 4°C (e.g., cold room) while shaking at 1,000 rpm on a horizontal shaker.
11. Wash Sepharose beads six times with 1.8 mL ice cold assay buffer per tube: Centrifuge tubes for 5 min at $500 \times g$ in a swing bucket centrifuge at 4°C to pellet the beads between washes. Carefully take off supernatants after each round of centrifugation by vacuum aspiration.
12. Cap each tube and count pellets for 9 min (e.g., γ-counter Cobra II, Packard) for measurement of the recovered counts per minute (cpm) of radio-labeled insulin.
13. Results are expressed as an index that is calculated in the following way: (cpm in the test serum – cpm of negative

serum)/(cpm of positive calibrator – cpm negative). The upper limit of normal needs to be determined from the 99th percentile values obtained in sera from non-autoimmune mouse strains.

3.2. Peptide Responsiveness of CD8+ T Cells Measured by ELISpot

Generally, all steps carried out before starting the cellular assay are performed in a sterile laminar flow work bench at room temperature using sterile, pyrogen-free consumables. Development of the ELISpot assay can be performed outside the laminar flow work bench.

1. Preparation of ELISpot plate (day −1)

    Pre-wet the required number of wells of the 96-well plate with 40 µL of sterile 35% ethanol. Cover the plate and incubate for 1 min (see Note 7).

    Shake out the ethanol and rinse wells two times with 200 µL sterile PBS-PF. In the meantime, dilute coating anti-IFNγ-antibody 1:100 in PBS-PF.

    Rigorously shake out the PBS-PF from wells and add 50 µL/well of coating antibody mixture per well. Cover the plate with a lid and seal the plate with parafilm. Incubate overnight at 4°C.

2. Setting up ELISpot assay (day 0)

    Shake out coating antibody and wash wells 5× with 200 µL PBS-PF. In the meantime, dilute Blocking stock solution (10×) in PBS-PF to obtain 1× Blocking buffer.

    Add 200 µL/well of 1× Blocking buffer. Cover the plate with a lid, seal the plate with parafilm, and incubate for 1 h at 37°C in the incubator.

    Adjust APCs to 2.5×10^6 cells/mL, CD8+ T cells to 1×10^6 cells/mL in culture media (see Note 8), and store them at 37°C in a CO_2 incubator until use (keep lid loose to allow gas exchange).

    Prepare 4× concentrated dilutions of stimulating peptides, solvents (negative controls), polyclonal stimulus (positive control) in culture medium and vortex (see Note 9).

    Transfer APCs and CD8+ T cells into liquid reservoirs (in case multichannel pipette use for transfer of cells into wells) or appropriate tubes (in case a multistep pipette is used) and mix cells carefully to achieve a uniform suspension.

    Remove Blocking buffer from the plate. Bring 100 µL of APC suspension and 50 µL of CD8+ T cell suspension into the appropriate wells using the multichannel or multistep pipette. Take care to mix cells from time to time in the reservoir/tube to maintain a uniform suspension.

    Carefully add 50 µL of peptide/control dilutions slowly to the wells. This must be done with care to avoid splashing of peptide into neighboring wells and to prevent the cells from being flushed to the edges of the well. Make sure to use a fresh pipette tip for every peptide dilution. If using activator beads, take care to vigorously vortex the bead containing dilution promptly before addition to the wells as the beads tend to sink to the bottom of the tube.

Cover the plate with a lid and incubate at 37°C in a CO_2 incubator for 15 h (see Note 10).

3. Development of ELISpot assay

Remove cells with a firm flick of the plate and wash wells five times with 250 µL PBS using the multichannel pipette. In the meantime, dilute an appropriate amount of biotin-coupled IFNγ detection antibody 1:100 in PBS 10 and mix.

Shake out PBS and add 100 µL detection antibody solution per well. Seal the plate with an adhesive sealing film and incubate the plate for 1 h at 37°C. Do not put the lid back on the plate at this stage as the resulting pressure will lead to leakage of the plate.

Remove the adhesive sealing film from the plate and flick and shake out the detection antibody solution. Detach the plastic underdrain of the plate and wash both sides of the membrane five times with PBS using a squirt bottle with a wide spout. Meanwhile, make a 1:5,000 dilution of Extravidin-AP in PBS 0.5 and mix.

Shake out PBS, place plate on top of an empty 96-well plate and add 100 µL of Extravidin-AP solution per well. Seal the plate with a fresh adhesive sealing film and incubate the plate for 1 h at room temperature without reattaching the plastic underdrain (see Note 11). Do not put the lid back on the plate.

Shake out Extravidin solution and wash both sides of the membrane five times with PBS. Meanwhile dissolve an NBT-BCIP tablet in 10 mL ddH_2O by vigorous vortexing.

As soon as the tablet is completely dissolved, pour the solution into a liquid reservoir. Shake out the PBS from the plate and remove the last drops by tapping the plate on a stack of non-fuzzing tissues. Place the plate on a fresh 96-well plate and add 100 µL of NBT-BCIP solution into each well. Incubate the plate in the dark and monitor spot development every 2–3 min. The formation of spots is expected to occur within the first 15 min. As soon as clear spots have developed, remove the NBT-BCIP solution and stop the reaction by rinsing both sides of the membrane with excessive ddH_2O (see Note 12).

Air dry the plate until the membrane is completely dry and count spots by use of an immunospot image analyzer (see Note 13).

4. Notes

1. Concentrated HCl (12 N) can be used at first and then 1 N HCl for last adjustments.
2. The purchase, shipment, and handling of iodine-125-labeled radioactive materials underlie national authorities and regulations. All specific rules need to be followed and appropriate precautions and good laboratory practices should be used in the storage, handling, and disposal of this material all the time. If Sanofi radio-labeled insulin is unavailable in your country, then it can be purchased from Perkin Elmer (Product number NEX420050UC).
3. Please include in the calculation about 10% on top of the actual tubes required.
4. The standard protocol described uses T cell depleted splenocytes as APCs as they are a natural source of APC and are usually accessible when mouse studies are carried out. T cell depletion of splenocytes can be easily achieved by labeling splenocytes with biotinilated antibodies towards the T cell markers CD3ε (clone 145-2C11), CD8α (Ly-2, clone 53-6.7) and CD4 (L3T4, clone GK1.5) and streptavidin coupled microbeads (Miltenyi). Subsequent negative selection using depletion columns leads to highly T cell depleted splenocytes. Alternatively, other APCs or cell lines that express the right MHC class I molecules can be used instead of splenocytes and may be suitable for your application (e.g., T2 cell lines expressing H-2Db or H-2Kb; MHC class I transfected RMA-S cells, K562/A*0201 cells for CD8+ T cells from HLA-A*0201 humanized mice).
5. Depending on the source of CD8+ T cells, magnetic bead enrichment might be counter productive. If the number of CD8+ T cells is small as for example after purification from pancreatic islets, we suggest staining cells for CD4 and CD8 and sorting CD8+ T cells. A detailed protocol for the isolation and propagation of CD8+ T cells from murine pancreatic islets has been recently published by others (21).
6. So far we used peptide purities >95% in case the epitope is known and purities >80% for screening purposes, but also lower purities may be sufficient for your purpose. We recommend ordering the lyophilized peptide in aliquots and storing them at −80°C until use. It is beneficial to reconstitute all the peptides at a standard concentration (e.g., 10 mg/mL or 10 mM) in the appropriate solvents to simplify assay setup. Preparation of small aliquots for single use will avoid freeze/thaw cycles.

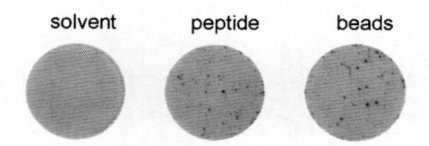

Fig. 1. Example of ELISpot CD8+ T cell responses towards peptide solvent alone (negative control), peptide of interest, and anti-CD3/anti-CD28/anti-CD137 stimulatory beads (positive control).

7. Take care that as soon as the membrane is activated with ethanol, it must never be allowed to dry until the end of the experiment as this will likely result in staining artifacts.

8. In our standard ELISpot protocol, we use 250,000 T cell depleted splenocytes as APCs and 50,000 CD8+ T cells in a final volume of 200 µL. Usually, CD8+ T cells are the limiting factor especially if they are isolated from mouse islets. Depending on the frequency of peptide-specific CD8+ T cells, also lower CD8+ T cell numbers may be sufficient for your experiment.

9. When using different solvents for your peptides, solvent controls for each solvent must be included. Additionally, we strongly recommend to include control wells that contain all components except the CD8+ T cells for all antigens tested. This will discriminate responses that arise from cytokine secreting non-CD8+ T cells. When using T-activator beads as positive control stimulus, we suggest using them at a concentration of 1 bead per CD8+ T cell as a rule of thumb.

10. Depending on the frequency of cytokine secreting cells, the optimal incubation time may vary. Too short incubation times result in weak staining, too long incubation times lead to a dark background as the secreted IFNγ will disperse throughout the whole well and bind to the capturing antibody.

11. As soon as the plastic underdrain is removed, contact with the membrane should be avoided. Especially contact to tissues will result in leakage of the plate through the membrane.

12. The first time one checks the development of spots can be difficult. Focus on the positive and negative control wells to get the right time point for clear staining with little background (Fig. 1).

13. There are various immunospot analyzers on the market. The main point is to achieve samples that allow a clear discrimination between background and spots and to analyze all wells of your experiment with the same software settings.

References

1. Atkinson MA, Eisenbarth GS (2001) Type 1 diabetes: new perspectives on disease pathogenesis and treatment. Lancet 358:221–229
2. Ziegler AG, Hummel M, Schenker M et al (1999) Autoantibody appearance and risk for development of childhood diabetes in offspring of parents with type 1 diabetes: the 2-year analysis of the German BABYDIAB Study. Diabetes 48:460–468
3. Kimpimaki T, Kulmala P, Savola K et al (2002) Natural history of beta-cell autoimmunity in young children with increased genetic susceptibility to type 1 diabetes recruited from the general population. J Clin Endocrinol Metab 87:4572–4579
4. Yu L, Robles DT, Abiru N et al (2000) Early expression of antiinsulin autoantibodies of humans and the NOD mouse: evidence for early determination of subsequent diabetes. Proc Natl Acad Sci U S A 97:1701–1706
5. Tian J, Chau C, Kaufman DL (1998) Insulin selectively primes Th2 responses and induces regulatory tolerance to insulin in pre-diabetic mice. Diabetologia 41:237–240
6. Muir A, Peck A, Clare-Salzler M et al (1995) Insulin immunization of nonobese diabetic mice induces a protective insulitis characterized by diminished intraislet interferon-gamma transcription. J Clin Invest 95:628–634
7. Bonifacio E, Atkinson M, Eisenbarth G et al (2001) International Workshop on Lessons From Animal Models for Human Type 1 Diabetes: identification of insulin but not glutamic acid decarboxylase or IA-2 as specific autoantigens of humoral autoimmunity in nonobese diabetic mice. Diabetes 50:2451–2458
8. Yu L, Eisenbarth G, Bonifacio E et al (2003) The second murine autoantibody workshop: remarkable interlaboratory concordance for radiobinding assays to identify insulin autoantibodies in nonobese diabetic mice. Ann N Y Acad Sci 1005:1–12
9. Bingley PJ, Bonifacio E, Mueller PW (2003) Diabetes Antibody Standardization Program: first assay proficiency evaluation. Diabetes 52:1128–1136
10. Schlosser M, Mueller PW, Torn C et al (2010) Diabetes Antibody Standardization Program: evaluation of assays for insulin autoantibodies. Diabetologia 53:2611–2620
11. Tsai S, Shameli A, Santamaria P (2008) CD8+ T cells in type 1 diabetes. Adv Immunol 100:79–124
12. Skowera A, Ellis RJ, Varela-Calvino R et al (2008) CTLs are targeted to kill b-cells in patients with type 1 diabetes through recognition of a glucose-regulated preproinsulin epitope. J Clin Invest 118:3390–3402
13. Anderson B, Park BJ, Verdaguer J et al (1999) Prevalent CD8(+) T cell response against one peptide/MHC complex in autoimmune diabetes. Proc Natl Acad Sci U S A 96:9311–9316
14. Brunner KT, Mauel J, Cerottini JC et al (1968) Quantitative assay of the lytic action of immune lymphoid cells on 51-Cr-labelled allogeneic target cells in vitro; inhibition by isoantibody and by drugs. Immunology 14:181–196
15. Prussin C, Metcalfe DD (1995) Detection of intracytoplasmic cytokine using flow cytometry and directly conjugated anti-cytokine antibodies. J Immunol Methods 188:117–128
16. Brosi H, Reiser M, Rajasalu T et al (2009) Processing in the endoplasmic reticulum generates an epitope on the insulin A chain that stimulates diabetogenic CD8 T cell responses. J Immunol 183:7187–7195
17. Trudeau JD, Kelly-Smith C, Verchere CB et al (2003) Prediction of spontaneous autoimmune diabetes in NOD mice by quantification of autoreactive T cells in peripheral blood. J Clin Invest 111:217–223
18. Williams AJ, Bingley PJ, Bonifacio E, Palmer JP, Gale EA (1997) A novel micro-assay for insulin autoantibodies. J Autoimmun 10:473–478
19. Naserke HE, Dozio N, Ziegler AG et al (1998) Comparison of a novel micro-assay for insulin autoantibodies with the conventional radiobinding assay. Diabetologia 41:681–683
20. Koczwara K, Schenker M, Schmid S et al (2003) Characterization of antibody responses to endogenous and exogenous antigen in the nonobese diabetic mouse. Clin Immunol 106:155–162
21. Jarchum I, Takaki T, DiLorenzo TP (2008) Efficient culture of CD8(+) T cells from the islets of NOD mice and their use for the study of autoreactive specificities. J Immunol Methods 339:66–73

Chapter 18

Positional Cloning of Diabetes Genes

Gudrun A. Brockmann and Christina Neuschl

Abstract

Several mouse strains are diabetic already at the juvenile age or develop diabetes mellitus during their life. Before these strains become diabetic, they often show several or all features of the metabolic syndrome, which is very similar to the etiology of diabetes in humans. Under the assumption that natural mutations are responsible for the development of diabetes in those mouse strains, they are valuable resources for the identification of diabetes genes and modifiers. Usually, several steps are necessary to detect the causative genes in the genome. These include the initial identification of the genomic regions contributing to the disease which is typically done by linkage mapping in an F_2 intercross or backcross population, fine mapping of the identified chromosomal interval to narrow down the target region carrying the causative genetic variation and subsequent functional and genetic characterization of the target gene or a small subset of genes. Here, we give a general overview on genetic models and the strategy for identifying diabetes genes and provide a specific protocol for the mapping and fine mapping of chromosomal regions carrying diabetes genes.

Key words: Linkage, Fine mapping, Intercross, Advanced intercross populations, Recombinant congenic strains, Recombinant inbred strains, Interaction

1. Introduction

Diabetes in mice is characterized by glucose dysregulation as a result of insulin failure or resistance which is accompanied by several components of the metabolic syndrome before diabetes becomes manifested. The features of the metabolic syndrome leading to diabetes are very similar in mice and human. Therefore, mouse strains that are prone to diabetes can serve as valuable genetic models to identify genes that contribute to high risk for becoming diabetic.

Because the risk for diabetes is a quantitative measure, the single genomic regions that harbor one or a few genes contributing to diabetes are called quantitative trait loci (QTL).

Environmental factors like diet composition or stress can interact directly or indirectly with those genes or gene products and trigger their activity in metabolic or regulatory pathways leading to diabetes. It is assumed that only a few genes are key determinants with major effects on diabetes, while many genes may contribute to diabetes as modifiers that can modulate the major gene actions. Those may enhance the development of diabetes or act protective. In addition to genes that interact with metabolic or environmental factors, we can assume interactions between genes that do not exert effects on diabetes themselves but contribute to a higher risk when interacting with specific alleles at other gene loci as it has been repeatedly shown for obesity (1–4). Furthermore, recent epidemiological data analyses in human populations and experiments in mice (5, 6) have provided evidence for parent-of-origin effects on increased diabetes risk for offspring of diabetic mothers or even fathers (7, 8). All possible gene actions should be considered in experiments that are performed to detect genetic entities contributing to diabetes.

During the past years, some diabetes genes have been found in human populations. Genetic variants associated with type 2 diabetes mellitus that were repeatedly confirmed by several studies are *TCF7L2*, *SLC30A8*, *HHEX*, *PPARG*, *KCNJ11*, and *FTO* (9). However, the significant contributions to understand the genetic determinants for diabetes come from mouse and rat experiments. Well-characterized mouse strains developing type 1 or 2 diabetes mellitus are, e.g., NZO, NOD, NSY, BKS, ThallyHo, LG, and SM (http://phenome.jax.org/). Using these mouse strains, many QTL and a few genes have been identified so far that cause type 1 or 2 diabetes mellitus or protect from it. Crosses with the obese db and ob mouse strains have shown that both mutant genes increase the diabetes risk. All identified mutant diabetes and modifier genes contributed in particular to enlighten our understanding of pathways that directly or indirectly interact with the regulation of glucose homeostasis.

1.1. General Strategy

The strategy for the identification of key diabetes or modifier genes consists of several genetic experiments to first map the regions in the genome where those genes reside, to secondly fine-map the initially identified chromosomal part carrying the target gene to a minimum size and to finally functionally and genetically annotate the gene or genes in the narrowed down fine-mapped region. This strategy has been repeatedly successfully applied, e.g., for the identification of the Rab-GAP *Tbc1d1* (10) and the transcription factor *Zfp69* (11) as genes controlling adiposity and the glucose level in the NZO mouse, which is a polygenic model of severe obesity and type 2 diabetes-like hyperglycemia. These results indicate that the dissection of the genome into single entities is a strong tool for the identification of genes and mechanisms that are relevant for the human disease. In addition, several QTLs were identified in different crossbred populations, for some of them candidate genes have been suggested (12).

The mapping of diabetes or modifier genes is performed in segregating populations of an initial cross between a diabetes-prone and a healthy or diabetes-resistant strain, or with strains that differ extremely in one or several features of the metabolic syndrome. Information about strain characteristics can be obtained from the Mouse Phenome Database, which is maintained by The Jackson Laboratory (Bar Harbor, ME) (http://phenome.jax.org/). This database stores different phenotypes for many inbred mouse strains. For example, sex-specific fasting insulin, glucose, triglyceride and lipid concentrations are given as characteristic factors of the metabolic syndrome for 43 mouse strains on a standard breeding and a high-fat diet (13). Mouse strains that differ extremely in the frequency of diabetes or, e.g., in the fasting glucose or insulin levels (Fig. 1) could be promising parental strains for finding genes contributing to differences in the risk for diabetes.

For the initial mapping of diabetes or modifier genes, we suggest the generation of an F_2 intercross or a backcross population. The frequency of diabetes in the F_1 population shows whether the contributing allele or alleles act in a recessive, dominant or additive manner. If no animal becomes diabetic, the mode of inheritance is very likely recessive. If a recessive mutation shall be identified, a backcross population is advantageous. In this case, the F_1 offspring are crossed back to the diabetes-prone strain that harbors the recessive allele. According to the Mendelian law, the advantage of this backcross population consists in the high proportion of offspring that can be expected to become diabetic, which is up to 50%, while the others are healthy. At this step, it is necessary to mention that the probability of those 50% for becoming diabetic is not 1 because the penetrance of the allele is lower (up to 64% in NZO, for example) and depends often on the degree of adiposity (15).

However, we suggest the generation of an F_2 intercross population with about 300–400 individuals to map diabetes genes and modifiers to specific chromosomal regions. This design allows for the simultaneous detection of recessive, dominant, and additive gene effects and permits the search for gene–gene interactions. For narrowing down the initially identified QTL region, we recommend the construction of recombinant congenic strains (RCS), recombinant inbred strains (RIS), and an advanced intercross line (AIL) (Fig. 2). In all those designs, recombination events in the target QTL region are used to physically dissect QTL haplotypes and to separate neighboring genes.

For constructing RCS, the positive and the negative QTL alleles are transferred to the background genome showing the opposite effect to control the compensatory or enhancing effect of the transferred QTL allele. Simultaneously, not only the whole QTL interval is transferred but also smaller regions of varying length.

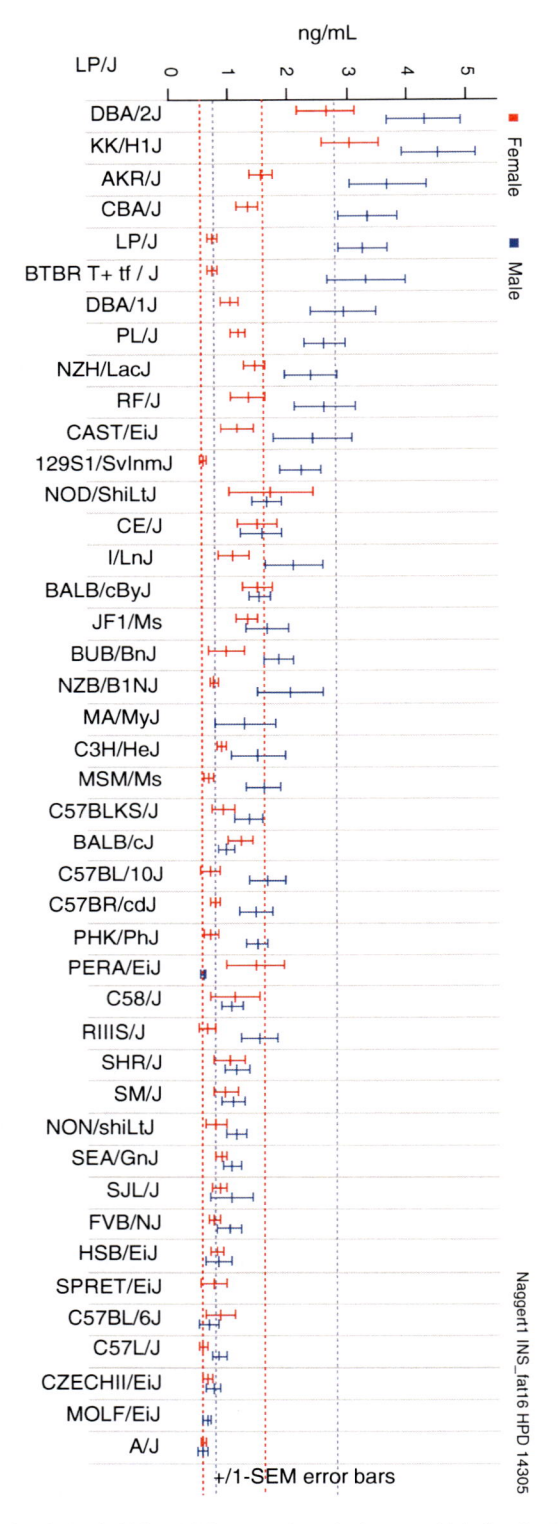

Fig. 1. Insulin levels (ng/mL) in 43 inbred strains of mice on a high-fat diet for 18 weeks. Mice were tested at 25–27 weeks of age. Insulin measurement was performed after a fasting period of 4 h, beginning 1 h after the start of the light cycle (food withheld at 0700 h; blood drawn at 1100 h). Males (*blue*), females (*red*) (13, 14) (*Source*: Mouse Phenome Database (http://phenome.jax.org/)).

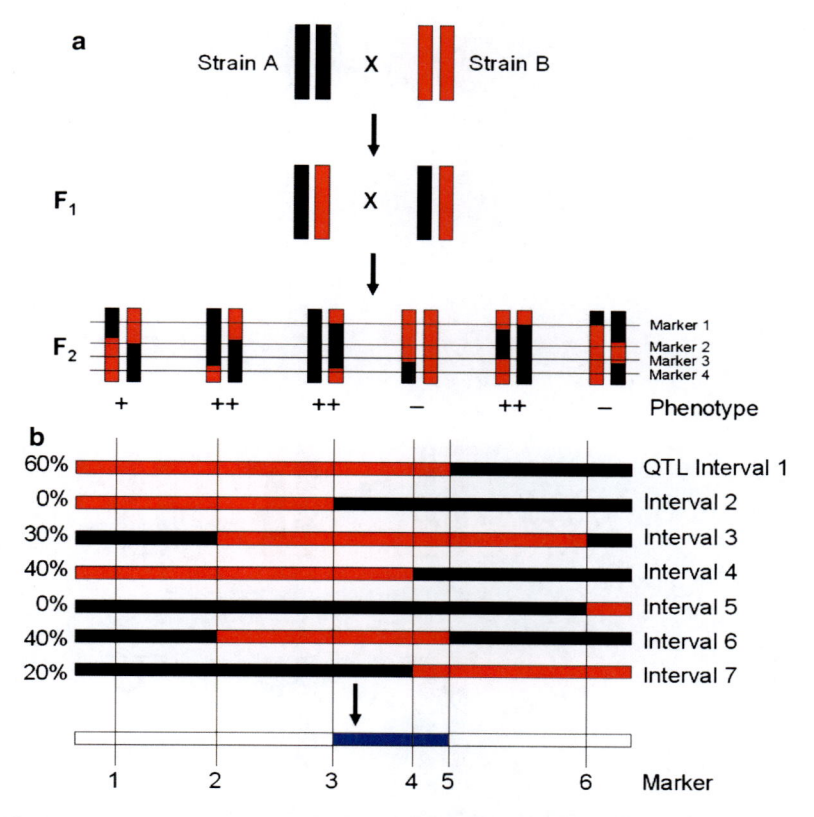

Fig. 2. Sketches for the generation and genomic composition of (a) an F_2 intercross population (F_2), (b) a set of recombinant congenic strains (RCS), (c) a set of recombinant inbred strains (RIS), and (d) an advanced intercross line (AIL). (a) A single pair of homologous chromosomes is shown. Genomic intervals derived from strain A are *black*, intervals derived from strain B are *red*. Using an F_2 intercross design by crossing individuals from two phenotypically and genetically diverse inbred strains, a pedigree has to be generated by repeated mating of the parents and subsequently by repeated matings within subfamilies of pairs of F_1 offspring (full-sib pairings). In the resulting F_2 population consisting of ideally >300 individuals, recombination events (change from *black* to *red* or vice versa) are traced by about 120 genetic markers evenly distributed across the whole murine genome. Each F_2 animal has to be genotyped at these markers and phenotyped for the trait of interest, e.g., diabetes by performing glucose and insulin tolerance tests ("high" phenotype indicated with "++," "medium" with "+" and "low" with "−"). Quantitative trait loci (QTL) mapping programs (e.g., GridQTL or R/qtl) use this information to link the genotypic and phenotypic data to detect chromosomal regions in which animals with the same genotype differ in their phenotype from animals with alternative genotypes. In this scheme, the region around markers 2 and 3 affect the risk for diabetes. Therefore, this region is likely to harbor one or several closely linked causal genes with different alleles in the parental strains. (b) In order to generate RCS, first, a decision has to be made of which QTL allele shall be transferred to which genetic background. Then, an F_2 individual has to be selected that carries the donor QTL interval with the allele that has to be transferred to the recipient inbred strain that carries the alternative QTL allele. In the sketch, a single chromosome is shown with the donor QTL interval derived from strain B (*red*) and the genome of the recipient inbred strain A (*black*). A cross has to be performed between a F_2 individual that carries the QTL-interval of donor strain B and an animal of the recipient strain A. All subsequent crosses are backcrosses to the recipient inbred strain A. At each generation, only those offspring who have received either the whole donor QTL interval or individuals that are recombinant in the QTL interval are selected as a parent for the next generation. Homozygous RCS are obtained ideally after ten generations of repeated backcrossing of mice that carry the whole or recombinant QTL interval. The inheritance of the targeted chromosomal region is traced by genetic markers. A comparison of phenotypes (in this case percentage of

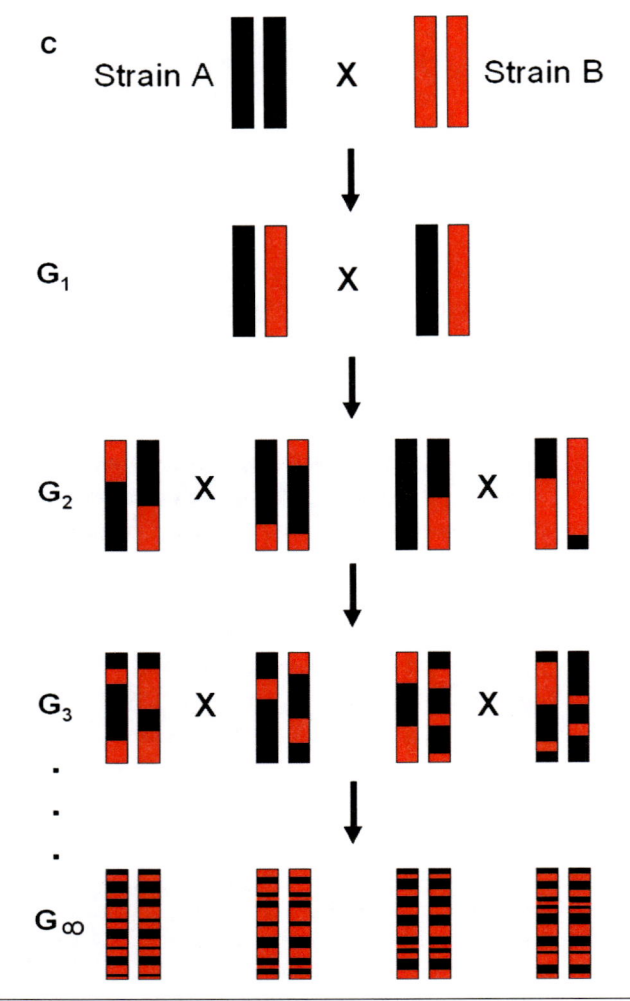

Fig. 2. (continued) diabetic mice (indicated on the *left*)) between the generated RCS harboring QTL intervals of different length provides information on which of the QTL interval is still showing the expected phenotype. This information enables a narrowing down of the candidate region on the chromosome (indicated in *blue*). (**c**) For the generation of RIS, first, a cross between two or several diverse inbred strains has to be performed. In the sketch, two inbred strains were used as founder strains, A (*black*) and B (*red*). In the G_2 generation, animals are not identical anymore due to the segregation and recombination of the alleles from the heterozygous G_1 parents. Each G_2 individual has a unique genotype with some loci homozygous for the allele originating from strain A, some homozygous for strain B and some heterozygous. Pairs of G_2 animals are now randomly chosen (e.g., by using the program RandoMate (20)) as founders for the new inbred strains. The offspring from each G_2 founder pair are maintained separately and mated to produce the next generation. In the subsequent 20 generations, brother–sister matings have to be further performed in order to generate inbred strains. In each G_∞ animal, many recombination events are accumulated resulting in a genetic mosaic of the two parental strains that lead to a RIS with unique genome composition. Each RIS can be expanded into as many animals as required at any time for phenotyping. It is only required to genotype each RIS once. Thus, a comparison of the phenotypes between different RIS enables the fine map (Fig. 2) ping

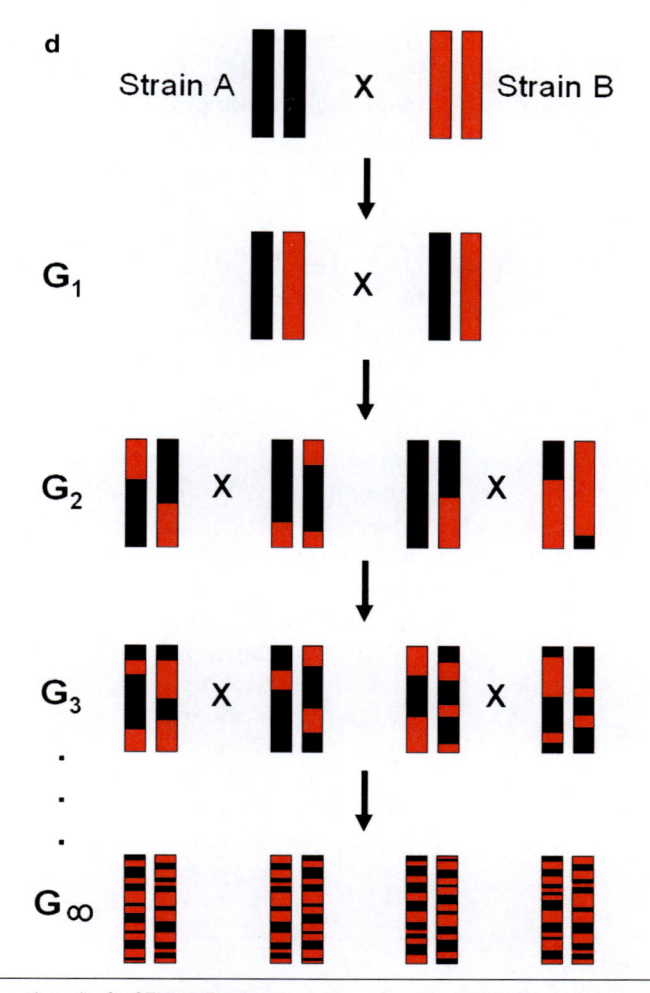

Fig. 2. (continued) of a QTL. (**d**) For the generation of an AIL, an initial F_2 cross as described in (**a**) is randomly crossed over many generations to produce an outcross population. During this process, random recombinations are accumulated in every individual. Thus, after many generations of random mating, a population is produced which consists of individuals that are all heterogeneous and contain a random mix of the parental genomes. Different from the RIS, the AIL individuals are not inbred.

Both the shorter QTL segments and the genomic overlap between those segments narrow-down the chromosomal fragment containing the causative gene or genes. The transfer of QTL alleles onto the opposite genetic background of one of the parental strains is controlled by strain specific marker alleles. This process is named marker-assisted introgression.

RIS are derived from inbreeding of randomly chosen pairs of full sibs from an initial cross between inbred strains. Well-characterized RIS with impact on the development of diabetes are the BXD (16, 17) and LGXSM (18) strain sets. Comprehensive information about the BXD and LGXSM RIS can be found in the

GeneNetwork (http://www.genenetwork.org/) and the Mouse Phenome Database (http://phenome.jax.org/) which store genotypes and phenotypes. An upcoming unique resource of RIS is the Collaborative Cross (CC) (19). This population, which has been generated from eight inbred mouse strains, permits fine mapping with a resolution of up to one single gene. For these CC strains, genotype data and sequence information will be publicly available.

If the QTL effect is large, advanced intercross populations can be used for fine mapping. They are generated by repeated random matings (20) over many subsequent generations. In every generation, additional recombinations are collected. Different from the RCS and RIS, where mouse strains with many identical individuals are being generated, every AIL animal carries a unique genome. In an AIL, imprinting effects can easily be tested by genotyping two subsequent generations, which gives information about the transmission of the paternal allele to the offspring. Evidence for imprinting is provided if the two groups of animals that received one and the same allele either from the mother or from the father differ significantly in their phenotype.

In all fine mapping designs, the overlap of haplotypes and QTL intervals of different length allow the reduction of the QTL region affecting the phenotype. The strategy for fine-mapping is the detection of all recombinations in the target QTL regions and the identification of those subregions that still show the alternative QTL allele effects to finally deduce a short chromosomal interval that ideally carries just one gene or only a few.

2. Materials

2.1. Animals

For genetic studies in diabetes research, the mouse lines used should be extremely different in respect to diabetes or diabetes risk factors. For example, mice that are diabetes-prone or develop features of the metabolic syndrome on the one hand and lines that are resistant on the other hand, are suitable. Such lines could be mouse strains with naturally occurring mutations or artificially modified mutant mouse lines. Information about phenotypes like glucose levels under different conditions, blood lipids, body fat content and more can be found for many mouse inbred strains in the Mouse Phenome Database (http://phenome.jax.org).

2.2. Diets

Some mouse lines develop diabetes on a standard breeding diet, others after challenge with a high fat diet. For experimental studies, the incidence of diabetes can be significantly increased under high fat diet feeding conditions. A standard breeding diet contains about

4.5% crude fat, 22.0% crude protein, 50% nitrogen free extract (starch and sugar), and other components. Such a diet contains about 14 MJ/kg metabolizable energy with 11% of its energy from fat, 36% from protein content, and 53% from carbohydrates. A high-fat diet typically contains 25–40% crude fat with 45–60% of its metabolizable energy from fat, respectively. The animals have ad libitum access to diets and water.

3. Methods

3.1. Generation of an Informative Mapping Population: F_2 Intercross (Fig. 2a)

1. Choose a diabetes-prone mouse strain and a healthy or diabetic-resistant strain.
2. Decide under which challenging conditions (diet, stress) the experiment shall be performed (see Note 1).
3. Decide which phenotypes are important for characterizing diabetes or the metabolic syndrome as precursor for diabetes in your study.
4. Decide if both or one specific sex shall be analyzed.
5. Find genetic markers that have different alleles in the two selected phenotypically diverse mouse strains either by looking up SNP or microsatellite allele information in the Mouse Genome Informatics (MGI) database (http://www.informatics.jax.org/) or by genotyping the parental strains genome-wide with for example SNP chips (21) or sequence analysis.
6. Choose informative markers across the whole genome having alternative alleles between the parental strains. An average distance between genetic markers of approximately 15–20 cM is recommended for a whole genome analysis in an F_2 population (22). This genetic distance refers to about 30–40 Mb in the physical map (23). About 120 markers label all linkage groups in the whole genome in an F_2 population. Chromosome ends should be covered with markers. Information on genetic variants between many mouse strains can be found for example at the MGI platform (http://www.informatics.jax.org) or the Ensembl Database (http://www.ensembl.org).
7. Mate the parental strains to produce F_1 offspring (see Notes 2, 3).
8. Choose random pairs of F_1 males and females and mate them to produce F_2 offspring (see Note 4).
9. If a high number of F_2 offspring has to be produced, same F_1 mating pairs can be mated repeatedly (see Notes 5–7).
10. Take tissue samples of every F_2 individual of the cross for DNA preparation and subsequent genotyping. These are preferably tail, toe, or ear clips.

11. Genotype all F_2 individuals at about 120 markers (from step 6).
12. Measure the phenotypes you are interested in of all F_2 individuals and in a subset of F_1 individuals. The measurements must include covariates like body weight that might influence the risk for becoming diabetic (see Note 8).
13. Check carefully the quality of collected phenotype data. Pay attention to outliers which may be erroneous data entries. Test the phenotypes for normal distribution. Non-normal distributed phenotypes should be transformed to obtain normal distribution.
14. Check carefully the quality of genotypes. Test the deviation of observed from expected genotype frequencies for every marker. Check for double recombinations for each marker position in all individuals. Check if the pedigree specific genetic map is consistent with the expected (public) genetic map. Solve inconsistencies.
15. Perform a linkage analysis using one of the many programs that are well suited for the analysis of crosses between inbred strains, e.g., R/qtl (24) or GridQTL (25, 26).
16. Use the best model for your data analysis which must include all experimental factors that significantly affect diabetes, e.g., sex, direction of cross, subfamily, pup size, number of mating, diet and age if different levels of those factors were used in the experiment, or body weight as a covariate, if body weight is correlated with the occurrence of diabetes.
17. Perform a one QTL scan assuming one QTL in a linkage group.
18. Test the influence of the fixed effects that were included into the model onto the QTL effect.
19. Perform a two QTL scan testing if two different QTLs occur in a linkage group.
20. Test the genetic interaction between different genomic loci.
21. Determine significance thresholds for the tests statistics accounting for multiple testing.
22. Collect peak positions for the test statistics and confidence intervals of the most likely QTL positions.
23. Determine the additive and dominance effects of the peak QTL positions and interacting QTLs.
24. Check the direction of allele effects by drawing effect plots showing the means and standard deviations of the three genotype classes AA, AB, and BB in the F_2 population (Fig. 3).
25. Use the confidence interval of the most significant QTL representing a diabetes predisposing or protecting gene for further fine mapping the target chromosomal region.

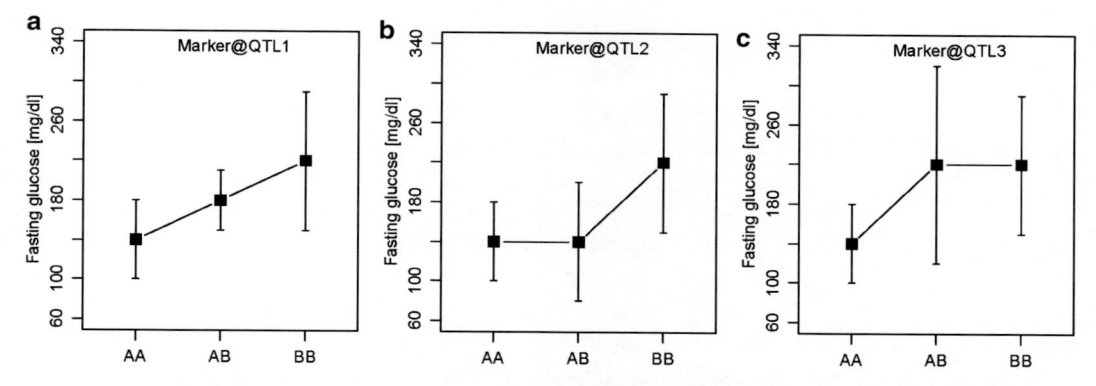

Fig. 3. Effect plots showing additive (a), recessive (b) and dominant (c) effects of the alleles A and B in an F_2 population. Depicted are the means and standard deviations of each of the three genotype classes AA, AB, and BB in an F_2 intercross between the strains A and B. Each plot represents a different QTL with the alleles at the marker position closest to the peak position of the test statistics.

3.2. Fine Mapping by Recombinant Congenic Strains (Fig. 2b)

1. See steps 1–22 in Subheading 3.1.
2. Identify single F_2 individuals that carry the donor QTL interval of interest, i.e., animals that are either homo- or heterozygous for the "high" or "low" allele, depending on which direction of effect you are interested in. In Fig. 2b, the donor "high" QTL allele originates from strain B (red).
3. Cross these individuals back to animals of the recipient inbred strain carrying the opposite QTL allele. In Fig. 2b, A is the recipient strain (black).
4. Follow the inheritance of the QTL interval by genotyping the offspring at the known markers embracing the QTL interval. Select those animals as parents for the next generation that have received the whole donor QTL-allele and all individuals showing recombination between the markers flanking the QTL interval.
5. Backcross these chosen animals to the recipient strain.
6. Follow the inheritance of the transmitted QTL interval by genotyping the offspring at the known markers embracing the QTL interval and choose additional informative markers within the QTL interval to detect further recombination events. Select those animals as parents for the next generation that have received the whole or recombinant donor QTL-allele.
7. Backcross these chosen animals to the recipient strain.
8. Repeat steps 6 and 7.
9. Cross most informative animals carrying interesting recombination break point repeatedly back to the recipient strain. After ten generations, these sub-strains are RIS.

10. You may want to phenotype recombinant animals during the process of generating these RCS to support decisions on most interesting QTL intervals.

11. Depending on the variance of your phenotypes, you should phenotype a certain number of males and/or females of every finished RCS. As phenotypes like fasting serum glucose, insulin concentrations, and responses to the glucose and insulin tolerance tests vary largely among individual mice, we recommend to phenotype at least ten males and/or ten females of each RCS to obtain representative means for every strain and enough power to detect significant differences between QTL intervals (see Notes 6–8).

12. Compare the phenotypes between the RCS harboring different QTL intervals via Analysis of Variance using standard statistical software. Conclude from the results, which narrowed down interval most likely contains the target QTL gene or genes.

3.3. Fine Mapping by Recombinant Inbred Strains (Fig. 2c)

1. See steps 1–8 in Subheading 3.1.
2. Choose brother–sister pairs of G_2 (equivalent to F_2) animals as founders for the new inbred strains.
3. Maintain the offspring from each G_2 founder pair separately and mate them brother × sister to produce the next generation.
4. Repeat full sib mating until the 20th generation. The generation of RIS takes 4–5 years, if four to five generations are produced per year.
5. Enlarge the size of each generated RIS as required for phenotyping.
6. Choose at least 25 strains of a set of RIS to fine-map your region of interest. Phenotype about ten males and females per strain (see step 11 in Subheading 3.2) (see Notes 6–8).
7. Check if dense marker information is publicly available. If so, you do not need to genotype the population. If not, choose genetic markers with a distance of about 1 Mb in your target QTL interval or across the whole genome and genotype one animal of each RIS at those markers.
8. Perform an association analysis between genotypes and phenotypes of the RIS using standard software to identify the most likely narrow QTL-region.

3.4. Fine Mapping by Advanced Intercross Lines

1. See steps 1–8 in Subheading 3.1.
2. Choose pairs of G_2 (equivalent to F_2) animals randomly as founders for the generation of the AIL.
3. Create a random mating scheme for the F_2 and every subsequent generation by using the program RandoMate (20) (http://www2.hu-berlin.de/wikizbnutztier/software/software_start.php) which avoids brother–sister pairing (see Note 9).

4. Following the suggestion of Darvasi and Soller (27), at least 50 different breeding pairs have to be used in each generation to ensure an effective population size of 100.

5. Repeat step 3 until the tenth generation or higher but try to enlarge the population size at each generation in order to get as many as non-directly-related (brothers and sisters) individuals as possible in the tenth generation or higher.

6. Measure the phenotypes you are interested in of all generated F_{10} or higher individuals (>400) (see Notes 6–8).

7. See step 6 in Subheading 3.1, but choose genetic markers with a distance of about 1 Mb or below either for your target QTL interval or across the whole genome.

8. Genotype all F_{10} or higher animals at these chosen markers.

9. Perform an association analysis between genotypes and phenotypes of the analyzed AIL generation using standard software. Consider hidden population substructures by identifying them using, e.g., GRAIP (28).

3.5. Conclusions

All above mentioned structured genetic models have contributed to map and fine-map obesity and diabetes-related genetic variation. Information on mapped QTLs can be found at the Mouse Genome Database. The positional candidate genes in the narrowed down interval are subject to further functional studies and mutation screens. Criteria for the further selection of the most likely candidate gene include the study of the gene expression in the tissues of interest in the parental, RCS, RIS or AIL animals, the density of non-synonymous SNPs and the occurrence of insertions and deletions within candidate genes present between the parental strains that were initially crossed to detect QTLs, potential functional changes in the protein as a consequence of the detected DNA variants, and lastly, the biological relevance of the most likely candidate gene with respect to effects on diabetes traits.

The physical dissection of the QTL together with subsequent in depth gene analyses led to the discovery of important diabetes or modifier genes like *Tbc1d1* and *Zfp69*. Additional naturally mutated genes like *Lep* and *Lepr* were identified that contribute to metabolic dysregulation and thus to increased risk for diabetes. These successful discoveries serve as proof of principle for the outlined strategy.

4. Notes

1. Fix the environmental conditions for husbandry during the whole experimental period (temperature, number of animals per cage, diet).

2. Note which parents gave birth to which F_1 offspring.
  3. Note the direction of cross, which could be either A×B or B×A with the father coming from the one or other strain and the mother coming from the opposite strain.
  4. Note which F_1 parents gave birth to which F_2 offspring, designate subfamily identifiers.
  5. Note the number of mating.
  6. Note the pup size.
  7. Note the number of animals per cage.
  8. Note which person measures which phenotype to account for subjective differences.
  9. Special Software

     RandoMate online tool: http://www2.hu-berlin.de/wikizbnutztier/software/software_start.php (20).

Acknowledgement

The project was supported by the National Genome Research Network (NGFNplus 01GS0829) and the German Research Foundation (DFG GRK 1208).

References

1. Brockmann GA, Kratzsch J, Haley CS et al (2000) Single QTL effects, epistasis, and pleiotropy account for two thirds of the phenotypic F_2 variance of growth and obesity in DU6i x DBA/2 mice. Genome Res 10:1941–1957
2. Brockmann GA, Tsaih S, Neuschl C et al (2009) Genetic factors contributing to obesity and body weight can act through mechanisms affecting muscle weight, fat weight or both. Physiol Genomics 36:114–126
3. Carlborg Ö, Brockmann GA, Haley C (2005) Simultaneous mapping of epistatic QTL in DU6i x DBA/2. Mamm Genome 16:481–494
4. Stylianou IM, Korstanje R, Li R et al (2006) Quantitative trait locus analysis for obesity reveals multiple networks of interacting loci. Mamm Genome 17:22–36
5. Reifsnyder PC, Churchill G, Leiter EH (2000) Maternal environment and genotype interact to establish diabesity in mice. Genome Res 10:1568–1578
6. Jarvis JP, Kenney-Hunt J, Ehrich TH et al (2005) Maternal genotype affects adult offspring lipid, obesity, and diabetes phenotypes in LGXSM recombinant inbred strains. J Lipid Res 46:1692–1702
7. Abbasi A, Corpeleijn E, van der Schouw YT et al (2011) Maternal and paternal transmission of type 2 diabetes: influence of diet, lifestyle and adiposity. J Intern Med 270: 388–396
8. Penesova A, Bunt JC, Bogardus C et al (2010) Effect of paternal diabetes on pre-diabetic phenotypes in adult offspring. Diabetes Care 33:1823–1828
9. Zeggini E, Scott LJ, Saxena R et al (2008) Meta-analysis of genome-wide association data and large-scale replication identifies additional susceptibility loci for type 2 diabetes. Nat Genet 40:638–645
10. Chadt A, Leicht K, Deshmukh A et al (2008) Tbc1d1 mutation in lean mouse strain confers leanness and protects from diet-induced obesity. Nat Genet 40:1354–1359
11. Scherneck S, Nestler M, Vogel H et al (2009) Positional cloning of zinc finger doma in transcription factor Zfp69, a candidate gene for

obesity-associated diabetes contributed by mouse locus Nidd/SJL. PLoS Genet 5:e1000541

12. Schmidt C, Gonzaludo NP, Strunk S et al (2008) A metaanalysis of QTL for diabetes related traits in rodents. Physiol Genomics 34:42–53

13. Svenson KL, von Smith R, Magnani PA et al (2007) Multiple trait measurements in 43 inbred mouse strains capture the phenotypic diversity characteristic of human populations. J Appl Physiol 102:2369–2378

14. Naggert J, Svenson KL, Smith RV et al (2011) Diet effects on bone mineral density and content, body composition, and plasma glucose, leptin, and insulin levels in 43 inbred strains of mice on a high-fat atherogenic diet. MPD:Naggert1. Mouse Phenome Database web site, The Jackson Laboratory, Bar Harbor. http://phenome.jax.org. Accessed June 2011

15. Plum L, Kluge R, Giesen K et al (2000) Type 2 diabetes-like hyperglycemia in a backcross model of NZO and SJL mice: characterization of a susceptibility locus on chromosome 4 and its relation with obesity. Diabetes 49:1590–1596

16. Peirce JL, Lu L, Gu J et al (2004) A new set of BXD recombinant inbred lines from advanced intercross populations in mice. BMC Genet 5:7

17. Taylor BA (1989) Recombinant inbred strains. In: Lyon ML (ed) Genetic variation in the laboratory mouse, 2nd edn. Oxford University Press, Oxford, pp 773–796

18. Hrbek T, de Brito RA, Wang B et al (2006) Genetic characterization of a new set of recombinant inbred lines (LGXSM) formed from the intercross of SM/J and LG/J inbred mouse strains. Mamm Genome 17:417–429

19. Churchill GA; The Complex Trait Consortium (2004) The collaborative cross, a community resource for the genetic analysis of complex traits. Nat Genet 36:1133–1137

20. Schmitt A, Bortfeldt R, Neuschl C et al (2009) RandoMate: a program for the generation of random mating schemes for small laboratory animals. Mamm Genome 20:321–325

21. Yang H, Ding Y, Hutchins LN et al (2009) A customized and versatile high-density genotyping array for the mouse. Nat Methods 6:663–666

22. Liu BH (1998) Multi-locus models, marker coverage and map density. In: Liu BH (ed) Statistical genomics—linkage, mapping, and QTL analysis. CRC Press, Boca Raton, pp 345–358

23. Cox A, Dumont BL, Ding Y et al (2009) A new standard genetic map for the laboratory mouse. Genetics 182:1335–1344

24. Broman KW, Wu H, Sen S et al (2003) R/qtl: QTL mapping in experimental crosses. Bioinformatics 19:889–890

25. Seaton G, Haley CS, Knott SA et al (2002) QTL express: mapping quantitative trait loci in simple and complex pedigrees. Bioinformatics 18:339–340

26. Seaton G, Hernandez J, Grunchec JA et al (2006) GridQTL: a grid portal for QTL mapping of compute intensive datasets. In: Proceedings of the 8th world congress on genetics applied to livestock production, Belo Horizonte, 13–18 Aug 2006

27. Darvasi A, Soller M (1995) Advanced intercross lines, an experimental population for fine genetic mapping. Genetics 141:1199–1207

28. Peirce JL, Broman KW, Lu L et al (2008) Genome Reshuffling for Advanced Intercross Permutation (GRAIP): simulation and permutation for advanced intercross population analysis. PLoS One 3:e1977

Chapter 19

Retinal Digest Preparation: A Method to Study Diabetic Retinopathy

Nadine Dietrich and Hans-Peter Hammes

Abstract

Retinal digestion is a commonly used method for studying experimental diabetic retinopathy in animal models. The method allows to assess qualitatively and quantitatively the morphology of the retinal vasculature, including characteristics of endothelial cells and pericytes. The digestion method uses the enzyme trypsin and enables the precise evaluation of venolar and arteriolar diameters, endothelial cell and pericyte numbers, and the formation of acellular capillaries.

Key words: Eye, Retina, Retinal vasculature, Acellular capillaries, Endothelial cell, Pericyte, Diabetic retinopathy, Digestion, Trypsin, Morphometry

1. Introduction

The characteristics of diabetic retinopathy are (1) increased vascular permeability, (2) loss of pericytes, and (3) acellular capillary formation. Pericyte loss begins at 2 months of diabetes and increases (in diabetic rat retina stronger than in mouse retina) with disease duration (1). Persistent hyperglycemia induces the additional loss of endothelial cells which causes capillaries to occlude. The formation of these acellular capillaries is the critical quantitative lesion that represents the most typical alteration in a diabetic retina, and the origin of retinal ischemia. Acellular capillaries start to become increased in specific strains of diabetic rats and mice at 4 months, but are most commonly analyzed at 6 months of disease duration (1–3). However, rodents may differ in their propensity to develop acellular capillaries, most likely because of genetic differences (2).

The technique to display the morphology and morphometry of the retinal vasculature is the retinal digest preparation, by which retinal cells are digested away using trypsin leaving the vasculature behind. Originally, different digest mixtures were used for the digest of rodent retinae, i.e., a combination of pepsin and trypsin (4). Pepsin's digestion properties are usually faster and stronger compared with trypsin. However, the advantage of pepsin is also the biggest disadvantage as vessels can be overdigested when a combination is used. On the other hand, using a combination of pepsin/trypsin may result in only partially digested retinae when exposure and concentrations are underused. Additionally, companies providing both chemicals have improved purification and activity of enzyme preparations. The retina contains little trypsin-resistant collagen and is therefore very easy to digest (5). We therefore developed a digestion protocol using trypsin only, in particular, for rat and mouse retinae. After culture dish exposure of the retina to the digestion solution, it is transferred to a glass slide and neuroglial cells are eliminated physical forces (dropping distilled water on the retina). The remaining vasculature is visualized using PAS staining, based on the abundance of mucopolysaccharides in the vessel walls of the retina.

2. Materials

Instruments
Stereomicroscope (×1 and ×2 magnification), cold light supply, incubator (37°C), electric pump, flexible infusion tube, culture dishes (35 × 10 mm and 60 × 15 mm), 5 mL syringe, 22G and 25G needles, fine forceps (e.g., Dumont No. 3 or No. 5), VANNAS scissors, fine spatula, aspirator, liquid blocker (e.g., Pap Pen), glass cuvettes, uncoated glass slides, and coverslips (Fig. 1).

2.1. Fixation

Caution! Formalin is toxic and it is necessary to work with a hood! 4% Formalin (phosphate buffered saline (PBS)): fill 100 mL PBS 10× (from company) in a 1 L graduated glass cylinder, add 100 mL of 37% formalin and fill up to 1 L with Aqua bidest.
The fixation solution can be stored at room temperature in a glass bottle indefinitely.

2.2. Retina Isolation

For the isolation of the retina, PBS 1× is needed. Dilute 10× PBS 1:10 with Aqua bidest.

2.3. Retina Digestion

1. Aqua bidest.
2. 0.2 M Tris–HCl, pH 7.45: dissolve 24.22 g Tris base in 500 mL Aqua bidest. Adjust pH to 7.45 with HCl, then fill up to 1 L

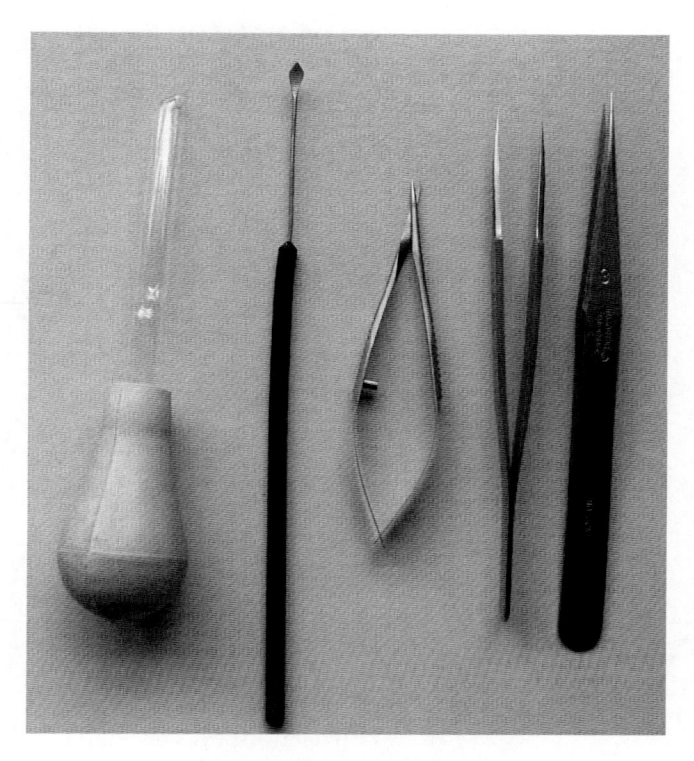

Fig. 1. Needed instruments for retina isolation. From *left to right*: Aspirator, spatula, scissors, two forceps.

with Aqua bidest, and check pH again. The solution can be stored at room temperature (see Note 1).

3. 3% Trypsin in 0.2 M Tris–HCl, pH 7.45. Prepare the solution fresh on the day of digestion.

2.4. PAS Staining

1. Aqua bidest.
2. Schiff's fuchsine-sulfite reagent (ready-to-use). Repetitive use (up to three times) possible.
3. 1% Periodic acid: for 200 mL final reagent, dissolve 2 g periodic acid in 20 mL Aqua bidest and fill up to 200 mL with 96% ethanol (see Note 2).

The solution is stored at 4°C and is used up to three times.

4. Mayer's hemalum solution 1:2 diluted with Aqua bidest. Store the solution at 4°C and filtrate (folded filters) it before use. Solution is used three to five times.
5. 70, 80, 96, and 100% ethanol.
6. Xylene.
7. Mounting medium based on xylene, e.g., Eukitt® or Depex®.

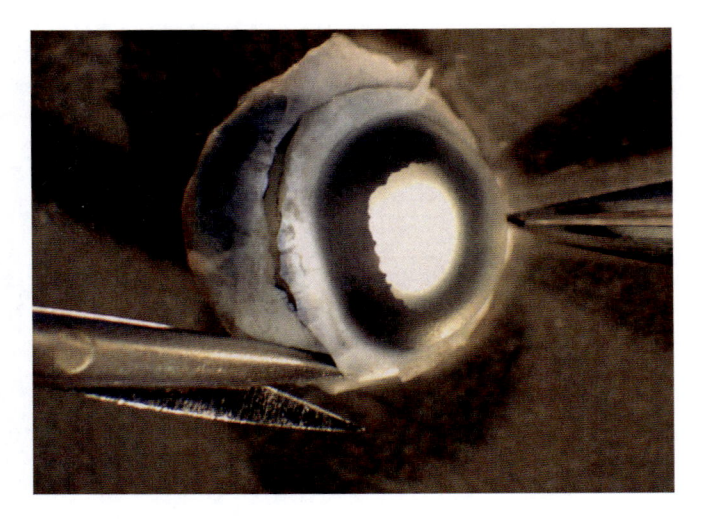

Fig. 2. Fixation and incision of the eye ball.

3. Methods

3.1. Fixation

After enucleation, eyes are fixed in 4% formalin for a minimum of 2 days at room temperature (see Note 3).

3.2. Retina Isolation

1. Wash the eye once in 1× PBS, and place the eye in a 35 mm culture dish under a stereomicroscope. The bulb should be covered with 1× PBS to avoid drying out during the retina isolation procedure (see Note 4).

2. Fix the eye with the forceps and cut with the scissors along the ora serrata. The cutting line is light gray in mice and rats with dark fur and white in albino mice and rats. It marks the border between retina and ciliary body (Fig. 2) (see Note 5).

3. Remove the cornea and the ciliary body. Occasionally, the lens will adhere to the eye cup. Remove the lens carefully using forceps, and allow the vitreous to become removed (see Note 6). Remaining parts of the ciliary body at the edge of the eye cup ought to be removed because retina may adhere and could be destroyed during subsequent preparations (Fig. 3).

4. Insert the small spatula between pigment epithelium and retina and split carefully around the eye cup, until the entire retina is removable. Dissect retina from optic nerve using the spatula as a scalpel. Caution! The retina is fragile! (Fig. 4) (see Note 7).

5. The retina is immersed in 4% formalin until digestion. From this step onward, use the aspirator to avoid rupture of the retina (Fig. 5) (see Note 8).

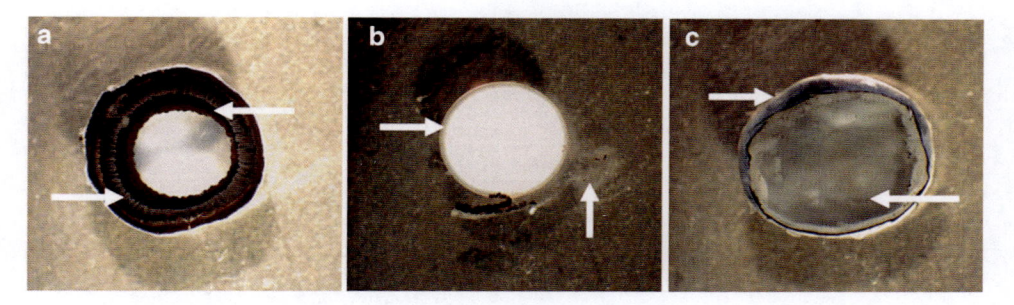

Fig. 3. Parts of the eye at various stages of preparation: (**a**) rear view of the cornea after dissection from the posterior globe. *Upper arrow*: iris, *lower arrow*: ciliary body. (**b**) Lens and vitreous after dissection. *Upper arrow*: lens, *lower arrow*: vitreous/membrane. (**c**) Posterior globe after dissection. *Upper arrow*: pigment epithelium, *lower arrow*: retinal surface.

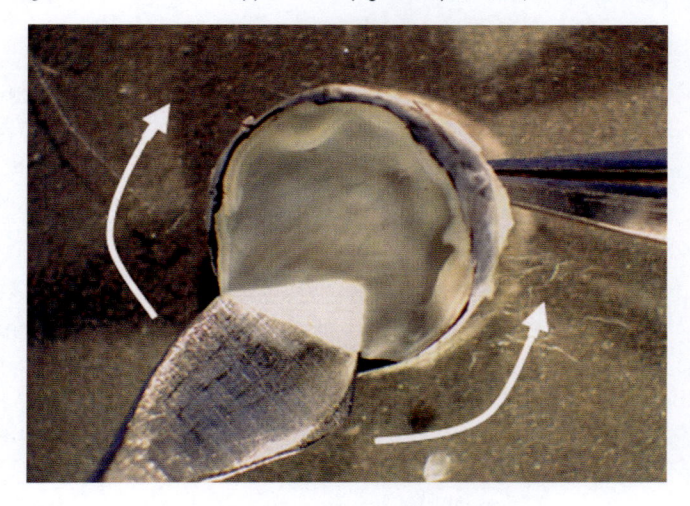

Fig. 4. Spatula between retinal pigment epithelium (*below*) and retina (*above*).

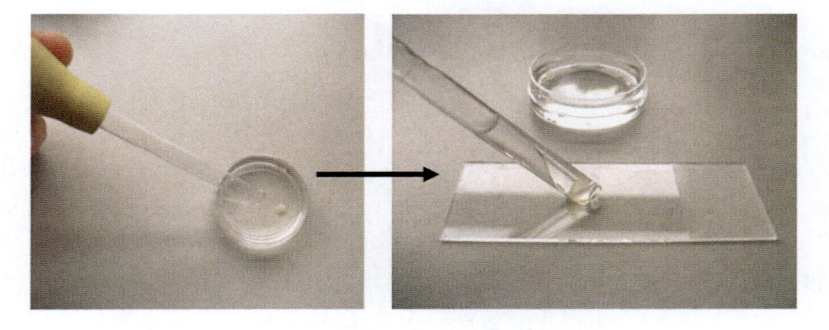

Fig. 5. How to use the aspirator: aspire the retina for transfer.

3.3. Retinal Digestion

1. Fill a 35 mm culture dish with aqua bidest and place the retina using the aspirator. Discard aqua bidest to remove formalin. Measures of precaution to keep the retina in the dish are summarized in Note 9. Refill the dish with aqua bidest. The retina should be entirely covered. Incubate at 37°C for 1 h.

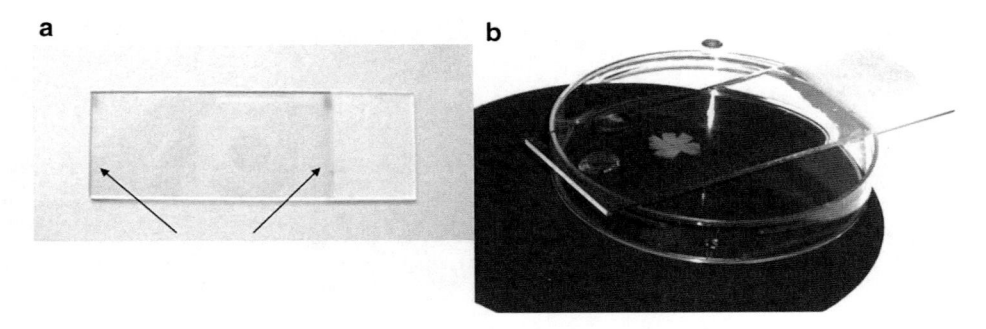

Fig. 6. (a) *Arrows*: PAP pen marks. (b) Equipment: glass slide on 60 mm culture dish.

2. Substitute the Aqua bidest with 3% Trypsin and put the dish back to 37°C. Trypsin exposure at this step is highly variable due to species, strain, and disease conditions. Usually, rat retina digestion occurs faster than mouse retina digestion.

3. Hourly inspection of the digestion progress under the stereomicroscope is mandatory! After 1–2 h, the vitreous/membrane (if still in place) scales off. Careful removal at the optic nerve disc using scissors is essential (see Note 6). At this point, "shamrock" incision is performed for flattening of the retina during on-glass-slide preparation (see Note 10). Incubation at 37°C progresses thereafter.

4. While waiting for the right time point, prepare your instruments:

   Connect the infusion tube on one side with a pump, preferably with a glass bottle for waste disposal interconnected, and with a 22G needle for aspiration on the other side. Fill fresh aqua bidest in a beaker, charge the 5 mL syringe, and attach the 25G needle.

   Needles are reshaped for better handling (Fig. 7).

5. The adequate time point for transfer from the digestion bath to the glass slide is given, when you observe the following changes:

   (a) The cell composition of the retina changes and tissue fragments can be located at the bottom of the dish.

   or

   (b) The retina is flattening (see Note 11).

6. Prepare the glass slide by applying two barrier lines with the PAP pen on each short side and place the slide on a 60 mm culture dish under the stereomicroscope (Fig. 6) (see Note 12).

7. Cover the slide with aqua bidest using the syringe, transfer the retina to the slide with an upside down orientation using the aspirator (photoreceptor layer up, ganglion cell layer down) (see Note 13).

19 Retinal Digests   297

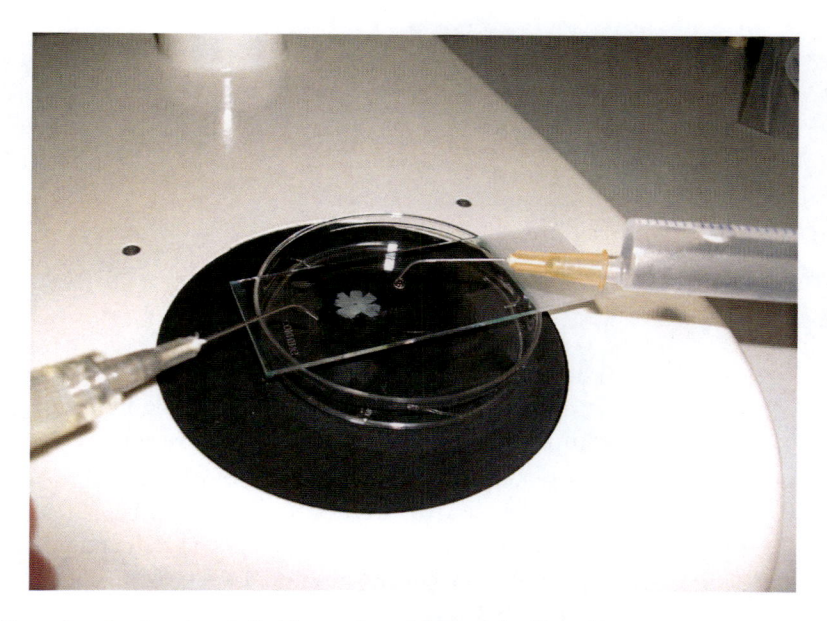

Fig. 7. *Right side*: syringe for dropping. *Left side*: needle on infusion tube for sucking.

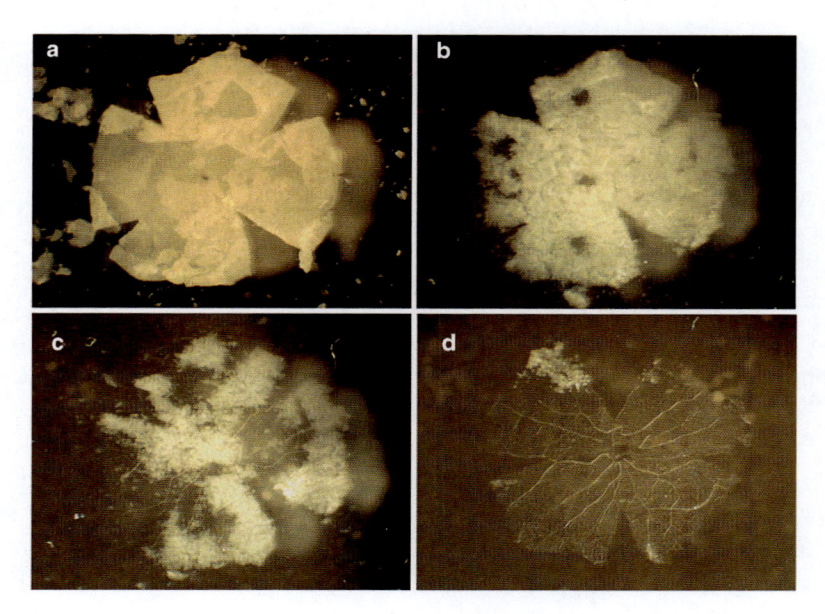

Fig. 8. (**a**) Photoreceptor layer disappear. (**b**, **c**) Smaller parts leaving the vasculature. (**d**) Cleared vasculature with one small indigestible part (*top left*).

8. Clear the vasculature from the cells through dropping aqua bidest with the syringe on the retina, while eliminating the disintegrating neuroglial cells away at the same time through water aspiration (see Note 14). This step must be carefully monitored under the stereomicroscope (Fig. 7).

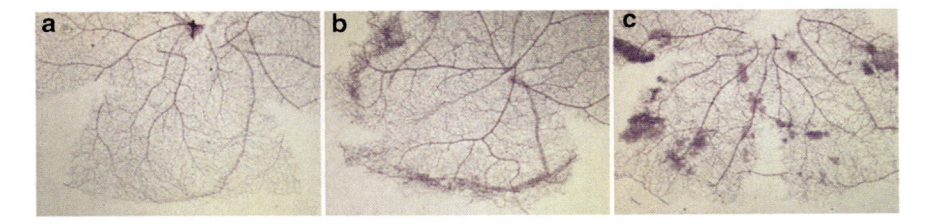

Fig. 9. Risk of producing artifacts (a) Normal leave. (b) Folded leave. (c) Leave with artifacts.

The first layer that disintegrates is the photoreceptor layer. Usually, it can be removed in large fragments (Fig. 8a). Other retinal layers cells disintegrate (Fig. 8b–d) (see Note 15).

With progressing digestion, the retina becomes adhesive to the glass slide and to dissecting instruments. Thus, it is strongly recommended to avoid contact of the retinal digests with forceps or needles! Any other material such as dust or hair also easily contaminates the preparations.

9. Wash digests repetitively! Remaining cell(s) aggregates may reattach to the isolated vasculature and cause artifacts during the drying process, even when distant to the sample.

Sometimes, parts of the retina resist to digestions (Figs. 8d and 9c) In this case, leave the undigested parts as injury or destruction of the retinal digest may occur.

10. Eliminate as much solution as possible by aspiration and air-dry the vasculature while carefully monitoring the specimen under a normal microscope. The four leaves must be completely spread (they should not fold) (Fig. 9a, b) (see Note 16).

3.4. PAS Staining

Fixation following the digestion procedure is unnecessary. Perform staining using glass cuvettes.

1. 1% Periodic acid: 15 min.
2. Wash briefly in Aqua bidest.
3. Schiff's fuchsine-sulfite reagent: 15 min.
4. Tap water (no Aqua bidest) until digests turn pink (~2 min).
   At this step, lukewarm tap water is used instead of flowing water.
5. Wash briefly in Aqua bidest.
6. Mayer's hemalum solution: 30 s (fresh solution) to 2 min (often used solution).
7. Tap water (no Aqua bidest) until digests turn blue (~2 min).
   Again, lukewarm tap water is used instead of flowing water.
8. Wash briefly in Aqua bidest.
9. 70% Ethanol: 1 min.
10. 80% Ethanol: 1 min.

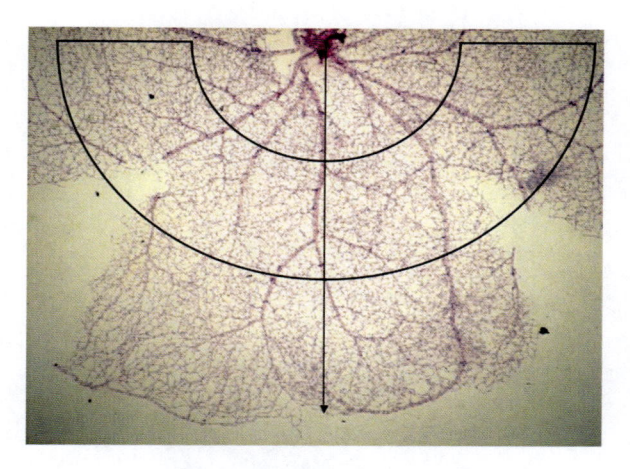

Fig. 10. Area of interest in which acellular capillaries are determined.

11. 96% Ethanol: 5 min.
12. 100% Ethanol: 5 min.
13. Xylene 5 min.
14. Xylene 5 min.
15. Mounting medium.

3.5. Quantification

We use a microscope and Cell-F software (Olympus Opticals, Hamburg, Germany).

For the quantification of acellular capillaries, we use an integration ocular and count segments of acellular capillaries in ten randomly selected fields within the intermediate circular segment of the retina (see Fig. 10 for localization).

The cell numbers are normalized to square millimeter of capillary area (AC/mm² cap. area) (Fig. 11).

Pericytes and endothelial cells are identified by shape of the nuclei and their localization in relation to the capillaries (Fig. 12) (6).

Cells are counted in ten randomly selected areas in a circular area of the intermediate third of the retina under ×400 magnification. The cell numbers are calculated relative to the retinal capillary area and expressed as numbers per square millimeter of capillary area (cells/mm² cap. area) (7).

4. Notes

1. It is possible to use Tris–HCl instead of Tris base and adjust the pH with NaOH. The solution sometimes forms a precipitate, which can be ignored. Exclude bacterial or fungal contamination!

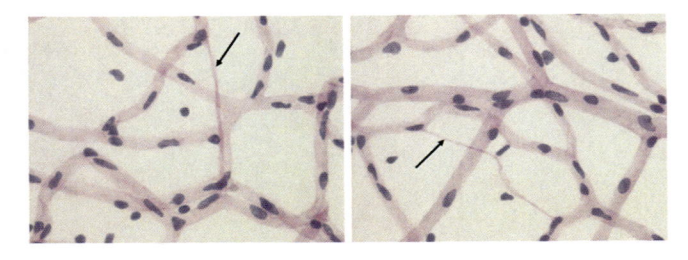

Fig. 11. Retinal digest preparation of diabetic rat. *Arrows* indicate acellular capillaries.

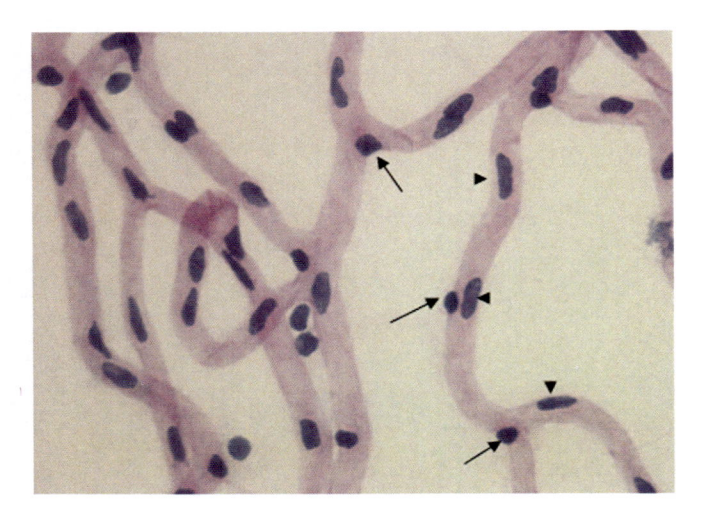

Fig. 12. Retinal digest preparation of a normal rat retina. *Arrows*: Pericytes with round shape and dark staining. *Arrowheads*: Endothelial cells with oval shape and lighter staining.

2. The periodic acid must be completely dissolved in Aqua bidest before adding 96% ethanol.
3. The minimum fixation time is 48 h. There is no maximum fixation time, since eyes which were stored for months in 4% formalin are still digestible and give good morphological results. Adjusting in the digestion period may be necessary. Eyes frozen in liquid nitrogen and stored at −80°C are transferred to 4% formalin and can be digested after 48 h.
4. PBS immersion is only necessary when inexperienced and slow in manipulating.
5. Never hold the entire eye between forceps. Inadequate pressure will cause impression of the lens onto the retina and subsequent damage or destruction! Use extraocular structures to hold the eye.
6. After fixation, the vitreous appears as a fine membrane. Occasionally, the vitreous is removed together with the lens. If not, there are two alternatives:

(a) The vitreous can be removed by soft traction; the risk of loosing the larger vessels is high if traction is too strong. Central adhesion (optic disc) can be released by careful incision. Larger defects increase the risk of total destruction during subsequent manipulation. However, if separation in the periphery between vitreous and retina is unsuccessful, go immediately to step (b).

(b) Let the vitreous come off during the digestion procedure (see step 3 in 3.3 digestion).

In mouse eyes, the lens "falls out" by itself and the vitreous cannot be identified. It is thus impossible to remove it before digestion. In rat eyes, the lens usually adheres to the corneal part and the vitreous can be removed or it adheres to the lens.

Removal of the vitreous is mandatory because vessel remnants may potentially interfere with the morphometry procedure.

7. Residual large pigment epithelium remnants can be removed by careful use of forceps. Small pieces will come off during the digestion procedure.

8. Never use forceps to transfer the retina! Always use the aspirator (see Figs. 1 and 5)!

9. While removing dispensable solution from the culture dish, make sure that the retina sticks to the rim. For waste disposal, use a beaker, so that the inadvertent misplaced retinae can be rescued with the aspirator.

10. Incisions should be limited to two-third of the retina' radius towards the disc. Otherwise, the risk of destruction is high during the digestion procedure.

11. From our experiences rat retinas need 2–6 h and mouse retinas 4–10 h. If there is nothing happening after 12 h, then a digestion is not possible.

12. Use 60 mm culture dish as slide carrier to avoid the loss of the retinal sample. When the retina is rinsed on the slide, it occasionally flows off. Rescue is possible if it flows into the culture dish, but impossible if it would be inserted between glass slide and microscope plate.

13. If digestion is too extensive at this point, the retina will completely disintegrate.

14. Be careful to use gentle drops rather than high flow to avoid holes in the vasculature.

When using a minipump to remove waste solution around the digest, avoid close contact.

15. If only the photoreceptors can be loosened, but no other layers, transfer the retina back to trypsin, incubate it for 1 h and try

again. As long as there is no part with "free" vessels, the procedure can be repeated.

16. Retinal leaves tend to move towards the retinal center. The vasculature will fold and be insufficiently spread quantitative analysis (e.g., see Fig. 9b). If the vessel net has dried out, correction is no longer possible. If the vessel net is still wet, you can try to spread it again with Aqua bidest.

References

1. Hammes HP, Lin J, Wagner P et al (2004) Angiopoietin-2 causes pericyte dropout in the normal retina: evidence for involvement in diabetic retinopathy. Diabetes 53:1104–1110
2. Kern TS, Miller CM, Tang J, Du Y, Ball SL, Berti-Matera L (2010) Comparison of three strains of diabetic rats with respect to the rate at which retinopathy and tactile allodynia develop. Mol Vis 16:1629–1639
3. Hammes HP, Federoff HJ, Brownlee M (1995) Nerve growth factor prevents both neuroretinal programmed cell death and capillary pathology in experimental diabetes. Mol Med 1:527–534
4. Buscher C, Weis A, Wohrle M, Bretzel RG, Cohen AM, Federlin K (1989) Islet transplantation in experimental diabetes of the rat: XII. Effect on diabetic retinopathy. Morphological findings and morphometrical evaluation. Horm Metab Res 21:227–231
5. Cogan DG, Kuwabara T (1984) Comparison of retinal and cerebral vasculature in trypsin digest preparations. Br J Ophthalmol 68: 10–12
6. Feng Y, Pfister F, Schreiter K et al (2008) Angiopoietin-2 deficiency decelerates age-dependent vascular changes in the mouse retina. Cell Physiol Biochem 21:129–136
7. Wang Q, Gorbey S, Pfister F et al (2011) Long-term treatment with suberythropoietic Epo is vaso- and neuroprotective in experimental diabetic retinopathy. Cell Physiol Biochem 27: 769–782

Chapter 20

Lineage Tracing of Pancreatic Stem Cells and Beta Cell Regeneration

Isabelle Houbracken, Iris Mathijs, and Luc Bouwens

Abstract

Restoring a functional β cell mass in diabetes patients by β cell transplantation or stimulation of β cell regeneration are promising approaches. It requires knowledge on the mechanisms of β cell neogenesis, an issue that is still quite controversial. Postnatal islet regeneration may or may not depend on an influx of new islet cells from adult progenitors. To solve this issue in animal models, genetic lineage tracing has become a crucial research method. This method allows to test the various hypotheses that have been proposed concerning β cell neogenesis and regeneration.

Key words: Pancreas, Lineage tracing, Islet neogenesis, Progenitor cells, Diabetes, Regeneration, β Cells, Cre recombinase, X-gal

1. Introduction

Diabetes researchers have always shown a lot of interest in the possibility to regenerate pancreatic β cells. Restoration of a functional β cell mass by cell transplantation from cadaveric organ donors was shown to restore glycaemic and metabolic control in Type 1 diabetes (T1D) patients (1–5). However, this therapeutic approach is hampered by insufficient supply of donor organs. Regeneration of endogenous β cells can represent a new therapeutic modality that is independent of transplantation or organ supply and is a potential target for pharmaceutical interventions. Moreover, Type 2 diabetes (T2D) patients, which represent the largest number of diabetes patients, may also benefit from regenerative therapy as there is evidence for a reduction in the β cell mass in T2D (6, 7).

As it will be discussed in this review, many studies have given compelling evidence that the β cell mass, at least in rodents, has regenerative capacity. Different cellular sources and mechanisms have been proposed, and in some cases shown to cause regeneration.

However, despite many research efforts it remains unclear whether adult stem cells reside in postnatal pancreas and to what extent they participate to β cell regeneration. As a new tool, genetic lineage tracing studies are now shedding light on a controversial issue.

2. Experimental Models for Beta Cell Regeneration

It is important to first consider the various existing experimental models to study regeneration. Mechanisms and cellular sources of regeneration can vary for different forms or extent of injury. Multiple experimental injury models may therefore be needed to consider the different mechanisms, key cells, and signals involved.

β Cell regeneration has been studied in different experimental models in rodents; they can be subdivided according to the nature and extent of tissue injury that is inflicted surgically, chemically, or genetically. First, there are models of general injury to the pancreatic tissue, namely partial pancreatectomy (Ppx), which can be performed to different extent, e.g., 50/70/95 %, and pancreatic duct ligation (PDL). After Ppx, the pancreas does not show the same extent of regeneration as is seen for example in the liver that completely restores its original organ volume. Nevertheless, a partial restoration of the β cell mass has been shown after Ppx. PDL is a special case, since ligation of the main pancreatic duct leads to massive death of acinar exocrine cells but it does not seem to affect the viability of the islet cells. In this model, injury leads to inflammation, acinoductal metaplasia (replacement of exocrine acini by ductal complexes), and islet hyperplasia. The β cell mass doubles approximately in 7 days (8).

A second type of injury model is alloxan- or streptozotocin-mediated destruction of β cells. These agents are selectively toxic to β cells, but the extent of β cell destruction depends on the dose and route of administration. For example, after intravenous administration of 70 mg/kg alloxan in mice, approximately 90–95 % of β cells are killed, as deduced from the reduction in insulin-immunostained cell surface (9, 10).

Whereas Ppx, PDL, and alloxan or streptozotocin are old models that have been used for many years, a third type of injury model has been introduced recently that is based on mouse transgenesis, namely genetic ablation of β cells. Two variants exist: β cells can be ablated with high specificity thanks to doxycycline-inducible expression of the Diphtheria toxin A subunit (DTA) under the control of insulin promoter (RIP) or via the use of RIP driving the expression of Diphtheria toxin receptor (DTR). In the first strain, the presence of doxycycline induces the expression of the toxin selectively in cells transcribing insulin, i.e., β cells, leading to about 70 % ablation of the β cells (11). Since the receptor for Diphtheria toxin is not present in mice; in the RIP-DTR transgenic strain, the receptor is only expressed in β cells. When the toxin is administered to these mice, it will therefore exclusively kill β cells. The latter strain has an ablation efficiency up to 99 % of the β cells (12).

3. Models and Strategies

3.1. Evidence for Adult Stem Cells in the Pancreas

The general definition of a stem cell is a cell that can continuously self-renew, and that also can produce daughter cells with the ability to differentiate into mature cell type(s). In the case of adult multipotent stem cells like the ones in bone marrow, skin, or small intestine, daughter cells are the different cell types that normally occur in the respective tissue.

During embryonic development, all pancreatic epithelial cell types, exocrine acinar cells, duct cells, and endocrine islet cells are of endodermal origin. They all arise from a common pool of multipotent stem cells that is characterized by the expression of a number of pancreas-specific key transcription factors, like *Pdx1*, *Ptf1a*, *Hnf1β*, *Cpa1,* and *Nkx6.1* (10, 13–15). There is no definitive evidence that such stem cells reside in the postnatal pancreas. This is complicated by the fact that, as it is generally the case, transcription factors that play a certain developmental role during embryogenesis, may have a different function in the adult organ. Therefore, it is not possible to prospectively identify adult stem cells in the postnatal pancreas by using these "embryonic" transcription factors as stem cell markers. For example, *Pdx1* and *Nkx6.1* are also expressed in mature β cells, *Ptf1a* and *Cpa1* in mature exocrine acinar cells, and *Hnf1β* in mature duct cells.

What is needed to conclusively demonstrate the presence of adult stem cells in a given tissue? For genuine adult stem cells, two strategies are followed:

1. Single cell cloning and generation of different cell types from a single cell either in vitro, or after transplantation in vivo (adoptive transfer).
2. Genetic lineage tracing based on a stem cell marker gene, for example driving Cre recombinase, and allowing to follow clonal offspring of stem cells over time, either during homeostasis or regeneration of a tissue.

These strategies have been applied successfully for the demonstration, amongst others, of haematopoietic, hair follicle, and intestinal stem cells (16–18).

However, so far they have not been demonstrated with cells from the pancreas as there are no published studies based on lineage tracing of adult stem cell markers in that organ. So, what is the evidence for adult stem cells residing in the postnatal and adult pancreas? Some studies have revealed cells with clonogenic property after isolation and culture from dissociated adult pancreas. Clonal growth can be considered an in vitro equivalent of self-renewal capacity. In one study, digested pancreatic tissue enriched in cells with ductal phenotype was obtained from prediabetic non-obese diabetic mice. It could be subcultured over a long period and the cells could be induced to produce functioning islets containing α, β, and δ cells (19). Others prospectively isolated cells expressing the c-Met receptor for hepatocyte growth factor and showed that these could form clonal colonies expressing markers of pancreas, liver, stomach, and intestine in vitro (20). Rovira et al. (21) sorted a cell preparation expressing aldehyde dehydrogenase enzymatic activity, and found that it was enriched in centroacinar and ductal cells. These cells were able to form self-renewing "pancreatospheres" in suspension culture. In these organoids, both endocrine and exocrine differentiation occurred. Others used *CD133* as a marker for stem cells. Based on this marker, cells were obtained from adult mouse pancreas that showed a high proliferative capacity, but that remained committed to the ductal lineage (22). Cells with similar characteristics, but isolated perinatally, showed some differentiation plasticity. *CD133* marker has been shown to be expressed on all differentiated centroacinar and duct cells in adult pancreas which means that it cannot be used for prospective isolation/lineage tracing of putative pancreatic stem cells (23). Mato et al. (24) purified a population of pancreatic stellate cells from lactating rats. These cells expressed the ATP-binding cassette transporter *ABCG2* that is frequently associated with stem cells. They could be grown for over 2 years as a fibroblast-like monolayer and retained the capacity to express phenotypic markers characteristic of β cells when cultured under specific conditions. Zulewski et al. (25) reported that nestin-positive cells isolated from pancreatic islets and ducts showed extended proliferative capacity, and were able to express both liver and exocrine pancreas markers, or to display a ductal/endocrine phenotype after differentiation.

Rare pancreas-derived cells have been found in the mouse that show clonal proliferation capacity and that could give rise to both neural and endocrine cells (26). These "multipotent precursor" cells were found to express insulin and could also be isolated from human pancreas (27).

It is unknown whether all or part of the above mentioned characteristics are common to one and the same type of progenitor cell. Even if they would indeed characterize the existence of one or more type(s) of progenitor cells, a contribution of these cells to β cell regeneration in vivo remains to be demonstrated. We must conclude at present that definitive proof for adult stem cells in the pancreas remains elusive due to the lack of specific markers for these cells.

3.2. Genetic Lineage Tracing to Test Neogenesis

Even if progenitor cells can be isolated from adult pancreas, this does not tell us whether and to what extent they may contribute to β cell regeneration. The problem is how to demonstrate or measure neogenesis of β cells from progenitor cells in vivo, in pancreas tissue following tissue injury. There are many studies that have proposed the existence of β cell neogenesis (i.e., the formation of new β cells from non-β cells) based on indirect evidence. Only recently methods allowing rigorous testing of the neogenesis hypothesis have been developed, namely based on genetic lineage tracing (see also Chapter 21). Whereas histological observations present snapshots from which it is difficult to objectively draw a whole picture, genetic lineage tracing represents a powerful tool to study tissue dynamics. The first study using this technology to test the hypothesis of β cell neogenesis is the study of Dor et al. (28). They used genetic pulse-chase labeling to obtain a cohort of labeled β cells at a chosen time and followed these cells over longer periods.

Their model consists of Insulin-CreER transgenic mice, in which the insulin promoter drives expression of tamoxifen-dependent Cre recombinase (CreER) in β cells. This strain was combined with the Z/AP reporter strain to generate Insulin-CreER:Z/AP mice. The injection of tamoxifen in these mice leads to the transient activation of Cre recombinase specifically in insulin-expressing cells, and not in putative progenitors since these are assumed not to transcribe insulin. This results in removal of a transcriptional stop sequence from the Z/AP transgene and constitutive expression of the human placental alkaline phosphatase (*HPAP*) reporter gene in β cells and their progeny. Thus, *HPAP* expression in cells born at any time after the tamoxifen pulse identifies these cells as the progeny of pre-existing Cre-expressing cells. Dilution of labeled preexisting β cells and their progeny by progenitor-derived, and hence unlabeled β cells, would indicate the occurrence of neogenesis. This study found that within a time window of 1 year following pulse labeling of 6–8-week-old mice, the proportion of labeled β cells remained constant. Since there was no dilution of labeled insulin-expressing cells, there was no evidence for β cell neogenesis. These data convincingly demonstrate that β cell growth during homeostasis after 6 weeks of age depends on their autoreduplication and not on neogenesis. The same conclusion is drawn during regeneration following partial Ppx (28) or partial genetic ablation (11). A possible hurdle for this lineage tracing approach is given by the recent observation of rare insulin-expressing "multipotent precursor" cells in the pancreas (27). This could flaw the lineage tracing of insulin-expressing cells since this is based on the assumption that insulin is only expressed by mature β cells and not by progenitor cells.

3.3. Genetic Lineage Tracing to Test the Ductal Hypothesis

The failure of the Dor (28) and Nir (11) studies to find evidence for neogenesis still leaves open the possibility that neogenesis may operate in other experimental models than those studied. Indeed,

Inada et al. (29) used another genetic lineage tracing model, with human carbonic anhydrase-II (*CAII*) promoter acting as a driver of a Cre-lox reporter system. This was used to trace the progeny of duct cells, which express *CAII*, during the first 4 weeks of life. The authors found a significant proportion of β cells that were labeled in normal neonates. In this study, they did not use a pulse-chase system (CAII-Cre instead of CAII-CreER), assuming that *CAII* enzyme is only expressed in duct cells with expression starting only at the end of gestation. They also studied PDL and then used a CAII-CreER pulse-chase system for tracing duct cell progeny. In this model, they also found that part of β cells were derived from *CAII* expressing cells, which is taken as evidence for neogenesis.

However, this observation was not confirmed by the lineage tracing study of Solar et al. (10). They used another genetic label to trace duct cells, namely hepatocyte nuclear factor 1β (*Hnf1β*). The advantage of this transcription factor as a marker is that it is expressed homogenously by all duct cells both in embryonic and postnatal pancreas (whereas *CAII* expression only starts at the very end of gestation). It was thus possible to compare pre- and postnatal derivation of cells from duct cells. The results demonstrate that early embryonic duct cells act as multipotent progenitors for all pancreatic lineages (duct, acinar, islet cells), but their differentiation potency becomes gradually restricted during development. At the end of gestation and after birth, duct cells are only capable of generating other duct cells, and they do not contribute further to β cell mass, or to other cell types. Also during regeneration or expansion of the β cell mass in two models, namely PDL and alloxan-destruction, no marked β cells could be found. This study thus finds no evidence for β cell neogenesis from *Hnf1β*+ duct cells postnatally, whereas it does confirm neogenesis before birth.

At present, the discrepancy between the Inada (29) and the Solar (10) studies is difficult to explain. It has been suggested that *Hnf1β* used in the Solar study (10) may be expressed at a lower level in a subset of duct cells that would represent progenitor cells (30). However, in the Solar study it was ascertained that both *Hnf1β* protein and *Hnf1β*-driven Cre enzyme are homogenously expressed in the duct cell population, even if the recombination efficiency is rather low (10). The existence of a very small subset of *Hnf1β*-negative duct cells is difficult to exclude, although it seems unlikely that before birth progenitor cells are *Hnf1β*-positive as shown in the Solar study, but after birth they would be *Hnf1β*-negative. Interestingly, another study appeared in which the *Mucin-1* gene was used to trace duct cells and a subset of acinar exocrine cells that express the gene (31). This study confirms the Solar study in that there was no evidence for derivation of β cells from duct cells postnatally. Two other studies independently generated Sox9-CreER mice to trace the fate of duct cells and both confirmed that β cell neogenesis takes place from duct cells before birth but not thereafter (32, 33).

Also after PDL they found no contribution of duct cells to the β cell mass. Furthermore, it was found that PDL induces *Ngn3* expression in both duct-derived and endocrine cells but that these ductal cells did not differentiate into endocrine cells (32).

How to explain the discrepancy between the Inada study and the other 4 studies using lineage tracing? A weak point of the Inada study is that they used CAII-Cre mice where recombination can take place constitutively before birth when there is still neogenesis taking place. Another drawback is that it made use of a human fragment of the *CAII* promoter to direct Cre recombinase expression in transgenic mice. It is more complicated to examine transcriptional activation of a human gene promoter in a mouse (e.g., *CAII* in the Inada study (29)), than the endogenous gene promoter (e.g., *Hnf1β* in the Solar study (10)). Indeed, it has been reported that the human *CAII* promoter in transgenic mice is expressed with a tissue specificity that differs from the normal mouse pattern of *CAII* expression (34). This opens the possibility of tracer misexpression in cell types other than duct cells.

Furthermore, the carbonic anhydrase family includes at least 14 isoenzymes expressed from different genes, with for example *CA-V* being expressed in β cells (35). It remains to be excluded that the human *CAII* promoter can be regulated by the same proteins that regulate expression of, for example, mouse *CA-V*. Otherwise, this could also lead to tracer misexpression in β cells. Furthermore, false-positive cells were noted in wild-type mice that were discounted as resulting from antibody binding to endogenous β-galactosidase expressed in β cells, which further complicated the analyses (29). It is therefore crucial to rely not only on immunohistochemical stainings to detect tracer expression, but also to perform enzyme histochemical stainings, with X-gal substrate in the case of LacZ (as, e.g., in the Solar study (10)) (see also Chapter 21).

The validity of genetic lineage tracing experiments is dependent on rigorous testing that the marker expression (e.g., *CAII*, or *Hnf1β*), the Cre enzyme, and the β-galactosidase or its reaction product, are initially restricted to the putative cell of origin.

3.4. Genetic Lineage Tracing to Test Acinar Transdifferentiation

As an alternative to stem cell-mediated regeneration, transdifferentiation was proposed as a mechanism of β cell neogenesis (36). Transdifferentiation is the stable conversion of a differentiated cell type into another differentiated cell type (37). For example, in vitro transdifferentiation was reported of rat (38) and mouse (39) acinar exocrine cells to β cells. This transdifferentiation was induced by *EGF*, *LIF*, and/or other extracellular factors and depends on activation of *STAT3* and *MAPK* pathways, and transient expression of *Ngn3*, whereas it is suppressed by *Notch* signaling (40, 41). In the latter study, nongenetic cell tracing was performed by specific labeling of acinar cells with a lectin, wheat germ agglutinin, to demonstrate that the newly formed β cells originated from acinar cells.

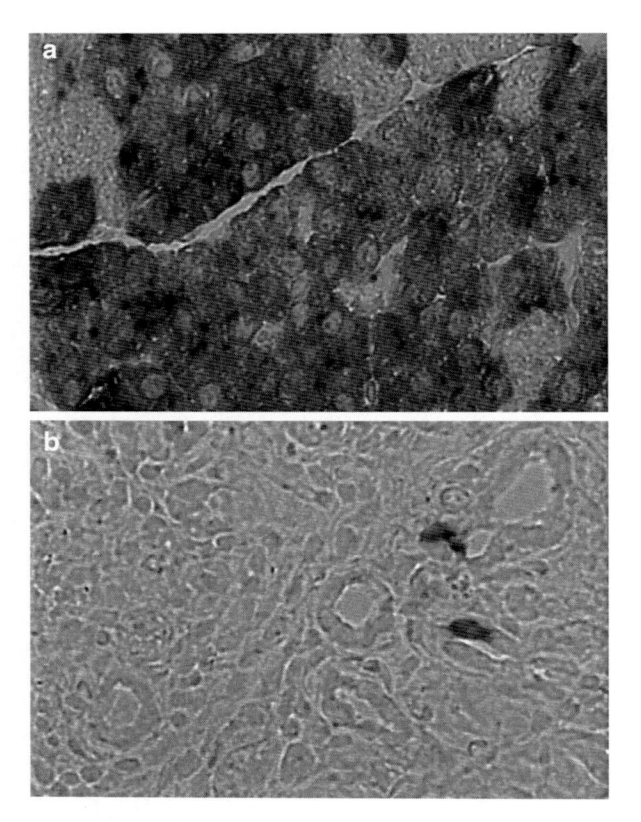

Fig. 1. X-gal enzyme histochemistry on non-ligated (**a**) and ligated (**b**) pancreas from Elastase-CreER R26R mice reveals efficient labeling of acinar cells in non-ligated pancreas, whereas almost no acinar cells survive or transdifferentiate to duct cells in the ligated pancreas.

This highly efficient lectin labeling system can also be applied to trace human acinar cells (42).

In vivo, it was shown that viral transduction to force overexpression of 3 transcription factors in adult pancreatic cells led to β cell neogenesis. Genetic lineage tracing with Cpa1-CreER demonstrated that it were acinar exocrine cells which transdifferentiated into β cells (43).

However, in the absence of genetic modification to induce transcription factor expression, a genetic tracing study using Elastase-CreER mice revealed no acino-insular transdifferentiation during β cell regeneration, after injury causing pancreatitis or PDL (44). We could confirm this observation, but noticed that after PDL almost no acinar cells survived (Fig. 1). Tamoxifen was administered to the Elastase-CreER mice and PDL was performed after a washout period of 3 weeks (see Chapter 21). Seven days later, in the ligated part, acinar cells had disappeared and were replaced by ductal complexes. More than a doubling of the β cell mass was observed in the ligated part compared to the unligated tail part of the pancreas and there was also a significant increase in

Ngn3 expression in the ligated portion of the pancreas, as described (10, 45). In these mice only acinar cells are labeled, but not duct cells (45). X-gal staining combined with immunohistochemistry revealed a mean labeling efficiency of nearly 50 % of acinar cells whereas in the ligated part of the pancreas, only 3.5 % of the duct cells were labeled with X-gal (Fig. 1). This means that if X-gal labeling is theoretically set at 100 %, maximally only 7–8 % of the ductal cells in PDL pancreas originated from acinar cells. Thus, PDL in our hands led to selective ablation of acinar cells and in such conditions it cannot be expected that these cells could contribute to the β cell mass (unpublished observations).

3.5. Genetic Lineage Tracing to Test Alpha Cell Transdifferentiation

Recently, the transdifferentiation from α cells to β cells has been reported (12). In this study RIP-DTR transgenic mice were used that express the DTR specifically in β cells. Administration of the toxin ablates nearly all β cells (>99 %). However, if the animals are kept alive by administering exogenous insulin, a partial regeneration of β cells ensues. By crossing these animals with glucagon reporter mice (tetracycline-dependent Cre-lox system), it was demonstrated that in the course of regeneration, α cells transdifferentiated into β cells. Lineage tracing also confirmed α-to-β-cell transdifferentiation in mice which overexpress *Pax4* in mature α cells (46). Indirect immunohistochemical evidence was also reported for a transdifferentiation of α-to-β-cells in mice treated with both PDL and alloxan (47).

3.6. Caveats Related to Lineage Tracing

Lineage tracing has become an indispensable tool to unequivocally prove the origin of cells. However, as indicated above, contradicting results can arise from studies using different tracing constructs and even from studies using identical tracing models. Before any solid conclusions can be drawn using this technique, some important controls should be kept in mind. It is important that experimental observations are reproducible and that alternative tracing models are able to confirm the same hypothesis. Furthermore, demonstrating the specificity of labeling, the extent to which the reporter faithfully recapitulates the wild-type pattern of gene expression is of crucial importance. The misexpression of the label in other cell types than the target cell population should be quantified after a short washout period after tamoxifen administration, since no transdifferentiation should have occurred yet but also no nuclear Cre expression should remain. If Cre recombinase is still nuclear, unlabeled cells may still become labeled.

Besides, one should confirm that recombination/labeling does not occur in a specific subpopulation of target cells, but instead occurs randomly. When labeling is not random, putative progenitor cells may be specifically spared from recombination, and therefore transdifferentiation may be missed. To this purpose, if the target population is not labeled at 100 % efficiency, as is mostly seen in CreER models, the labeled and unlabeled cells of the target population should be compared to ascertain that they represent the same cell type with respect to expression of cellular markers, morphology, proliferation rates, and levels of CreER. Furthermore, the detection of the label should be optimal. Immunohistochemical detection of the β-gal enzyme may be biased by non-specific immunostaining. So, enzyme histochemistry using X-gal staining represents a valid complement to this technique, as X-gal staining is able to distinguish between endogenous and bacterial β-galactosidase activity (48) (see also Chapter 21).

Another issue that should be addressed is whether the experimental model is still valid in the transgenic mice and after tamoxifen administration e.g., is the β cell mass, glycaemia, morphology, gene expression still as expected? In addition, leakiness of the reporter in animals not treated with tamoxifen with or without application of the experimental model should be analyzed. The significance of this caveat is depending on the tracing model used. When transdifferentiation of cell X to cell Y is to be confirmed in a model where the cell population of X is being labeled initially, activation of the label in X cells in the absence of tamoxifen still allows for the demonstration of transdifferentiation of X to Y. However, the analysis is then no longer quantitative. However, misexpression of the label in non-X cells in the absence of tamoxifen seriously complicates the interpretation of the experiment. On the other hand, when neogenesis from X to Y cells is to be confirmed in a model where Y cells are being labeled at start (by showing dilution of the label in Y cells), non-specific activation of the label in the absence of tamoxifen even in Y cells hampers drawing conclusions. This is because dilution of the label in Y cells by transdifferentiation of non-labeled cells may be missed, since extra labeling of Y cells may still occur during the experimental model when tamoxifen is already washed out.

So, although Cre/lox genetic lineage tracing is a powerful and sophisticated method to follow the fate of cells, the correct validation of controls remains essential.

4. General Conclusions

β Cell regeneration research has somewhat lagged behind embryological research. The latter is now making available advanced tissue- and cell-specific tools, for example, those based on the control of Cre recombinase that will aid future regeneration studies. It is germane to know from which cellular sources new β cells originate and to unravel the regulation of regeneration in order to develop potential regenerative therapies. From the available evidence, it is clear that mechanisms and cellular sources can vary for different forms or extent of injury to the β cells. It appears that β cell autoreduplication by mitosis can lead to regeneration of a functional cell mass when still 20–30 % of the β cells remain present after injury. When more than 95 % of the β cells have been destroyed by the injury, mitosis is insufficient but α cell transdifferentiation may partly regenerate the β cells. Multiple experimental injury models are therefore needed to consider the different mechanisms, key cells, and signals involved. Neogenesis of β cells from stem/progenitor cells remains controversial. Rigorous lineage tracing studies should finally clarify this issue provided that reliable stem/progenitor cell markers are found that may allow genetic tracing. The duct cell (transdifferentiation) hypothesis is under serious attack and the bulk of experimental evidence is now against this hypothesis. The potential involvement of acinar cells in β cell regeneration deserves to be further explored as proof-of-concept for this transdifferentiation has been obtained. What is particularly clear at present is that lineage tracing as a method is absolutely required for any future study of β cell neogenesis.

References

1. Keymeulen B, Ling Z, Gorus FK et al (1998) Implantation of standardized beta-cell grafts in a liver segment of IDDM patients: graft and recipients characteristics in two cases of insulin-independence under maintenance immunosuppression for prior kidney graft. Diabetologia 41:452–459
2. Ryan EA, Lakey JR, Rajotte RV et al (2001) Clinical outcomes and insulin secretion after islet transplantation with the Edmonton protocol. Diabetes 50:710–719
3. Shapiro AM, Lakey JR, Ryan EA et al (2000) Islet transplantation in seven patients with type 1 diabetes mellitus using a glucocorticoid-free immunosuppressive regimen. N Engl J Med 343:230–238
4. Street CN, Lakey JR, Shapiro AM et al (2004) Islet graft assessment in the Edmonton protocol: implications for predicting long-term clinical outcome. Diabetes 53:3107–3114
5. Warnock GL, Kneteman NM, Ryan EA et al (1992) Long-term follow-up after transplantation of insulin-producing pancreatic islets into patients with type 1 (insulin-dependent) diabetes mellitus. Diabetologia 35:89–95
6. Butler AE, Janson J, Bonner-Weir S et al (2003) Beta-cell deficit and increased beta-cell apoptosis in humans with type 2 diabetes. Diabetes 52:102–110
7. Jurgens CA, Toukatly MN, Fligner CL et al (2011) beta-Cell loss and beta-cell apoptosis in human type 2 diabetes are related to islet amyloid deposition. Am J Pathol 178:2632–2640
8. Wang RN, Kloppel G, Bouwens L (1995) Duct- to islet-cell differentiation and islet growth in the pancreas of duct-ligated adult rats. Diabetologia 38:1405–1411
9. Rooman I, Bouwens L (2004) Combined gastrin and epidermal growth factor treatment induces islet regeneration and restores normoglycaemia in C57Bl6/J mice treated with alloxan. Diabetologia 47:259–265
10. Solar M, Cardalda C, Houbracken I et al (2009) Pancreatic exocrine duct cells give rise to insulin-producing beta cells during embryogenesis but not after birth. Dev Cell 17:849–860
11. Nir T, Melton DA, Dor Y (2007) Recovery from diabetes in mice by beta cell regeneration. J Clin Invest 117:2553–2561
12. Thorel F, Nepote V, Avril I et al (2010) Conversion of adult pancreatic alpha-cells to beta-cells after extreme beta-cell loss. Nature 464:1149–1154
13. Gu G, Dubauskaite J, Melton DA (2002) Direct evidence for the pancreatic lineage: NGN3+ cells are islet progenitors and are distinct from duct progenitors. Development 129:2447–2457
14. Kawaguchi Y, Cooper B, Gannon M et al (2002) The role of the transcriptional regulator Ptf1a in converting intestinal to pancreatic progenitors. Nat Genet 32:128–134
15. Zhou Q, Law AC, Rajagopal J et al (2007) A multipotent progenitor domain guides pancreatic organogenesis. Dev Cell 13:103–114

16. Sato T, Vries RG, Snippert HJ et al (2009) Single Lgr5 stem cells build crypt-villus structures in vitro without a mesenchymal niche. Nature 459:262–265
17. Spangrude GJ, Heimfeld S, Weissman IL (1988) Purification and characterization of mouse hematopoietic stem cells. Science 241:58–62
18. Barker N, Clevers H (2010) Lineage tracing in the intestinal epithelium. Curr Protoc Stem Cell Biol Chapter 5:Unit5A.4
19. Ramiya VK, Maraist M, Arfors KE et al (2000) Reversal of insulin-dependent diabetes using islets generated in vitro from pancreatic stem cells. Nat Med 6:278–282
20. Suzuki A, Nakauchi H, Taniguchi H (2004) Prospective isolation of multipotent pancreatic progenitors using flow-cytometric cell sorting. Diabetes 53:2143–2152
21. Rovira M, Scott SG, Liss AS et al (2010) Isolation and characterization of centroacinar/terminal ductal progenitor cells in adult mouse pancreas. Proc Natl Acad Sci U S A 107:75–80
22. Oshima Y, Suzuki A, Kawashimo K et al (2007) Isolation of mouse pancreatic ductal progenitor cells expressing CD133 and c-Met by flow cytometric cell sorting. Gastroenterology 132:720–732
23. Lardon J, Corbeil D, Huttner WB et al (2008) Stem cell marker prominin-1/AC133 is expressed in duct cells of the adult human pancreas. Pancreas 36:e1–e6
24. Mato E, Lucas M, Petriz J et al (2009) Identification of a pancreatic stellate cell population with properties of progenitor cells: new role for stellate cells in the pancreas. Biochem J 421:181–191
25. Zulewski H, Abraham EJ, Gerlach MJ et al (2001) Multipotential nestin-positive stem cells isolated from adult human pancreatic islets differentiate ex vivo into pancreatic endocrine, exocrine, and hepatic phenotypes. Diabetes 50:521–533
26. Seaberg RM, Smukler SR, Kieffer TJ et al (2004) Clonal identification of multipotent precursors from adult mouse pancreas that generate neural and pancreatic lineages. Nat Biotechnol 22:1115–1124
27. Smukler SR, Arntfield ME, Razavi R et al (2011) The adult mouse and human pancreas contain rare multipotent stem cells that express insulin. Cell Stem Cell 8:281–293
28. Dor Y, Brown J, Martinez OI et al (2004) Adult pancreatic beta-cells are formed by self-duplication rather than stem-cell differentiation. Nature 429:41–46
29. Inada A, Nienaber C, Katsuta H et al (2008) Carbonic anhydrase II-positive pancreatic cells are progenitors for both endocrine and exocrine pancreas after birth. Proc Natl Acad Sci U S A 105:19915–19919
30. Bonner-Weir S, Li WC, Ouziel-Yahalom L et al (2010) Beta-cell growth and regeneration: replication is only part of the story. Diabetes 59:2340–2348
31. Kopinke D, Murtaugh LC (2010) Exocrine-to-endocrine differentiation is detectable only prior to birth in the uninjured mouse pancreas. BMC Dev Biol 10:38
32. Kopp JL, Dubois CL, Schaffer AE et al (2011) Sox9+ ductal cells are multipotent progenitors throughout development but do not produce new endocrine cells in the normal or injured adult pancreas. Development 138:653–665
33. Furuyama K, Kawaguchi Y, Akiyama H et al (2011) Continuous cell supply from a Sox9-expressing progenitor zone in adult liver, exocrine pancreas and intestine. Nat Genet 43:34–41
34. Erickson RP, Grimes J, Venta PJ et al (1995) Expression of carbonic anhydrase II (CA II) promoter-reporter fusion genes in multiple tissues of transgenic mice does not replicate normal patterns of expression indicating complexity of CA II regulation in vivo. Biochem Genet 33:421–437
35. Parkkila AK, Scarim AL, Parkkila S et al (1998) Expression of carbonic anhydrase V in pancreatic beta cells suggests role for mitochondrial carbonic anhydrase in insulin secretion. J Biol Chem 273:24620–24623
36. Bouwens L (1998) Transdifferentiation versus stem cell hypothesis for the regeneration of islet beta-cells in the pancreas. Microsc Res Tech 43:332–336
37. Tosh D, Slack JM (2002) How cells change their phenotype. Nat Rev Mol Cell Biol 3:187–194
38. Baeyens L, De Breuck S, Lardon J et al (2005) In vitro generation of insulin-producing beta cells from adult exocrine pancreatic cells. Diabetologia 48:49–57
39. Minami K, Okuno M, Miyawaki K et al (2005) Lineage tracing and characterization of insulin-secreting cells generated from adult pancreatic acinar cells. Proc Natl Acad Sci U S A 102:15116–15121
40. Baeyens L, Bonne S, Bos T et al (2009) Notch signaling as gatekeeper of rat acinar-to-beta-cell conversion in vitro. Gastroenterology 136:1750–1760 e1713
41. Baeyens L, Bonne S, German MS et al (2006) Ngn3 expression during postnatal in vitro beta cell neogenesis induced by the JAK/STAT pathway. Cell Death Differ 13:1892–1899
42. Houbracken I, Waele ED, Lardon J et al (2011) Lineage tracing evidence for transdifferentiation

of acinar to duct cells and plasticity of human pancreas. Gastroenterology 141(2):731–741
43. Zhou Q, Brown J, Kanarek A et al (2008) In vivo reprogramming of adult pancreatic exocrine cells to beta-cells. Nature 455:627–632
44. Desai BM, Oliver-Krasinski J, De Leon DD et al (2007) Preexisting pancreatic acinar cells contribute to acinar cell, but not islet beta cell, regeneration. J Clin Invest 117:971–977
45. Xu X, D'Hoker J, Stange G et al (2008) Beta cells can be generated from endogenous progenitors in injured adult mouse pancreas. Cell 132:197–207
46. Collombat P, Xu X, Ravassard P et al (2009) The ectopic expression of Pax4 in the mouse pancreas converts progenitor cells into alpha and subsequently beta cells. Cell 138: 449–462
47. Chung CH, Hao E, Piran R et al (2010) Pancreatic beta-cell neogenesis by direct conversion from mature alpha-cells. Stem Cells 28:1630–1638
48. Inada A, Nienaber C, Bonner-Weir S (2006) Endogenous beta-galactosidase expression in murine pancreatic islets. Diabetologia 49: 1120–1122

Chapter 21

Genetic Lineage Tracing of Beta Cell Neogenesis

Iris Mathijs, Isabelle Houbracken, and Luc Bouwens

Abstract

Genetic lineage tracing is an invaluable tool to demonstrate and measure neogenesis of beta cells from putative precursor cells. Cre-Lox recombination technology can be used for indelible labeling of a cohort of cells and following the fate of these cells and their progeny in animal models. Here, the combination is described of beta-galactosidase enzymatic staining with immunohistochemical staining to demonstrate labeled cells. This technique is performed in tissue cryosections.

Key words: Beta cell, Lineage tracing, Neogenesis, Regeneration, X-gal, Beta-galactosidase

1. Introduction

The protocol described here outlines the procedure of a genetic pulse-chase labeling approach to measure β cell neogenesis after an experimental procedure or treatment. For this purpose, mice carrying the RIPCreER trangene, in which the insulin promoter drives the expression of tamoxifen-dependent Cre recombinase (CreER) in β cells, are crossed with a Rosa26R-loxP-stop-loxP-LacZ reporter strain. In these mice, tamoxifen administration results in a transient nuclear translocation of the CreER protein, which leads to the Cre-mediated removal of a stop sequence and the expression of the *lacZ* reporter. The *lacZ* gene codes for beta-galactosidase and is enzymatically detected using X-gal, resulting in a blue staining. Cells with an active insulin promoter at the time of tamoxifen administration and their progeny will indelibly be labeled, while β cells that arise later from a non-β cell source will remain unlabelled. If the labeled β cell population becomes diluted after an experimental procedure involving injury-induced regeneration or growth, neogenesis contributes to the newly formed β cells. If not, β cell replication is the primary mechanism for the formation of new β

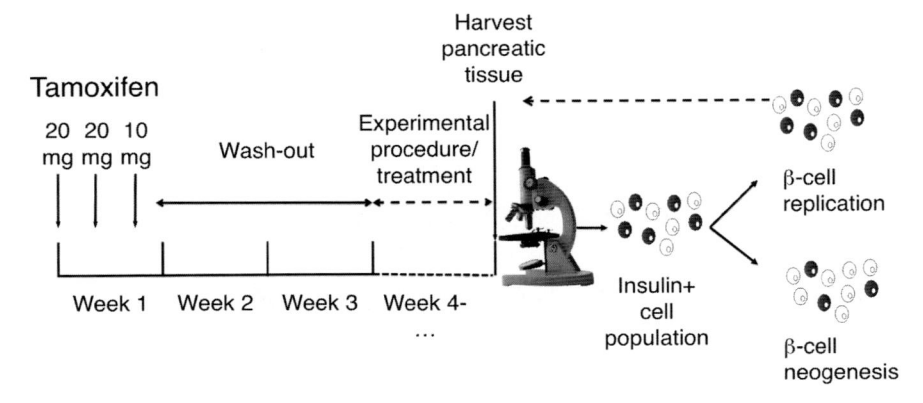

Fig. 1. Experimental setup of a lineage tracing protocol.

cells (see Chapter 20). Figure 1 shows the experimental setup of a lineage tracing protocol with RIPCreER; R26R-LacZ double transgenic mice.

2. Materials

2.1. Tamoxifen Administration

1. Tamoxifen (Sigma).
2. 99.8% Ethanol absolute (Fluka).
3. 0.9% NaCl solution (Baxter).
4. Mice: RIPCreER; R26R-LacZ double transgenic mice.
5. Feeding needle and 0.5 mL syringe.

2.2. Tissue Processing

1. Prepare stock solution of 20% paraformaldehyde (PFA): Add 50 g PFA in 250 mL phosphate buffered saline (PBS), add 6.25 mL 1 M NaOH. Dissolve until the solution is clear in a warm water bath at 65°C (see Note 1) Cool on ice. Adjust the pH at 7.5 (see Note 2). Store at −20°C per 10 mL (see Note 3).
2. Prepare 4% PFA working solution (see Note 4): Add 40 mL PBS to 10 mL 20% PFA, heat in a water bath at 60°C (see Note 5) until a clear solution is obtained and cool on ice before use.
3. 20% Sucrose: Dissolve 20 g of sucrose in 100 mL of ultra pure water.
4. OCT compound (Tissue-Tek).
5. Liquid nitrogen.

2.3. X-gal and Insulin Staining

1. 0.1 M Sodium phosphate buffer: Mix 230 mL 0.2 M $NaH_2PO_4 \cdot 2H_2O$ and 770 mL 0.2 M Na_2HPO_4 with 1 l of

ultra pure water. Bring pH to 7.3 using the acidic 0.2 M $NaH_2PO_4 \cdot 2H_2O$ and the basic 0.2 M Na_2HPO_4 (see Note 6).

2. X-gal washing buffer: 0.1 M sodium phosphate buffer with 0.02% IGEPAL CA-130 (Sigma) and 2 mM $MgCl_2$.

3. X-gal staining buffer: X-gal washing buffer with 5 mM $K_3[Fe(CN)_6]$, and 5 mM $K_4[Fe(CN)_6] \cdot 3H_2O$. Dissolve 10 mg X-gal in 400 µL DMSO for 10 mL of staining buffer. Heat the buffer to 37°C and add the X-gal solution (see Note 7).

4. PBS.

5. 2% Donkey serum diluted in PBS.

6. Anti-insulin antibody.

7. Fluorescently labeled secondary antibody that recognizes the primary antibody (e.g., from Jackson ImmunoResearch Laboratories).

8. Mounting medium for fluorescence with 4′,6-diamidino-2-phenylindole (DAPI) (see Note 8) (e.g., *Vectashield*® (Vector Labs)).

3. Methods

3.1. Tamoxifen Administration

1. Add 100 µL ethanol to 100 mg tamoxifen and make sure the ethanol is in contact with all of the tamoxifen before adding 900 µL 0.9% NaCl solution (see Note 9). Sonicate the emulsion three times for 20 s to remove clumps (see Note 10).

2. Vortex the emulsion shortly right before administration to avoid separation of the different phases. Feed 200 µL of the emulsion orally to the mice using a feeding needle (see Note 11). This procedure is repeated 2 and 4 days later with, respectively, 200 and 100 µL of the emulsion. The RIPCreER; R26R-LacZ mice receive in total 50 mg of tamoxifen.

3. Because it is not possible to obtain 100% labeling efficiency, it is important to compare the labeling efficiency with control littermates that receive the same tamoxifen emulsion but are not subjected to the experimental procedure or treatment.

4. A 2-week wash-out period between the last administration and the experimental procedure or treatment should be honored to be assured that no nuclear Cre-recombinase is present at the time of the experimental procedure or treatment.

3.2. Tissue Processing

The X-gal staining protocol described here is only suitable for cryosections, not for paraffin-embedded sections.

1. After the experimental procedure or treatment, euthanize the animals by cervical dislocation; remove the pancreas, cut into

pieces of approximately 4 mm^3 and fix for 4 h in 4% PFA solution at 4°C.
2. Rinse the tissue with ice-cold PBS three times for 15 min and incubate the tissue with 20% sucrose solution overnight at 4°C.
3. Embed the tissue in OCT compound and freeze in liquid nitrogen (see Note 12). Store at −80°C.
4. Cut cryosections of 7 μm using a cryotome. Use three sections that are separated by at least 150 μm. Cryosections should be stored at −20°C.

3.3. X-gal and Insulin Staining

1. Dry cryosections 30′ on room temperature.
2. Wash 5′ with PBS (see Note 13).
3. Wash three times for 5′ with X-gal washing buffer.
4. Cover the sections with X-gal staining buffer and incubate overnight at 37°C in a humified chamber (see Note 14).
5. Wash three times for 5′ with X-gal washing buffer.
6. Wash two times for 5′ with PBS.
7. Block nonspecific binding with 2% donkey serum for 30′ at room temperature.
8. Incubate with anti-insulin antibody diluted in PBS overnight at 4°C in a humified chamber (see Note 15).
9. Wash three times for 5′ with PBS.
10. Incubate with appropriate fluorescent secondary antibody for 30′ at room temperature.
11. Wash three times for 5′ with PBS.
12. Wash 5′ with ultra pure water.
13. Mount with mounting medium for fluorescence with DAPI (e.g., *Vectashield*® (Vector Labs)).

3.4. Image Analysis

1. Take pictures of all insulin positive cells (see Note 16) in the stained sections using imaging software such as NIS Elements with a 20× objective. Make a merged picture of three channels: brightfield (to visualize X-gal) and two fluorescence channels (to visualize insulin and DAPI or Hoechst).
2. Count the amount of insulin positive cells and X-gal/insulin double positive cells. Labeling efficiency is the proportion of double positive cells in the insulin positive cell population.
3. Compare the labeling efficiency of the treated group with that of the control animals to assess dilution of the labeled β cell population. If the labeling efficiency remains the same, proliferation is the main source of new β cells, if it is lower in

the treated group than in the control group, it suggests neogenesis.

4. Some caveats should be taken into account when applying lineage tracing (see Chapter 20).

4. Notes

1. Preparation of 4% and 20% PFA solution should be done in a fume hood to avoid inhalation of toxic fumes.
2. Make sure the solution is at room temperature before making final pH adjustments.
3. Stored at −20°C, the stock solution can be used for several months. Avoid repeated freeze/thaw cycles.
4. The 4% PFA working solution should be prepared freshly.
5. Precipitation of PFA will occur with insufficient heating.
6. Failure to adjust the pH may result in nonspecific staining since endogenous and bacterial (transgenic) beta-galactosidases have a different optimal pH (1).
7. To avoid precipitation of X-gal, the buffer should be properly heated to 37°C and the X-gal solution should be added dropwise.
8. Alternatively, sections can be stained with 1/250 Hoechst solution for 10 min prior to mounting. This has the advantage of being distributed more evenly throughout the tissue, whereas the mounting medium with DAPI stains the nuclei closest to the edges of the tissue the most and is less intensive in the middle of the tissue.
9. The tamoxifen solution should be prepared freshly each time.
10. Make sure the tamoxifen does not heat. The vial with the tamoxifen solution should be kept in ice-cold water while sonicating and in ice in between two sonication steps.
11. Be gentle. The tube should be inserted in the esophagus and not in the trachea to avoid suffocation.
12. Remove excess sucrose solution from the tissue with a paper towel. Put the tissue at the bottom of the cassette. Add OCT without creating air bubbles, since they will hinder the cryo-sectioning later. Slowly freeze at the liquid–air interface of nitrogen.
13. Washing steps can be prolonged for up to several hours.
14. The volume of this chamber should be small. Incubation at 37°C can lead to evaporation of the buffer and wrong concentration of the X-gal solution, which will lead to an incorrect

staining. Further, the X-gal solution can evaporate entirely and no staining will be detected in that case.

15. The volume of this chamber can be higher since cold incubation has less evaporation.

16. It is of vital importance to picture all insulin positive cells, including the single cells and the small clusters, since it is hypothesized that more small clusters are formed during neogenesis.

Reference

1. Inada A, Nienaber C, Bonner-Weir S (2006) Endogenous beta-galactosidase expression in murine pancreatic islets. Diabetologia 49:1120–1122

INDEX

A

ACE2. *See* Angiotensin converting enzyme 2 (ACE2)
Acellular capillaries 291, 299, 300
Advanced intercross populations 282
Albuminuria 19–21, 24, 150
Alloxan 163, 164, 171, 304, 308, 311
Amphotericin B 207, 209, 213, 214
Angiotensin converting enzyme 2 (ACE2) 21, 23
Animal model 23, 35, 38, 85, 90, 97, 100, 117, 125, 137, 162, 163, 171, 189, 251, 256, 266, 268
Autoimmune diabetes 31–40
Autoimmune diseases 6, 9, 32, 35, 265
Autoimmune manifestations 7

B

BB rat 31–40
BCM. *See* Beta (β)-cell mass (BCM)
Beta (β) cells 4, 18, 33, 48, 65, 75, 78, 89, 104, 127, 162, 189–200, 203–215, 219, 265–273, 303–313, 317–322
    autoimmunity 265–273
    dysfunction 75, 81, 89, 90, 92, 97–99, 108, 133, 139, 162, 167, 170, 171
    neogenesis 129, 138, 307–310, 313, 317–322
    regeneration 303–313
Beta-cell degranulation 78, 129, 130
Beta (β)-cell mass (BCM) 65, 90, 92, 94, 95, 97–99, 108, 109, 116, 117, 129, 130, 138, 141, 142, 145, 146, 151, 164, 165, 170, 171, 303, 304, 308–312
Beta (β)-galactosidase 309, 312, 317, 321
Bradykinin receptor 21–22

C

Cardiomyocytes 54
Catheterization 230, 234–239, 249
CD137 .... 8–12, 268, 273
CD8+ T cell 33, 37, 266–268, 270–273
Cell attached 205, 207–211
Collagenase 129, 130, 190, 191, 193, 195, 198, 199
Collagenase digestion 190, 192–195, 198, 199

Complications 19, 24, 49, 75, 79, 115–117, 126, 141, 147–151, 166, 169–171
    of diabetes 181
    of overt type 2 diabetes 178
Congenics 7–10, 60, 67–69, 83–85, 104, 142, 143
CreER. *See* Cre recombinase (CreER)
Crelox reporter system 308
Cre recombinase (CreER) 305, 307–312, 317, 319
CTLA4 .... 8, 9
Cynomolgus 177, 179, 180

D

Diabetes 3–13, 17, 31–40, 47–55, 59–70, 75–85, 89–100, 103–117, 125–151, 161–172, 177–184, 219, 251, 265, 275, 291, 303
    complications 126, 147, 151, 164
    nephropathy 17–28, 66, 148, 149, 181
    retinopathy 291–302
Diet-induced hyperglycemia 91, 92, 97, 99
Digestion 190, 193–195, 198, 199, 292–296, 298, 300, 301
Digests 191, 291–302
Ductal injection 193–195, 199

E

Echocardiography 50, 51
Electrical activity 204
ELISpot 266, 268, 270–271, 273
Endothelial cells 21, 22, 147, 291, 299, 300
Endothelial nitric oxide synthase (eNOS) 22, 149
Enteroviruses 34
Epigenetic 70, 146
Eye 115, 181, 294, 295, 300

F

fa gene mutation 103, 104
Fine mapping 143, 282, 284–287
Fructose 111, 113, 163, 166–167, 171

G

Genetic susceptibility 19
Gerbils 90, 96, 100

GFR. *See* Glomerular filtration rate (GFR)
GK Rat 113, 125–151
Glomerular filtration rate (GFR) 17, 19, 20, 22
Glucokinase 95, 111, 131, 163
Gluconeogenesis 63, 108–110, 250
Glucose
    clamp 63, 64, 230, 241–245
    effectiveness 230, 250, 251
    intolerance 67, 77, 104, 107–114,
        117, 126, 127, 137, 139, 142, 145, 168
    phosphorylation 95, 110–114
    production 63, 78, 108–114, 135–137,
        139, 141, 220, 228, 230, 248–250, 252
    tolerance 60, 77, 81, 113, 126–128, 139,
        142, 165, 167–170, 179, 180, 220, 221, 226, 227
    tracers 230
    transport 54, 107, 115, 136, 163, 225, 256, 261
Glucotoxicity 98, 99, 114–115, 117, 134, 146

H

Hepatic glucose production 63, 109–114, 135, 137, 250
High-fat (HF) diet 50, 62, 64, 67, 68, 132, 163,
    165–168, 277, 278, 282, 283
Hyperglycemia 4, 18, 31, 47, 59, 76,
    89, 103, 127, 163, 276, 291
Hyperglycemic 64, 76, 91, 95, 98, 104,
    105, 111, 117, 129, 130, 140, 141, 144, 145, 163, 164
Hyperinsulinemia 47, 48, 77–79, 90–92,
    104, 110–112, 114, 116, 117, 137, 166, 167, 169, 171
Hyperinsulinemic-euglycemic 136, 241–245
Hyperlipidemia 79, 81–83, 98,
    105, 106, 117, 146, 163, 166, 167, 171
Hypertension 19, 24, 49, 50, 60,
    66, 80, 115, 148, 150, 151, 166, 170

I

Idd. *See* Insulin dependent diabetes loci *(Idd)*
Innate immunity 38
Insulin action 78, 114, 135–137,
    139, 141, 144, 162, 250
Insulin autoantibodies 266–270
Insulin content 65, 94–96, 98, 108,
    115, 127, 129, 130, 150, 192, 197, 198, 200
Insulin deficiency 92, 95, 99, 141
Insulin dependent diabetes loci *(Idd)* 7, 8, 10
Insulin ELISA 192, 197–198, 200, 222, 223
Insulin resistance 47, 48, 54, 59,
    62–66, 75, 77–79, 84, 89, 90, 92, 96, 98, 103, 104,
    106, 107, 113, 114, 116, 117, 136, 137, 139, 141,
    143, 162, 163, 165–171, 255
Insulin RIA 92, 94, 192
Insulin secretion 47, 48, 77, 78, 81, 92, 94–96, 106,
    109, 126, 130, 132, 135, 137, 139, 140, 142–144,
    146, 151, 170, 179, 189–200, 219, 220, 251

Insulin sensitivity 60, 63, 64, 116,
    139–141, 220, 221, 225, 228, 230, 250, 255–262
Insulin therapy 181, 182
Insulitis 4, 6, 32, 33, 35, 37, 39, 40
Interaction 10, 60, 69, 84, 85, 104,
    148, 178, 276, 277, 284
Intercross 20, 60, 68, 69,
    85, 144, 277, 279, 282–287
Intrauterine growth retardation (IUGR) 163, 170–172
IUGR. *See* Intrauterine growth retardation (IUGR)

K

Ketogenic diet 23–24
Kilham rat virus (KRV) 36–40

L

Leptin 40, 49, 63, 66, 67, 79, 103,
    116, 117, 140
Leptin receptor 49, 63, 66, 67, 103, 116–117
Lineage tracing 303–313, 317–322
Linkage 6, 7, 9, 66, 81, 82, 142, 143, 283, 284
Lipotoxicity 99, 146
Liver 63, 78, 84, 85, 106, 109–117, 135–137,
    141, 144, 163, 164, 169–171, 182, 193, 195, 220,
    238, 242, 244, 247, 248, 250, 251, 304, 306
Liver glucotoxicity 114–115
Lymphopenia 32, 33, 37

M

Magnetic resonance imaging (MRI) 50, 51
Major histocompatibility complex (MHC) 32, 33,
    35, 128, 266, 272
    genes 4, 8, 32
Membrane potential 203, 209, 210
Metabolic cage 25, 26, 233, 240, 241
Metabolic syndrome 59–70, 255, 275, 277, 282, 283
MHC. *See* Major histocompatibility complex (MHC)
Mice 3, 18, 32, 47–55, 60, 75, 96,
    162, 190, 220, 230, 258, 266, 275, 291, 304, 317
MIN6 cells 196, 200
MIN6 pseudo-islets 196
Monosodium glutamate (MSG) 163, 169–170, 172
Morphometry 291, 301
Mouse metabolic cage 25
Mouse model of type 1 diabetes 22
Mouse phenotype 221
MRI. *See* Magnetic resonance imaging (MRI)
MSG. *See* Monosodium glutamate (MSG)

N

Neogenesis 109, 110, 129, 138,
    307–310, 312, 313, 317–322
Neuromedin U 69

Neuromedin U receptor 66, 69
Nicotinamide 39, 163, 165, 168–169, 171
NOD. *See* Non-obese diabetic (NOD)
Nonhuman primates..162, 177–184
Non-obese diabetic (NOD).................... 3–13, 32, 265, 306

O

Obesity..47–55, 59–70, 75–77, 79,
83–85, 89, 92, 96, 97, 100, 103–107, 113, 116, 117,
140, 149, 151, 165, 166, 169–171, 183, 255, 276, 287
Oxidative stress (OS)............................. 23, 80, 97, 109, 129,
133, 135, 148–150, 163, 170

P

Pancreas...32, 34, 35, 84, 96, 98,
108, 109, 125, 128–131, 134, 135, 138, 139, 141,
142, 144–146, 164, 165, 170, 190–192, 194, 195,
198, 199, 230, 251, 304–308, 310, 311, 319
Pancreatic beta-cell... 40, 47, 65,
162–165, 167, 168, 170, 171, 219, 265
pancreatic-blood glucose clamp.......................230, 241–243
Pancreatic duct ligation (PDL)........................ 304, 308–311
Pancreatic islets... 9, 11, 32–33, 35,
40, 128–135, 143, 189, 191, 199, 266, 272, 306
Partial pancreatectomy (Ppx)............................162, 164, 165,
172, 304, 307
Patch-clamp technique 204, 208
PDL. *See* Pancreatic duct ligation (PDL)
Perforated-patch.............................. 207, 209–211, 213–215
Pericytes 147, 291, 299, 300
Positional cloning 275–288
Ppx. *See* Partial pancreatectomy (Ppx)
Prediabetes 34, 138–141, 178, 179, 182
Prevention of diabetes 4, 12, 33–34, 180
Progenitor cell 147, 306–308, 311, 313
Proinsulin
 biosynthesis 95, 130
 conversion intermediates 92, 94
Psammomys obesus...89–100

Q

Quantitative trait loci (QTL) 6, 66–70,
81–84, 142, 144, 275–277, 279–282, 284–287

R

Radio-binding assay 266, 268–270
Recombinant congenic strains (RCS)..............277, 279, 280,
282, 285–287
Recombinant inbred strains (RIS) 277, 279–282, 285–287

Regeneration 164, 172, 303–313, 317
Regulatory T cell (Treg) 7, 9–11, 33–38
Retina.. 147, 291–301
Retina digestion...292–293, 296
Retinal digests 291–302
Retinal vasculature...291
Rhesus 177, 179, 181–183
RIS. *See* Recombinant inbred strains (RIS)

S

Sand rat...89–100
Single channel current 208, 210
Skeletal muscle 68, 78, 84, 107,
114–116, 136, 137, 242, 244, 248, 255–262
Skeletal muscle glucotoxicity..115
Standard whole-cell.................................. 207, 210, 211, 214
Stem cell 303–313
Streptozotocin (STZ) 18–19, 35, 65,
163–165, 167–169, 171, 304

T

TALLYHO 59, 66, 68, 75–85
T1D. *See* Type 1 diabetes (T1D)
T2D. *See* Type 2 diabetes (T2D)
TLR. *See* Toll-like receptor (TLR)
Toll-like receptor (TLR) 35–38
Tracing 308–313
Treg. *See* Regulatory T cell (Treg)
Trypsin 292, 293, 296, 301
24-hour urine collection 18, 25–27
Type 1 diabetes (T1D) 3–13, 18, 20–24,
31–40, 65, 163, 165, 265, 266, 303
Type 2 diabetes (T2D) 22, 23, 49, 50,
59–60, 64–65, 69, 70, 75–85, 89, 100, 104,
107–111, 113–115, 117, 125–151, 161–172,
177–184, 219, 220, 251, 276, 303

V

Vasculature 22, 79, 292, 297, 298, 301, 302
Virus infection..35–39

X

X-gal..309–312, 317–322

Z

ZDF. *See* Zucker diabetic fatty (ZDF)
ZF. *See* Zucker fatty (ZF)
Zucker diabetic fatty (ZDF)................................... 103–117
Zucker fatty (ZF) 103, 104, 116, 117

Printed by Books on Demand, Germany

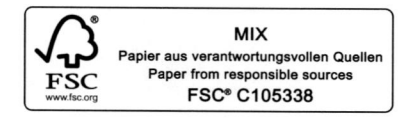